The 1990 Sandoz Lectures in Gerontology

Challenges in Aging

The 1990 Sandoz Lectures in Gerontology

Challenges in Aging

edited by

M. Bergener
M. Ermini
H.B. Stähelin

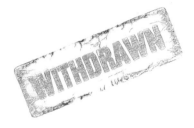

1990

ACADEMIC PRESS

HARCOURT BRACE JOVANOVICH, PUBLISHERS
LONDON   SAN DIEGO   NEW YORK   BOSTON
SYDNEY   TOKYO   TORONTO

ACADEMIC PRESS LIMITED.
24/28 Oval Road,
London NW1 7DX

United States Edition published by
ACADEMIC PRESS INC.
San Diego, CA 92101

British Library Cataloguing in Publication Data
Challenges in aging
  1. Man. Aging
  I. Bergener, M.   II. Ermini, M. (Marco) III. Stähelin, H.
  B. IV.   Series
  612.67

ISBN 0–12–090163–3

Typeset by Photo·graphics, Honiton, Devon
and printed in Great Britain by St Edmundsbury Press Ltd, Bury St Edmunds, Suffolk

Contributors

M. Bergener *Rheinische Landesklinik Köln, Wilhelm-Griesinger-Str. 23, D–5000 Köln 91, FRG.*

C. Bertoni-Freddari *Gerontological Research Department INRCA, Via Birarelli 8, I–60121 Ancona, Italy.*

J.E. Birren *Brookdale Distinguished Scholar, Ethel Percy Andrus Gerontology Center, University Park-MCO191, Los Angeles CA 90089-0191, USA.*

J.C. Brocklehurst *Withington Hospital, Nell Lane, West Didsbury, Manchester M20 8LR, UK.*

T. Casoli *Centre for Surgical Research, INRCA Research Department, Via Birarelli 8, 60121 Ancona, Italy.*

J.R.M. Copeland *Department of Psychiatry, University of Liverpool, Royal Liverpool Hospital, POB 147, Liverpool L69 3BX, UK.*

D. Danon *The Weizmann Institute of Science, Center for the Biology of Aging, Rehovot 76100, Israel.*

M. Ermini *Foundation for Experimental Aging Research, Felix-Platter-Spital, CH–4055, Basle, Switzerland.*

A.V. Everitt *The Ageing and Alzheimer's Disease Research Institute, University of Sydney, Concord Repatriation General Hospital, Sydney, New South Wales 2139, Australia.*

P. Fattoretti *Centre for Surgical Research, INRCA Research Department, Via Birarelli 8, 60121 Ancona, Italy.*

L.M. Fisher *Brookdale Distinguished Scholar, Ethel Percy Andrus Gerontology Center, University Park–MCO191, Los Angeles, CA 90089–0191, USA.*

J.F. Fries *Department of Medicine, Stanford University School of Medicine, Stanford, CA 94305, USA.*

V.V. Frolkis *Institute of Gerontology of the USSR, Vyshgorodskaya Street 67, Kiev 114 252655, USSR.*

C.G. Gottfries *University of Gothenburg, Department of Psychiatry and Neuro-chemistry, St. Jorgen's Hospital, S–42203 Hisings Backa, Sweden.*

C. Hesse *Carl Korth Institut, Rathsberger Str. 10, D–8520 Erlangen, FRG.*

J.A. Joseph *Department of Health and Human Services, National Institutes of Health and Human Services, National Institute on Aging, Gerontology Research Center, 4940 Eastern Ave, Baltimore, MD 21224, USA.*

M.H. Liang *Harvard University Medical School, Brigham and Women's Hospital, Robert B. Brigham Multipurpose Arthritis Center, Department of Rheumatology/Immunology, 75 Francis Street, Boston, MA 02115, USA.*

M. Link, *Managing Director, Sandoz Pharma Ltd, CH–4002 Basle, Switzerland.*

W. Meier-Ruge *Division of Neuropathology, Institute of Pathology, University of Basel, Basel CH–4057, Switzerland.*

F.H. Messerli *Ochsner Medical Institutions, 1514 Jefferson Highway, New Orleans, LA 70118, USA.*

A.G. Need *Institute of Medicine and Veterinary Science, Frome Road, Adelaide SA5000, Australia.*

B.E.C. Nordin *Institute of Medicine and Veterinary Science, Frome Road, Adelaide SA5000, Australia.*

H. Orimo *University of Tokyo, Faculty of Medicine, Department of Geriatrics, 7-3-1 Hongo, Bunkyo-ku, Tokyo, Japan.*

Y. Ouchi *Department of Geriatrics, Faculty of Medicine, University of Tokyo, Tokyo 113, Japan.*

B. Roos *Managing Director, Federal Office of Public Health, PO Box 2644, CH–3000 Berne, Switzerland.*

L. Rosenmayr *Institute of Sociology, University of Vienna, Alser Str. 33, A–1080 Vienna, Austria.*

G.S. Roth *Department of Health and Human Services, National Institutes of Health and Human Services, National Institute on Aging, Gerontology Research Center, 4940 Eastern Ave, Baltimore, MD 21224, USA.*

H.B. Stähelin *Head of the Geriatric Clinics, Felix-Platter-Spital and Kantonsspital Basle, CH–4055 Basle, Switzerland.*

J. Ulrich *Division of Neuropathology, Institute of Pathology, University of Basel, Basel CH–4057, Switzerland.*

M. Vercruyssen *Ethel Percy Andrus Gerontology Center, University Park–MCO191, Los Angeles, CA 90089-0191, USA.*

J.A. Yesavage *Stanford University Medical Center, Department of Psychiatry and Behavioral Sciences, Psychiatric Intensive Care Unit (Ward 5C4), Veteran's Administration Medical Center, Palo Alto, CA 94304, USA.*

Preface

The 1990 Sandoz Lectures in Gerontology are the fourth in this series of biennial events established for the promotion of interdisciplinary exchange among gerontologists. The rising number of the old and very old is no longer only of concern to industrialized nations but a world-wide phenomenon. Social and psychological as well as biological factors of mutual interdependence contribute to this development which for the majority of the population is associated with health and independence, for a minority, however, with impairment and disablement. Hence, it was the goal of the Editors and the Scientific Board of the Lectures to focus on factors important for disablement and handicap in old age.

The understanding of cognitive and behavioural alterations in aging, the response to a rapidly changing environment and the adaptive responses of the old individual has to be seen in the light of the knowledge of decreasing capacity of regulatory cell functions of different organs during aging. The biological basis of the old differs from the young, a fact which has to be taken into account when dealing with social and medical problems of the greying population. Thus, substantial benefits for the individual and the society may be expected if common disabling conditions are postponed or even altogether avoided.

In former Lectures much emphasis was given to degenerative brain disease. The present Lectures focus on disability due to musculoskeletal and vascular impairment. Also the order of the Lectures was changed in as much as the first chapter deals with psychosocial issues, the second is devoted to a better understanding of molecular biological age-related changes and the last chapter focuses on medical and epidemiological approaches in the management of disability and handicap in the old.

As in the case of previous Sandoz Lectures in Gerontology, the faculty and the organizers met at the beginning of the Lectures in an informal "trigger meeting" to initiate an interdisciplinary dialogue among the participants (see pp. xv–xvi).

We are very much indebted to the generous support by Sandoz Pharma Ltd. of Basel which guaranteed the realization of this outstanding meeting. Special thanks go to the members of the organizing committee Dr. L. Abisch, A. Booz, Dr. C. Hesse and G. Nussbaumer, who assured together with the Editors the success of the 1990 Sandoz Lectures. Special thanks go to Dr. V. Biro and M.-P. Giesen who carefully edited the discussion.

The Editors are confident that the 1990 Sandoz Lectures in Gerontology continue a series of highly respected and authoritative publications in gerontology and will serve the reader as useful references in the fields discussed.

M. Bergener, Cologne (FRG)
M. Ermini, Basle (CH)
H.B. Stähelin, Basle (CH)

Welcome Address

M. Link

*Managing Director, Sandoz Pharma Ltd, Basle,
Switzerland*

I welcome you on the occasion of the opening of the 1990 Sandoz Lectures in Gerontology. For the fourth time in a row, researchers and doctors are gathering in Basel in order to listen to the presentations of scientists of various disciplines about their latest results. You are coming from many countries of the world, and you have various interests, but the common denominator of all of us is the interest in elucidating some more secrets of the aging process and especially to find better ways of helping the elderly men and women who are sick and in distress.

The title of this year's Sandoz Lectures is "Challenges in Aging". It is, indeed, not one challenge which we are facing, but many challenges.

We certainly need to further intensify research in all areas. This means to build on the many exciting results which have been achieved over the last few years, and to draw the right conclusions.

We have to develop a better understanding of the elderly. We must let them feel that we owe them all the economic well-being which we are enjoying today, and that we still can learn a lot from them.

We, the representatives of the industrialized world, have to transfer our knowledge of gerontology and geriatric medicine to the developing nations where prolonged life expectancy is creating new and special problems.

These are just a few of the challenges which we have to face. We can still win this uphill battle if we can win the support of the decision makers, the politicians, and the public at large. Therefore, with the Sandoz Lectures we do not only want to spread scientific knowledge among the scientists, but to develop also the public opinion. In this respect we are happy that more representatives of the media than ever from all over the world are covering the 1990 Sandoz Lectures. Please, let your readers and listeners at home feel some of the spirit of the symposium, and let them understand the need for action.

It is a special pleasure and honour for us to welcome the Rector Magnificus of the Basle University, Dr. Carl Rudolf Pfaltz.

Since the beginning of this series, the Sandoz Lectures have taken place under the auspices of the Swiss Society for Gerontology. We want to express our gratitude to this society.

We also want to welcome the president of the International Association of Gerontology, Dr. Samuel Bravo Williams from Mexico, and with him the past president of this society, Dr. Ewald W. Busse from Durham, N. C., and the president elect, Dr. Edit Beregi from Budapest who will organize the next International Congress of Gerontology in 1993.

Two years ago, Dr. Manfred Bergener from Cologne was honoured on this spot as the "spiritual father of the Sandoz Lectures". Dr. Bergener was the chairman of the Organizing Committee of this symposium since the beginning, and I would like to highlight his merits once more.

We are also very happy that we have with us the chairmen of the regional committees of the Sandoz Foundation for Gerontological Research, Dr. Robert N. Butler from New York, Dr. Eurico de Carvalho Filho from Sao Paulo, Dr. Michael Hall from Southampton, Dr. Jerzy Hildebrand from Brussels, Dr. Christopher Nordin from Adelaide and Dr. Hajime Orimo from Tokyo. The President of the Board of Trustees of this Foundation, Dr. Paul Kielholz cannot be with us because of health reasons.

We are very honoured by the presence of Dr. Kazuo Hasegawa from Kawasaki, chairman of the International Psychogeriatric Association and honorary member of the regional committee for Japan of the Sandoz Foundation. A special welcome goes to Dr. T. Franklin Williams, Director of the American National Institute on Aging in Bethesda.

Within only a few years, the Sandoz Prize for Gerontological Research has gained a world-wide reputation. All the speakers of the Sandoz Lectures had applied for the Prize. All of them would have deserved it, but the jury could award the 1989 Prize only to a restricted number of persons, namely Dr. James Birren from Los Angeles, Dr. J.C. Brocklehurst from Manchester, Dr. David Danon from Rehovot and to the team Dr. G.S. Roth and James A. Joseph from Baltimore.

From all of the speakers we expect to learn a lot during today and tomorrow.

On behalf of the management of Sandoz Pharma Ltd I welcome all of you. I am sure that you will have two interesting, stimulating days, and a lot of discussions. I am sure that you will also have fun. But all the time we should think of the challenges we are facing, the "Challenges of Aging".

Contents

Regulatory Factors of Cell Function during Aging

Chronic Illness in the Elderly: Clinical Strategies

Aging in the Nineties and Beyond: What is Necessary in Research and Practice?

M. Bergener, M. Ermini and C. Hesse

This "trigger meeting" meant an attempt at and a chance of true interdisciplinarity since representatives of transcultural sociological research were on the table as well as classical experimental psychologists, geriatricians, psychiatrists and scientists engaged in morphometric research and biologists studying subtle changes in neuronal transmission.

As to the first part of the question: much more knowledge is needed in neurophysiology and the interplay between neurophysiology and other physical functions. For example, the changes in postural stability with age are still only poorly understood in spite of the frequency of falls in the elderly. There are findings that oestrogens seem to be affecting dopaminergic neurons in the brain and therefore also the control of motor performance. This may possibly lead to changes in the processing of feedback impulses from the ankle to the brain. This promising clue to a link between clinical observation and cell biological findings should be followed as well as many others.

Although a considerable part of aging research has for the last years turned into research in Alzheimer's disease there are still substantial shortcomings in understanding the different types of dementia, partly due to the lack of autopsies but also due to problems in clinical research. Much insight has been gained in molecular biology and neurochemistry of dementing processes but attempts to correlate the clinical picture with these findings are scarce at the best. This implies for instance that clinical criteria for the definition of Alzheimer's disease are still imprecise.

However, despite the general importance of senile dementia the concern was expressed that the favourization of Alzheimer's disease over other topics may lead to a narrowing of research interests in gerontology.

One single factor for the extension of life has been identified in the last

xv

decade: food restriction which could possibly be complemented by hypophysectomy. This seems to extend life span at least in rodents although the way of action is not yet understood. One possibility could be to view aging as a process which exposes the organism to many influences, e.g. to the prolonged action of hormones but also of substances such as lipids or glucose, which might trigger the aging process in a dose- and time-related manner. So, the introduction of time instead of age could lead us to further research.

There is broad consent that there is a big deficit in theoretical gerontology. This leads to increasing specialization with the emergence of microfacets which in themselves cannot bear a relation to the whole. For example, in experimental psychology it could be demonstrated that motor skills decrease during the aging process in such a way that smooth movements degenerate into single small parts but at present nobody knows whether this fragmentation is related to aging *per se* or to underlying pathological conditions, whether there is one reason or whether there are multiple convergent causes.

Furthermore, a generally accepted definition for age-related changes is still lacking. If it is possible to prevent an "age-related" condition by any kind of intervention, this condition slips out of the context of age-related changes. The crisis in theory described by these examples could be a chance and a challenge for a more integrated theory of aging or one that is of a higher degree of sophistication. It could lead to more knowledge by combining age with other environmental factors, e.g. social status, education, life style. We find increased chances of integration in later adulthood in education, e.g. to integrate issues of prevention and self-control into life style. So, possibly a combination of biological and sociopsychological research could promote gerontology further in the future. This makes it necessary to understand the language of at least one different discipline.

Research into the processes of aging will also be stimulated when the focus is turned from the sick people seen by doctors and nurses to the more healthy ones and when it is possible to separate the influences of time and of the aging process which should not be confused. The balance of destructive and repair processes as well as that between destruction and compensation should be studied more intensely to understand the general phenomenon of reduced adaptive capacity.

Opening Address: the Demographic Structure of the Swiss Population and its Implications for Public Health

B. Roos

Managing Director, Federal Office of Public Health, Berne, Switzerland

It was with great pleasure that I agreed to deliver the opening address at the 1990 Sandoz Lectures in Gerontology. Although I have decided to speak on the topic of the demographic structure of the Swiss population and its implications for public health, I would like to stress right from the beginning that I am not an expert on questions of social policy or demography. However, in my position as Director of the Federal Office of Public Health, compatible with what is called in the USA Surgeon General, I have to deal with such health policy problems too. As you know, the health care system in Switzerland, which is a federalistic country composed of 26 individual states, is characterized by clear divisions of power between the Cantons and the Confederation. In our country, curative medicine as well as medical care of the elderly is the responsibility of Cantons and communities. The central government, that is the Confederation, is the competent authority for health protection in accordance with the law.

At the outset of my address I would like to state the following. For all of us, health is the greatest good and a gift which we hope to preserve until ripe old age. The state of health is largely influenced by individual life styles. Many of our fellow beings, however, expect state and community to protect their health during their entire life. To live longer and reach a ripe old age has always been one of the dreams of mankind. It cannot be denied that in our so-called "post-industrial" era this dream has in part been fulfilled. It is a truism that the average life expectancy at birth has increased quite considerably since the beginning of this century and is approaching what might be the maximum from a biological point of view. Since the beginning of the century, life expectancy in Switzerland has increased for men from 49 to 75 years and for women from 52 to 80 years. The increase is longevity is mainly due to a marked reduction in the mortality rate of the younger population and is the result of improvements in our living conditions. More attention to hygiene, better nutrition and improved working conditions as well as the elimination of infectious diseases mainly through vaccinations and better preventive measures in general resulted in ever more people reaching old age. Only time will tell whether it is possible to go even beyond what seems to be the maximum life expectancy as mentioned above. In this connection I would like to mention the research results of Professor Gehring from the Biocenter in Basle, indicating that the lack of certain proteins may be responsible for a limitation of the life span.

At this point, I would like to add that the figures on average life expectancy should not blind us to more urgent questions, namely the question concerning quality of life. In other words, are we doing enough to provide the elderly with structures that are adapted to their individual needs and that enable them to pass the rest of their lives in peace and without undue worries?

The structure of our population is changing not only due to an increase in the average life expectancy. In addition, the reproductive rate of the Swiss population plays an important role. It is another truism that the rate has decreased during the last decades. Thus, a rough estimate will tell us that the Swiss population is approaching a steady state or may even start to decrease. The consequences are that not only the number, but also the percentage of elderly people in the entire population will continue to increase. Already during the first years of the third millenium, there will be about the same number of elderly people and of adolescents and children, that is, around 20% each. The development of the population can easily be forecast, but the economical, social and moral problems which may result are difficult to judge. We do not know yet how we will react to the situation and how we will tackle the many new problems. Our lack of knowledge in this respect shows already in the use of words: the German word "Ueberalterung" implies in my view the notion that there are too many elderly people. This notion seems linked with the hope that probably one day, there will be less again. Furthermore, we have difficulties with the word "old" and prefer to use "aged", since being old is seen today as rather negative. In colloquial usage, "old" means worn out, decrepit, useless. We therefore have to be vigilant that in our throw-away mentality we do not start to look upon the elderly as a population group which can be passed over, put into state-owned institutions, "withdrawn from service", so to speak, and finally be forgotten.

The official language used in this connection isn't better either: people over 65 are called "aged"—but is it true that everybody who has reached 65 is indeed old, worn out and in need of assistance? We should not forget that retirement age has arbitrarily been set at 65. It is interesting to know that the age of 65 was decided upon as retirement age by the German invalidity and old age insurance agency already in 1916, that is, at a time when the average life expectancy amounted to about 50 years. At that time only about 38% of the male and 45% of the female population in Switzerland reached the retirement age of 65, while today 75 and 85%, respectively, do so. Or, to put it in other words, a 65-year-old man today has an average life expectancy of over 15 years as compared to only about 10 at the beginning of this century. These comparisons show that there has to be a marked difference between the vitality of 65-year-old people of today and those of bygone days. In my view, it is therefore entirely arbitrary to label everybody over 65 as "aged". Therefore, taking 65 as the basis for the planning of future health care needs, as is usually done, is in contradiction to the facts. If we rigidly stick to it, we run the risk of misjudging the situation and making decisions based on wrong forecasts. In addition, we should keep in mind that the age structure of those over 65 is changing too. The number of people over 80 will increase considerably in the coming years. In 1980, 2.6% of the Swiss population belonged to this age group, in 2015 the figure will have increased to about 6%.

Now I would like to turn to the needs of the elderly and to try and show how they can be integrated in the future planning. It is a fact that health care needs and demands for assistance increase with age. However, there are large differences between individuals with regard to quality, onset and duration of the assistance required. The utilization of health care services does definitely not increase in a linear fashion in relation to age, but rather exponentially, due to the disproportionate increase in needs.

With regard to the various diseases which appear with old age, we may assume that they will remain more or less the same. What we can expect, however, is an increase in the number of cases of disease or disability which you will be discussing during the Congress.

As mentioned earlier, the individual life style has an important influence on the physical and psychological condition in which an individual reaches a certain age. Thus, it is highly advisable to promote, in the population at large, everything which contributes to a healthy life style. In doing so, the fact should be kept in mind that disease and disability due to old age cannot be eliminated. However, it may be possible to postpone the onset of such disease and disability to ever later years. In other words, we should concentrate our efforts on an increase in the number of years spent in good health. It is here that I see an important task for the health care authorities, namely, not to discharge their duty towards the elderly merely by providing public assistance, but rather by helping them to improve their state of health. For this to come true, we have to be able to better assess the needs of old age which in turn calls for innovations and more studies in the field of social and preventive medicine.

As mentioned earlier, the state of health of the older population depends not only on biological factors which determine the aging process, but to a considerable degree on the social and physical environment in which the individual lives. Important factors in this connection are life style, nutritional habits and working environment as well as the attitude of society towards health. I am convinced that it is possible to influence these factors in such a way that disease and disability due to old age are less severe and, most importantly, their onset delayed as compared to the past. As far as pharmaceutical research is concerned, it should be possible to develop drugs which help to further improve the state of health of the elderly.

Let us now turn to some of the questions in connection with health care costs. It cannot be denied that the costs for medical and health care needs increase with age. Unfortunately, some of the discussions on these problems give the impression that elderly people are considered by many as unscrupulous consumers of health care services. Old and sick people are accused of being unable to defray the costs incurred for their care. This is a completely distorted view and would be similar to accusing young people of causing too high costs for education, which is not done of course; rather, we have got used to it due to the introduction of compulsory education over one hundred years ago. The fact that the health care costs are incurred largely by the older population, in particular during the last few years of life, is in itself an indication of an improvement of the health status during the earlier years of life. If appropriate preventive measures can contribute to a reduction in the health care costs incurred during the earlier periods of life, then there should be enough means to pay for the unavoidable health care costs of old age. As an example I would like to mention heavy smokers who cause considerable health care costs already at an early age.

We can be sure of one thing, namely that all well-intentioned appeals to cut down on expenses will not reduce the ever-increasing number of elderly people. Therefore, it would be more realistic to speak about problems of financing health care due to demographic changes instead of referring to cost explosion. In fact, it should be clear to everybody that a longer life will inevitably mean that larger provisions for the future have to be made. Or, in other words, we have to lay aside during younger, healthier years what we may need during old age and show solidarity with the elderly by providing the necessary financial means for their needs. A sense of responsibility to provide as far as possible for one's own old age should be promoted actively with all generations. The functioning of the social system remains closely linked to a favourable economic development in our country.

The future health care costs depend not only on the number of elderly people but also on the manner in which we organize medical care. What is required most is the development of services according to needs. Services provided outside hospitals through community nurses and lay personnel should, in order to be taken seriously, not be cheaper than those provided by old people's and nursing homes. In my opinion, the responsibility to provide for the elderly should not be left to the state alone. Instead, I believe that we ought to try and live up to our social responsibility and that the young people should show their solidarity with the elderly. This has been the case for centuries, e.g. in the Canton of Berne where the parents continue to stay on the farm in a tiny house, the so-called "Stöckli", even after the son has taken over the farm and the large house. It is in this area where the most urgent problems have to be solved in order to ensure an efficient co-ordination of the efforts of the various institutions concerned with out-patient care. I would like to repeat that it is above all solidarity which is required and which will help us solve the problems.

ACKNOWLEDGEMENT

The author wishes to acknowledge the help of Stephanie Zobrist, Ph.D. in the preparation of this address.

Part I

Human Competence: Changes under Normal and Pathological Conditions

Aging and Speed of Behaviour: its Scientific and Practical Significance

*James E. Birren, Max Vercruyssen and Laurel M. Fisher

Ethel Percy Andrus Gerontology Center, Los Angeles, USA

INTRODUCTION

One of the most reliable findings in the behavioural sciences is the slowing of behaviour with increasing age. Older adults are significantly slowed relative to younger adults across many different types of tasks (e.g. Dustman *et al.* 1984, 1989). For example, results from 26 studies showed that simple reaction time (RT) slows by about 20% between 20 and 60 years of age (Vercruyssen *et al.* 1988a). Large population studies continue to show a significant relationship of speed of performance with age, and that the age and speed factor is embedded in a matrix of relationships with physiological and behavioural parameters (Era *et al.* 1986, Era 1987). Older adults seem to be particularly slowed in tasks requiring rapid processing of stimuli and activation of appropriate motor programs (Botwinick 1964). However, age-related slowing of behaviour does not seem to translate into a qualitatively different type of information processing (Birren *et al.* 1980). Research prior to 1980 (reviewed in Birren *et al.* 1980) indicates that there may be few age differences in *how* young and older adults process information (see also Birren 1964, Welford 1977, Botwinick 1978, Salthouse 1982).

In recent years, research into age-related slowing has investigated several questions, two of which are: (1) what are the antecedents or causes of age-related slowing?; (2) is slowing truly general, affecting all components of information processing without prejudice or does it affect discrete components? This brief paper will not be a comprehensive survey but will review pertinent research published during the 1980s and describe some of the recent research conducted at the University of Southern California's Laboratory of Attention and Motor Performance (USC-LAMP).

RECENT EXAMINATION OF CONTRIBUTING FACTORS

A number of different factors, including subject characteristics as well as experimental manipulations, have been shown to have an impact on speed of behaviour. Age, gender, cognitive capacity, physical fitness of the subject, how much practice subjects have prior to the critical measurement of speed, and the task itself, all contribute to the observed changes in speed of behaviour. Any theoretical statements made about one of these factors should be qualified by statements about the other critical factors.

Speed and Stages of Information Processing

A number of investigations during the 1980s have continued to search for the cognitive processes or stages of information processing which slow more than other stages or processes. It appears that speed of lexical access or semantic activation is relatively intact with age (Bowles and Poon 1981, Howard et al. 1986, Balota and Duchek 1988). Central cognitive processes seem to be more slowed with age than initial perceptual processes (Salthouse and Somberg 1982a). Age differences in reaction time can be minimized if older adults limit the amount of processing needed to complete the task (Cohen and Faulkner 1983). Complex tasks put older adults at a distinct disadvantage (Corpolongo and Salmon 1981), even if initial performance levels among the age groups are equated. Movement time seems to be markedly slowed with age (Stelmach et al. 1986, Balota and Duchek 1988).

One common method of isolating stage-specific differences in information processing is Sternberg's (1969) additive factor method (AFM). Simon and Pouraghabagher (1978) used the AFM to isolate the stage(s) at which information processing is differentially slowed by age. By loading early and central stages, they found only an age by stimulus degradation interaction. The interaction indicated that concentrated slowing is found during early stages of processing. However, Salthouse and Somberg (1982b) used AFM in a reaction time study of speed and found that age interacted with each stage of processing from encoding to response preparation. Salthouse and Somberg (1982b) concluded that age-related slowing was indeed a general phenomenon and not specific to any one information-processing stage. In yet another application of the AFM involving older subjects, Moraal (1982a, b) conducted a series of three reaction time experiments and concluded that there was not sufficient evidence for supporting either generalized or stage-specific slowing with age.

Certainly, the question of whether aging affects specific stages or generally affects all stages of information processing was not clearly answered by these studies. Therefore, several studies carried out by USC-LAMP have applied the AFM in order to resolve the conflict (Carlton *et al.* 1989, Vercruyssen *et al.* 1989a). The studies involved manipulating intratask factors including stimulus degradation, stimulus–response (S–R) compatibility, and response–stimulus interval (RSI), over 2 days of testing. As seen in previous experiments, practice significantly improved reaction time (RT) and different results were produced when subjects were naive compared to when they had large amounts of practice. Since the AFM requires the use of skilled subjects, the results reported here will be the data from the second day, after RT performance had stabilized. The extent to which slowness may be more manifest in unfamiliar tasks, rather than practised tasks, limits the interpretation of results from the AFM relative to the general or specific character of slowness.

Young subjects performed faster than the older adults across all RT conditions. Reaction time for the compatible S–R condition was about half of the time required to respond in the incompatible S–R condition, a significant effect. Older adults were disproportionately slower in the incompatible S–R condition compared to young adults.

In the RSI = 5 s condition, older subjects were disproportionately slowed by the low S–R compatibility condition. Older adults were not disproportionately slowed relative to young adults in the degraded stimuli condition. These results indicate that older adults may experience greater slowing in central decision-making processes (Figure 1). When RSI = 0 s, there was no interaction of age and response compatibility or degradation (Figure 2). Further analyses of these data to clarify the results are now in progress, but it is becoming clear that many of the equivocal findings can be explained in terms of RSI, practice, physical fitness, and attention.

Taken together, the studies of information processing by USC-LAMP and others seem to indicate some disproportionate slowing which is stage specific. This is especially true when older subjects are under conditions of stimulus degradation and stimulus–response incompatibility. However, it is clear that older adults also tend to be generally slowed across stages of information processing.

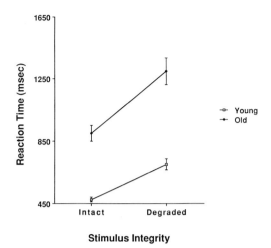

Fig. 1. Mean reaction time in ms for RSI = 5 for young ($n=10$) and older adults ($n=10$) on intact and degraded stimuli.

Longitudinal Studies

The previous studies demonstrate age-related slowing within cross-sectional designs. Recent results from longitudinal studies further demonstrate age-related slowing in a within-subjects design. Longitudinal studies also shed light on when the slowing occurs in the life span and at what magnitude.

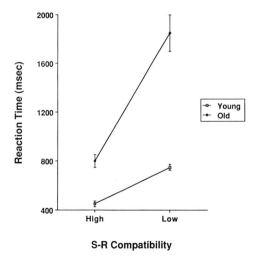

Fig. 2. Mean reaction time in ms for RSI = 0 for young ($n=10$) and older adults ($n=11$) by high and low stimulus–response compatibility.

Reaction time data from the Baltimore Longitudinal Study of Aging were analysed by Giambra and Quilter (1988; see also Quilter *et al.* 1983, Shock *et al.* 1984). Giambra and Quilter (1988) used the Mackworth clock test to measure vigilance and reaction time in 53 men first tested during 1962–1964 and then retested 18 years later. In the Mackworth clock test, subjects are instructed to observe a second hand of a clock for unusual jumps and press a button as soon as they observed such a jump. Over the 18-year period separating test occasions, the subjects showed no overall decrease in vigilance. However, subjects who were young (27–39) at the time of initial testing showed a decrease in reaction time, whereas those who were older (50–74) showed an increase in reaction time at the second administration. This finding suggested that reaction time for vigilance monitoring decreases from youth to midlife, but begins to increase somewhere between the ages of 55 and 60 (Giambra and Quilter 1988).

Giambra and Quilter (1988) report additional results from the Baltimore Longitudinal Study on the amount of slowing over the life span using a measure of psychophysiological arousal, skin potential response latency (SPRL). SPRL showed lowered levels of arousal with age. Older men showed longer response latencies at the second test session, indicating they required more time to show autonomic arousal. It appears that the time taken to show autonomic arousal also increased with age, as well as overt reaction time. Thus, the subjects showed slowing on a behavioural and a psychophysiological measure.

Cardiovascular Function and RT

Speed of behaviour may not only be useful as a marker of the integrity of the central nervous system (CNS), but may also be an indicator of cardiovascular health. In a Swedish longitudinal study (Berg 1980), participants with diastolic blood pressure over 115 mmHg had significantly lower scores on the Perceptual Speed (Identical Forms) test relative to those with blood pressure under 115 mmHg. Berg (1980) concluded that the greatest impairment among those with cardiovascular disease is on the speeded tests, but this relationship tended to hold for males only.

Wilkie and Eisdorfer (1973, cited in Siegler 1983) analysed the reaction time data from the Duke Longitudinal Study in relation to blood pressure. Participants ranged in age from 60 to 90 years of age. At the time of first measurement, RT was not related to blood pressure. While there were no subjects with high blood pressure remaining in the sample by the fourth wave, those with borderline high blood pressure showed slowing of RT. In contrast, 70-year-old subjects with normal blood pressure showed little change in RT over test occasions.

Nowlin and Siegler (1985) studied longitudinal change on a continuous

performance task (CPT) and cardiovascular disease. They divided participants in the Duke Longitudinal Study into three groups: (1) those without
heart disease; (2) those with hypertension; (3) those with evidence of
atherosclerosis. All three groups were slowed about the same amount over
time. That is, the three groups retained their relative rank over time.
Individuals with atherosclerosis had significantly slower reaction times
than the other two groups. Nowlin and Siegler (1985) concluded that
cardiovascular fitness is intimately related to cognitive performance,
specifically from the middle-age years and beyond.

Efforts to Alter Speed of Behaviour

Efforts to alter the speed of response in older adults via behaviour
modification methodologies have not met with much success. Denney
(1981/2) and Hoyer et al. (1978/9) attempted to train older adults to
respond quickly in a reaction time task. Hoyer et al. (1978/9) found that
a young group evidenced larger gains from the training than did an older
group (although the older subjects were able to increase their speed
somewhat). Denney (1981/2) found only one experimental manipulation in
three experiments which affected older adults' response time. Older adults
who were forced to respond quickly were able to respond more quickly.

Drug studies attempting to decrease reaction time have yielded equivocal
results. When older adults are given amphetamine their reaction time does
not generally increase, while reaction time was speeded in the young
(Halliday et al. 1986). Methylphenidate did increase older adults' response
processing in one of two experiments utilizing that drug. In the young,
amphetamine generally speeds movement time but not RT (Frowein and
Sanders 1978, Frowein 1981a,b).

The results from the longitudinal studies, the work on cardiovascular
patients, and the efforts to alter speed of response, as well as the work
from USC-LAMP, all point to the conclusion that speed of behaviour is
biologically based. For example, one sobering statistic observed in the
Swedish longitudinal study was the high correlation of 0.54 ($P < 0.05$)
between the number of months to death after the first test occasion and
Perceptual Speed (Identical Forms) test (PS-IF) score at age 70 (Berg
1980). PS-IF was one of the few cognitive subtests to correlate with time
to death and was also the subtest with the highest correlation with time to
death. Subjects with lower PS-IF scores had the fewest months to death,
while those with higher scores had more months before death.

In a general sense, speed of behaviour arises from the operation of the
CNS. Indeed, speed is not a narrow factor related solely to movement but
can be viewed as broadly reflective of many types of processing by the
CNS. Various oscillations of CNS electrophysiology may be related to

movement timing and sleep/wake cycles (Llinas 1988). Prinz *et al.* (1990) provide a more complete review of changes in EEG patterns with age. Hicks and Birren (1970) suggested that damage to the basal ganglia, a brain stem structure with diffuse cortical projections, may result in a slowed organism. Ivry and Keele (1989) noted that increased variability in older adults' ability to accurately time movements and perceive the passage of time may reflect on the integrity of the cerebellum and may also involve basal ganglia functioning (see also Freed and Yamamoto 1985).

If one considers the role of the CNS as a regulatory organ, utilizing both "software" and "hardware" principles of operation (including the interactions of the software and hardware), changes in the speed of CNS processing may be a good marker of the aging process. In short, speed of behaviour may be one of the best indicators of the integrity of the CNS, especially under different stressors, such as age, damage to the brain, drugs, etc. This line of reasoning raises the possibility of using measures of speed of behaviour in situations where a quick assessment of CNS functioning is required.

Effects of Physical Fitness

Clarkson-Smith and Hartley (1989) administered a battery of cognitive ability measures, including a reaction time measure, to 62 older adults who exercised regularly and 62 older adults who did not exercise regularly. Overall, they found significantly better performance on all measures by the exercisers compared to the non-exercisers. Specifically, reaction time for the exercisers was significantly faster compared to the non-exercisers. Stones and Kozma (1989) also found enhanced performance on two-digit symbol reaction time tasks for older adults who exercised compared to older adults who did not exercise.

Dustman *et al.* (1984) also conducted an aerobic training study, employing a battery of neuropsychological tests, and found similar improvements for simple RT, the Stroop Colour Word test, critical flicker fusion, digit symbol, and dots (errors). However, they found no improvements for depression scores, sensory thresholds and visual acuity. They speculated that aerobic training promoted increased cerebral metabolic activity which resulted in improvements in neuropsychological test scores (Dustman *et al.* 1984).

USC-LAMP research in the last few years has focused on elucidating the effects of age, gender, arousal, physical fitness, practice, and task loading on speed of behaviour. Maintaining physical fitness certainly plays a significant role in retarding some of the decline in speed of response in older adults. It appears that increasing the level of arousal, as in standing and mild exercise during administration of a task, improves RT. This is

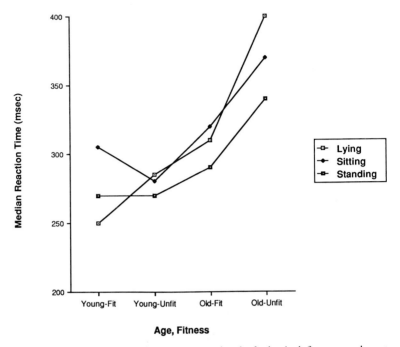

Fig. 3. Median reaction time by age group, level of physical fitness, and postural position. Reaction time was significantly faster in the standing postural position for all subjects (Woods 1981).

particularly the case when CNS speed has been temporarily slowed, e.g. time-on-task, fatigue, drowsiness, lethargy, boredom, and lack of concentration.

In order to separate out the effects of generalized arousal and increased cardiovascular activity on reaction time, Woods (1981) devised a unique study. She tested young and older adults in a simple and complex reaction time setting while manipulating postural position and intensity of exercise. The old and young subjects were categorized at the start of the experiment as physically fit or unfit. On the first day the subjects performed the reaction time tasks in each of three postural positions: lying, sitting, and standing. This manipulation was presumed to alter systemic arousal. On the second day of testing, cardiovascular activity was manipulated by having the subjects freely pedal a bicycle ergometer, pedalling at 20% of maximum heart rate (HRmax), and at 40% HRmax, while performing simple and choice reaction time tasks.

As expected, older adults were significantly slower than young subjects in both RT and movement time (MT). Older adults were disproportionately slower on the complex two-choice RT task. Unfit older adults were especially slow on the complex RT task relative to younger adults. The physically fit older adults had significantly faster RT and MT than the unfit older adults. In fact, fit older adults more closely resembled unfit young adults in speed of response.

The reaction time of young adults did not differ with postural position. However, there were significant differences in the older adults. Older subjects were faster when standing than when they were sitting or lying. The largest postural improvements in RT were observed in the unfit older adults, who significantly decreased their reaction time by 16% while standing relative to sitting (Woods 1981).

Results of the exercise intensity manipulation support the notion that acute exercise elevated arousal in the underaroused. Woods (1981) found that young adult reaction time did not differ across exercise intensity condition. However, fit older adults did best during free pedalling, whereas unfit older adults had the fastest reaction time during the 20% condition HRmax (Woods 1981).

Presumably, reaction time is most improved by exercise in relation to age, with improvement in reaction time being proportional to the amount of possible improvement in the subject. It is assumed that the young subjects improve little because they are already at an optimal level of tonic arousal. The old unfit, on the other hand, are the most underaroused and, therefore, require more cardiovascular stimulation to elevate their tonic arousal and improve RT.

Using simple and two-choice RT tasks, Woods (1981) found posture effects only in the older adults. Using a much more difficult manipulation of a four-choice RT task, Vercruyssen *et al.* (1988a) found posture effects for both young and older adults. Young and older adults participated over 2 days in serial choice reaction time (SCRT) and variable choice reaction time (VCRT) tasks using both intact and degraded stimuli. The general level of arousal was manipulated by testing the subjects while either standing or sitting.

The young subjects were faster than the older subjects and all subjects had faster RT with intact stimuli relative to degraded stimuli. Older adults were disproportionately slowed during the degraded task condition compared to the young. There was an interaction between gender and degradation. Females were faster on the degraded task condition compared to males, but there were no differences between males and females with intact stimuli (see Vercruyssen *et al.* 1989b). While all subjects on Day 2 were faster than on Day 1, the older adults improved more on the second day than the younger subjects.

Degradation interacted with practice for VCRT. On the second day the differences between the intact and degraded condition were less, although the intact condition still produced faster RTs overall. Similar to previous studies, fastest RTs during the VCRT task were obtained with RSIs of 2 s when stimuli were presented randomly at RSIs of 0, 1, 2, 3, and 6 s. Particularly, older adults were at a disadvantage when the stimuli are degraded and the task is unfamiliar (see Cann 1990 for a review of this research).

Woods (1981) found that changing posture from lying to sitting to standing consistently improved RT in older adults. This may indicate that the general level of arousal influences the changes in RT seen with age. The fit older adults had considerably faster RT and MT than the unfit older adults regardless of postural position. Cross-sectional and aerobic training studies have shown that physical fitness is a very important variable in determining the extent of age-related slowing. Older physically fit individuals have faster RTs than their sedentary counterparts and are often as fast as, or faster than, young sedentary (or below average fitness) individuals (Clarkson-Smith and Hartley 1989, Dustman *et al.* 1989). Thus, data from our lab and elsewhere point to the general benefit of exercising in mitigating the slowing which accompanies age (see also Rikli and Busch 1986, Spirduso and MacRae 1990, Vercruyssen *et al.* 1988). The effects of arousal, activation, and attention and the limits of their relevance to slowing with age need further investigation.

MODELLING AND DATA STIMULATIONS

Modelling

The research on speed of behaviour has proceeded on several fronts, both in the empirical reaction time arena and in the more theoretical and statistical arenas. Cerella (1985) and Salthouse (1988) have each applied widely different techniques to model reaction time data in order to test several hypotheses about the nature of age-related slowing. Cerella (1985) performed a meta-analysis on nearly 190 different reaction time tasks found in 18 studies. He tested a multiplicative model of slowing (one general factor) and an additive model of slowing (many slowing factors). The means from young and older adults were plotted, the older scores against younger. Regression lines were then calculated. The best fitting model was the multiplicative model with two factors (age of subjects: under 60, over 60; task type: sensory–motor, experimental). Cerella suggests that slowing occurs on two levels: one slowing coefficient applies to those under 60, another, with a steeper slope, to those after 60. In addition, the slowing seen for control conditions is less than what is seen for the experimental conditions. Cerella concluded that differences in reaction time with age appear to be due to general slowing factors and that different experimental

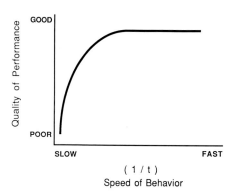

Fig. 4. Hypothetical relationship between speed of behaviour and quality of performance.

results across studies are due to differences in the "ratio of sensory–motor and computational components in the experimental conditions" (Cerella, 1985, p. 81).

In a computer simulation of information processing, Salthouse (1988) was able to mimic the response time data in older adults by specifying slower propagations through nodes in a computational type of network. Salthouse noted several ways in which a network could be altered to produce inefficient processing. Slowing of propagation across the network resulted in a gradual decline, not a sudden sharp decrement, in functioning. Merely slowing speed of transmission did not alter the network structurally and the processing still occurred in the same manner as before. The inefficiencies of the computational network processing under reduced speed only became more evident under complex tasks. However, any limitation on activation time would result in the curtailment of interactive processing or parallel processing. Making distinctions among theories explaining the age-related declines in memory and attention, such as reduced capacity in older adults, reduced number of nodes, or slowing of message transmission speed, is especially difficult, as these limitations appear quite similar at certain levels of analysis. While Salthouse makes no claim for evidence for a general slowing hypothesis from these simulations, the results of slowing speed of propagation certainly mimic many of the predicted effects of the general slowing hypothesis.

Factor Analyses of Attention and Intelligence

Factor analyses of speeded psychometric tests also reveal a general speed factor of intelligence across age groups (Cornelius *et al.* 1983, Hertzog *et al.* 1986, Horn 1982, 1988, Stankov 1988). Horn (1982, 1988) has defined a general speed factor, Gs, in his fluid-crystallized theory of intellectual abilities. Gs seems to load on the second order factor, Gf, fluid intelligence. Fluid intelligence is thought to be linked closely with physiological functioning of the person (Horn, 1982, 1988). This supports the notion that speed of response is biologically based and is most affected by the physiological changes that come with age.

When the effects of an age-related decline in speed and attention are partialled out of the fluid intelligence factor, the decline seen in fluid intelligence with age disappears (Horn 1982, Stankov 1988). It seems that speed of response is fundamental to attention and fluid intelligence and, as speed declines, so do attention and fluid intelligence scores.

Surprisingly, the increase in crystallized intelligence seen with age increases even more if the decline in the speed of response factor is partialled out (Stankov 1988). It seems as though the speed of response factor has a dampening effect on the accumulated information and expertise which comes with age. Thus, speed of response differentially affects fluid intelligence and crystallized intelligence as one ages.

Age and Attention

Stankov (1988) identified a separate attention factor which was affected by a speed of behaviour factor. USC-LAMP has been investigating different aspects of attention in an effort to understand how speed of behaviour might relate to attentional processes. McDowd *et al.* (submitted) recently investigated how often young and older adults experience lapses of attention in everyday life. For example, throwing away a piece of gum and chewing on the wrapper would be a common lapse of attention. A self-report questionnaire describing various types of lapses was administered to 364 subjects between the ages of 17 and 84. It was thought that due to age-related slowing, older adults would report a greater frequency of attentional lapses than young adults. In addition, a factor analysis was performed on the questionnaire items as a replication of a previous study using the questionnaire by Reason (1984).

Surprisingly, the number of reported lapses decreased with increasing age, i.e. young adults reported a far greater number of lapses than older adults. The factor analysis revealed a two-factor solution, consisting of an Action factor and a Memory factor. These two factors replicated Reason's (1984) findings. About half of the older adults' scores tended to load on the Action factor and half loaded on the Memory factor. For the young subjects, more items tended to load on the Action factor than on the Memory factor.

It seems that some types of lapses which loaded on the action factor in young adults shifted to loading on the memory factor in older adults. Age-related slowing in speed of behaviour may assist in interpreting these results. In young adults, with quicker responses, certain types of lapses may be more related to functions which require action. In contrast, in older adults, who respond slower, those same types of lapses may have come to depend more on memory functions than action.

The data on attentional lapses reveal how fundamental and pervasive the loss of speed with age can be. Slowing of behaviour is not simply a robust laboratory finding to tickle scientific curiosity. It is expressed in the daily life of older adults, from small unintentional lapses of attention to slowed reactions while driving on a busy freeway (Vercruyssen *et al.* 1988b).

IMPLICATIONS

Applications

There are many important implications of the slowing of behaviour with age in daily life, ranging from automobile driving and pedestrian safety to design of consumer products (Charness and Bosman 1990, Parmelee and Lawton 1990). Research on speed of behaviour has progressed to the point where we can begin to make suggestions about the use of measures of speed of behaviour: as a measure of CNS integrity, to facilitate older adults' use of environments, and possibly point to some measures to prevent some of the consequences of slow behaviour.

Architects, engineers, and others who design products and environments for older adults could use knowledge about the changes in speed of behaviour to design buildings, e.g. the timing of elevator door closing, so as to minimize the effects of slowness of the older user. Traffic engineers could program traffic light changes to allow for the older adults' slower walking pace.

If one takes seriously the hypothesis that speed can be used as a general indicator of the integrity of the CNS, it has enormous practical significance for those desiring to test new drugs designed for older adults. Simple and complex reaction time measures could be taken before, during, and after drug administration. The speed of behaviour can serve as a measure of change in function due to the drug. Speed of behaviour can be used to assess the status of patients after surgery or damage to the brain. It can also be used as one index when evaluating personnel for positions requiring quick decisions and actions.

Increasingly we are becoming aware of the benefits of aerobic exercise for older adults. Since physically fit older adults are faster in their behaviour than are the unfit, reaction time measures can play a role in assessing the physical status of older adults and the changes brought about by exercise programs (Prinz *et al.* 1990, Spirduso and MacRae 1990). Greater education is needed about the benefits of exercise for adults and the relationship of fitness to speed of behaviour.

Future Research

Given the established background of research and the high reliability of the observations of the slowness of behaviour with age, research is needed that will provide further knowledge about the causes of the slowness with age as well as its consequences for complex behaviour. While past research suggests that slowness of behaviour reflects the likelihood of survival, little is known about the biological and behavioural processes involved (Birren *et al.* 1980). Research efforts should be directed toward elucidating the behavioural consequences of slowing, the antecedents of slowing, and the development of methods to attenuate slowing with age.

Presently numerous hypotheses may be advanced to account for the causes of the slowness of behaviour with age. Slowing may reflect the non-specific vulnerability of the neuron over the life span such that as the population of cells declines, the efficiency and capacity of neuronal transmission becomes increasingly limited. Alternatively, specific subsystems of the CNS may be responsible, e.g. the norepinephrine system and the locus coeruleus (Bondareff 1985); the basal ganglia (Hicks and Birren 1970), the reduction of dopamine levels; and the cerebellum and the extra-pyramidal motor system (Woodruff-Pak 1989).

Suggestions about the origins of slowness with age linked to levels of CNS arousal are contradictory. Some investigators have hypothesized that age-related reduction in speed is due to an overaroused CNS and others have hypothesized an underaroused CNS is the culprit (Woodruff 1985). Clearly, different avenues of intervention would follow from these two opposing hypotheses. One possible reason for the contradictory hypotheses may be a confusion of CNS arousal with autonomic nervous system (ANS) activity. Generally, measures of ANS activity may suggest a high level of arousal, but in older adults this may not reflect CNS arousal. It may be that as one ages, there is an uncoupling of CNS–ANS function (March and Thompson 1977). It is possible that older adults can show overarousal in the ANS and be underaroused in the CNS. Future research should use multiple measures of arousal, including both CNS and ANS measures.

Related to the hyperarousal hypothesis is the idea that the older nervous system is more noisy. In other words, the signal-to-noise ratio is altered with age, such that the information signal competes with a higher background level of noise (Welford 1977). Results from electrophysiological studies suggest that there is a lower level of excitability with age (Prinz *et al.* 1990). These findings do not clearly address the question of signal-to-noise ratio changes with age as they did not determine the relative level of signal strength to noise with age.

One of the most general hypotheses about aging and the rising probability of death is related to the brain/body weight ratio (Sacher 1977). Evolution has resulted in primates possessing a large brain relative to body size. While the relatively larger brain may confer a survival advantage, it may also dictate that the involution of the nervous system will ultimately end the life of the organism, with slowness appearing as an early manifestation of the aging organism and its survival fitness. This pattern of thinking places slowness of behaviour in the forefront of the quest for markers of aging. It also raises perplexing questions about the role of the concept of time in scientific explanations (Schroots and Birren 1988).

The previous discussion relates to the probable biological basis of slowness in behaviour with age. Research is also required in the task of describing and explaining the consequences of slowness for complex behaviour. In analytical terms, slowness in behaviour can be regarded as a dependent variable, which is to be explained by other independent variables. However, slowness can, in turn, be regarded as an independent variable upon which more complex behavioural processes depend (e.g. complex decision-making processes; Birren 1988, Birren and Birren 1990).

One can assume that functioning of the organism, particularly of the brain, must in some way be hierarchically organized. Some functions must be dependent upon the integrity of subordinate systems. In this sense, the components of intellectual abilities are more complex than the speed of behaviour, but may in fact be limited by speed (Horn 1982). In a dynamic system with decay processes, such as short-term memory and processes of habituation, speed may be a limiting factor in all of their component processes. Thus, research is needed which will help delineate the significance of speed in complex cognitive performance of older adults. Presumably, speed of functioning will be of greater significance for some aspects of intellectual abilities than others, e.g. fluid intelligence (Horn 1982). In contrast, recalling events in long-term memory should be little influenced by slowing of behaviour. The hierarchical significance of speed within other cognitive abilities is a prime topic for research.

Another area of research concerns the adaptations that older adults may make as a consequence of their expectations, resulting in slowness of behaviour. In other words, the social expectation that older adults should be slow in manner and behaviour may result in older adults who *are* slow (Botwinick 1978). Such social behavioural interactions with age require research before one concludes that all slowness rests upon a biological basis and/or is the consequence of irreversible disuse.

The above complexitites require sophistication in research methodology if we are to specify with assurance the causes and consequences of slowness of behaviour with age, and the range of its modification through optimum life style and interventions. Future research should specify in detail the subject characteristics, task characteristics, and the statistical analyses used in studies (Vercruyssen *et al.* 1990b). Many calls for greater sophistication in research methods on aging have been made (Schaie *et al.* 1988). It is too much to expect that a single piece of research will answer many of the issues raised here. However, it is desirable that future research be more additive, in the sense that we desire to integrate findings into an increasingly broader picture of the causes and consequences of slowness in behaviour with age.

Conclusions

1. Slowing of behaviour with age is a well-established observation. It is a robust phenomenon with many research implications awaiting investigation.
2. The weight of present evidence suggests that slowness of behaviour with advancing age is a general process which is most likely of a biological nature.
3. Slowing of behaviour appears to have hierarchical consequences limiting complex functioning such as attention and fluid intelligence.
4. General slowing of behaviour with age is moderated by exercise and an active life style. In contrast, cardiovascular disease is related to disproportionate slowing with age.
5. Since slowness of behaviour with age appears to be related to individual longevity and biological changes in the CNS, research should be pursued which will integrate the behavioural and biological knowledge domains. Such knowledge should be useful in improving the quality of life in advanced age.

ACKNOWLEDGEMENTS

The authors appreciate comments made on an earlier draft of this manuscript by M.T. Cann and K. Hashizume. This manuscript is based on invited papers by the first author at the 1989 International Congress on Gerontology,

June 18–23, in Acapulco, Mexico, as well as the Conference über Altern und Leistung, October 1989 in Hamburg, Germany (proceedings in German, Finnish and English).

REFERENCES

Balota, D. and Duchek, J. (1988). Age-related differences in lexical access, spreading activation, and simple pronunciation. *Psychology and Aging* **3**, 84–93.

Berg, S. (1980). Psychological functioning in 70- and 75-year-old people. *Acta Psychiatrica Scandinavica* **62**, suppl. 288.

Birren, J. E. (1964). "The psychology of aging". The University of Chicago Press, Chicago, IL.

Birren, J. E. (1988). A contribution to the theory of aging: As a counterpoint of development. In "Emergent theories of aging" (J. E. Birren and V. L. Bengtson, eds) pp. 153–176. Springer, New York.

Birren, J. E. and Birren, B. A. B. (1990). The concepts, models, and history of the psychology of aging. *In* "Handbook of the psychology of aging" 3rd edn (J. E. Birren and K. W. Schaie, (eds) pp. 3–20. Academic Press, New York.

Birren, J. E., Woods, A. M. and Williams, M. V. (1980). Behavioral slowing with age: Causes, organization and consequences. *In* "Aging in the 1980s: psychological issues" (L.W. Poon, ed.) pp. 293–308. American Psychological Association, Washington, DC.

Bondareff, W. (1985). The neural bases of aging. *In* "Handbook of the psychology of aging" 2nd edn. (J. E. Birren and K.W. Schaie, eds) pp. 95–112. Van Nostrand Reinhold, New York.

Botwinick, J. (1964). Theories of antecedent conditions of speed of response. *In* "Behavior, aging, and the nervous system" (A.T. Welford and J. E. Birren, eds). Charles Thomas, Springfield, IL.

Botwinick, J. (1978). "Aging and behavior" 2nd edn. Springer, New York.

Bowles, N. and Poon, L. (1981). The effect of age on speed of lexical access. *Experimental Aging Research* **7**, 417–425.

Cann, M. T. (1990). "Age and speed of behavior: effects of gender, postural arousal, and task loading". Master's thesis, Human Factors Department, University of Southern California, Los Angeles, CA.

Carlton, B. L., Vercruyssen, M., McDowd, J. M. and Birren, J. E. (1989). Effects of age and practice on stages of information processing. Presented at Western Psychological Association–Rocky Mountain Psychological Association Conference. "Symposium on Attention and Memory in Cognitive Aging", Reno, NV.

Cerella, J. (1985). Information processing rates in the elderly. *Psychological Bulletin* **98**, 67–83.

Charness, N. and Bosman, E. A. (1990). Human factors and design for older adults. *In* "Handbook of the psychology of aging" 3rd edn. (J. E. Birren and K. W. Schaie, eds). pp. 446–464. Academic Press, New York.

Clarkson-Smith, L. and Hartley, A. A. (1989). Relationships between physical exercise and cognitive abilities in older adults. *Psychology and Aging* **4**, 183–189.

Cohen, G. and Faulkner, D. (1983). Age differences in performance on two information-processing tasks: Strategy selection and processing efficiency. *Journal of Gerontology* **38**, 447–454.

Cornelius, S., Willis, S., Nesselroade, J. and Baltes, P. (1983). Convergence between attention variables and factors of psychometric intelligence in older adults. *Intelligence* **7**, 253–269.

Corpolongo, M. and Salmon, P. (1981). Comparison of information-processing capacities in young and aged subjects using reaction times. *Perceptual and Motor Skills* **52**, 987–994.

Denney, N. (1981/2). Attempts to modify cognitive tempo in elderly adults. *International Journal of Aging and Human Development* **14**, 239–254.

Dustman, R. E., Ruhling, R. O., Russell, E. M., Shjearer, D. E., Bonekat, H. W., Shigeoka, J. W., Wood, J. S. and Bradford, D. C. (1984). Aerobic exercise training and improved neuropsychological function of older individuals. *Neurobiology of Aging* **5**, 35–42.

Dustman, R. E., Ruhling, R. O., Russell, E. M., Shjearer, D. E., Bonekat, H. W., Shigeoka, J. W., Wood, J. S. and Bradford, D. C. (1989). Aerobic exercise training and improved neuropsychological function of older individuals. *In* "Aging and motor behavior" (A.C. Ostrow, ed.) pp. 67–83. Benchmark, Indianapolis, IN.

Era, P. (1987). Sensory, psychomotor, and motor functions in men of different ages. *Scandinavian Journal of Social Medicine* Suppl. 39.

Era, P., Jokela, J. and Heikkinen, E. (1986). Reaction time and movement times in men of different ages: A population study. *Perceptual and Motor Skills* **63**, 111–130.

Freed, C. and Yamamoto, B. (1985). Regional brain dopamine metabolism: A marker for the speed, direction, and posture of moving animals. *Science* **229**, 62–65.

Frowein, H. W. (1981a). Selective effects of barbituates and amphetamine on information processing and response execution. *Acta Psychologica* **47**, 105–115.

Frowein, H. W. (1981b). "Selective drug effects on information processing". Thesis for doctor in de sociale wetenschappen (Ph.D. in Social Sciences) at de Katholieke Hogeschool, Tilburg, The Netherlands.

Frowein, H. W. and Sanders, A. F. (1978). Effect of amphetamine and barbituate on serial reaction time under paced and self-paced conditions. *Acta Psychologica* **42**, 263–276.

Giambra, L. and Quilter, R. (1988). Sustained attention in adulthood: A unique, large-sample, longitudinal and multicohort analysis using the Mackworth Clock-Test. *Psychology and Aging* **3**, 75–83.

Halliday, R., Callaway, E., Naylor, H., Gratzinger, P. and Prael, R. (1986). The effects of stimulant drugs on information processing in elderly adults. *Journal of Gerontology* **41**, 748–757.

Hertzog, C., Raskind, C. and Cannon, C. (1986). Age-related slowing in semantic information processing speed: An individual differences analysis. *Journal of Gerontology* **41**, 500–502.

Hicks, L. H. and Birren, J. E. (1970). Aging, brain damage, and psychomotor slowing. *Psychological Bulletin* **74**, 377–394.

Horn, J. L. (1982). The aging of human abilities. *In* "Handbook of developmental psychology". (B. B. Wolman, ed.) pp. 847–870. Prentice Hall, New York.

Horn, J. L. (1988). Cognitive diversity: A framework of learning. *In* "Learning and individual differences". (P. Ackerman, R. Sternberg and R. Glaser, eds) Freeman, New York.

Howard, D., Shaw, R. and Heisey, J. (1986). Aging and the time course of semantic activation. *Journal of Gerontology* **41**, 195–203.

Hoyer, F., Hoyer, F., Treat, N. and Baltes, P. (1978/9). Training response speed in young and elderly women. *International Journal of Aging and Human Development* **9**, 247–253.

Ivry, R. and Keele, S. (1989). Timing functions of the cerebellum. *Journal of Cognitive Neuroscience* 1, 136–152.

Llinas, R. (1988). The intrinsic electrophysiological properties of mammalian neurons: Insights into central nervous system function. *Science* 242, 1654–1664.

March, G. R. and Thompson, L. M. (1977). Psychophysiology of aging. In "Handbook of the psychology of aging" 2nd edn (J.E. Birren and K.W. Schaie, eds) pp. 219–248. Van Nostrand Reinhold, New York.

McDowd, J. M., Birren, J. E., Taylor, A. and Gutacker, P. (submitted). Every day lapses of attention and memory across the lifespan.

Moraal, J. (1982a). Age and information processing. "Proceedings of the Human Factors Society 20th Annual Meeting" pp. 184–188.

Moraal, J. (1982b). "Age and information processing: An application of Sternberg's Additive Factors Method". Technical Report No. IZF 1982-18, Soesterberg, Netherlands: TNO Institute for Perception.

Nowlin, J. and Siegler, I. (1985). Psychomotor performance and cardiovascular disease. In "Normal aging III" (E. Palmore, E. Busse, G. Maddox, J. Nowlin and I. Siegler, eds). pp. 43–50. Duke University Press, Durham.

Parmelee, P. A. and Lawton, M. P. (1990). The design of special environments for the aged. In "Handbook of the psychology of aging" 3rd edn (J. E. Birren and K. W. Schaie eds) pp. 465–479. Academic Press, New York.

Prinz, P., Dustman, R. and Emmerson, R. (1990). Electrophysiology and aging. In "Handbook of the psychology of aging" 3rd edn (J. E. Birren and K. W. Schaie, eds) pp. 135–149. Academic Press, New York.

Quilter, R. E., Giambra, L. M. and Benson, P. E. (1983). Longitudinal age changes in vigilance over an eighteen year interval. *Journal of Gerontology* 38, 51–54.

Reason, J. (1984). Lapses of attention in everyday life. In "Varieties of attention" (R. Parasuramen and D. R. Davies, eds) pp. 515–549. Academic Press, New York.

Rikli, R. and Busch, S. (1986). Motor performance of women as a function of age and physical activity level. *Journal of Gerontology* 41, 645–649.

Sacher, G. E. (1977). Life table modification and life prolongation. In "Handbook of the biology of aging" (C. Finch and L. Hayflick, eds) pp. 582–638. Van Nostrand Reinhold, New York.

Salthouse, T. A. (1982). "Adult cognition". Springer, New York.

Salthouse, T. A. (1988). Initiating the formalization of theories of cognitive aging. *Psychology and Aging* 3, 3–16.

Salthouse, T. A. and Somberg, B. (1982a). Isolating the age deficit in speeded performance. *Journal of Gerontology* 37, 59–63.

Salthouse, T. A. and Somberg, B. (1982b). Time-accuracy relationships in young and old adults. *Journal of Gerontology*, 37, 349–353.

Schaie, K. W., Campbell, R. C., Meredith, W. and Rawlings, S. W. (eds) (1988). "Methods of research on aging". Springer, New York.

Schroots, J. J. F. and Birren, J. E. (1988) The nature of time: Implications for research on aging. *Comprehensive Gerontology, C* 2, 1–29.

Shock, N., Greulich, R., Andres, R., Arenberg, D., Costa, P., Lakatta, E. and Tobin, J. (1984). "Normal human aging: the Baltimore longitudinal study of aging". US Department of Health and Human Services, NIH Publication No. 84-2450.

Siegler, I. (1983). Psychological aspects of the Duke Longitudinal Studies. In "Longitudinal studies of adult psychological development", (K.W. Schaie, ed.) pp. 135–190. The Guilford Press, New York.

Simon, J. R. and Pouraghabagher, A. (1978). The effects of aging on stages of information processing in a choice reaction time task. *Journal of Gerontology* **33**, 553–561.

Spirduso, W. W. and MacRae, P. G. (1990). Motor performance and aging. *In* "Handbook of the psychology of aging" 3rd edn (J. E. Birren and K. W. Schaie, eds) pp. 184–200. Academic Press, New York.

Stankov, L. (1988). Aging, attention and intelligence. *Psychology and Aging* **3**, 59–74.

Stelmach, G. E., Goggin, N. and Garcia-Colera, A. (1986). Movement specification time with age. *Experimental Aging Research* **13**, 39–46.

Sternberg, S. (1969). The discovery of processing stages: Extensions of Donder's method. *Acta Psychologica* **30**, 276–315.

Stones, M. and Kozma, A. (1989). Age, exercise, and coding performance. *Psychology and Aging* **4**, 190–194.

Vercruyssen, M., Cann, M. T., McDowd, J. M., Birren, J. E., Carlton, B. L., Burton, J. and Hancock, P. A. (1988a). Effects of age, gender, activation, and practice on attention and stages of information processing. Presented at "Proceedings of the 1988 Human Factors Annual Meeting", pp. 203–207. Santa Monica, CA.

Vercruyssen, M., Ynclino, V., Hancock, P. A., McDowd, J. M. and Birren, J. E. (1988b). Human attention: Implications for health and society. "Proceedings of the American Industrial Hygiene Conference", Akron, OH.

Vercruyssen, M., Carlton, B. L. and Buckles, V. (1989a). Specific effects of age and practice on stages of information processing. "Proceedings of the Human Factors Society—33rd Annual Meeting", Santa Monica, CA: Human Factors Society.

Vercruyssen, M., Cann, M. T. and Hancock, P. A. (1989b). Posture effects on gender differences in speed of behavior. "Proceedings of the Human Factors Society—33rd Annual Meeting", Santa Monica, CA: Human Factors Society, pp. 896–900.

Vercruyssen, M., Cann, M. T., Birren, J. E., McDowd, J. M. and Hancock, P. A. (1988). Effects of aging, physical fitness, gender, and neural activation on CNS speed of functioning. "Proceedings of the International Council for Physical Fitness Research, Osaka Symposium", Osaka, Japan.

Vercruyssen, M., McDowd, J. M. and Birren, J. E. (1990b). Age, divided attention, and dual-task performance. *In* "Multiple-task performance" (D. Damos, ed.), Taylor & Francis, London, in press.

Welford, A. T. (1977). Motor performance. *In* "Handbook of the psychology of aging" 2nd edn (J. E. Birren and K. W. Schaie, eds) pp. 450–496. Van Nostrand Reinhold, New York.

Woodruff, D. S. (1985). Arousal, sleep, and aging. *In* "Handbook of the psychology of aging" 2nd edn (J. E. Birren and K. W. Schaie, eds) pp. 261–295. Van Nostrand Reinhold, New York.

Woodruff-Pak, D. S. (1989). Neurobiological models of learning, memory, and aging. *In* "The course of later life" (V. L. Bengtson and K. W. Schaie, eds) pp. 107–134. Springer, New York.

Woods, A. M. (1981). "Age differences in the effects of physical activity and postural changes on information processing speed". Doctoral dissertation, Psychology Department, University of Southern California, Los Angeles, CA.

Discussion

Williams: What about the variability in older people? Are there in your studies some older people who do as well as younger ones? I have been examining several data very closely in relation to a very practical question: that is the age discrimination of airline pilots in the USA who have to stop piloting commercial planes at the age of 60. I think there is plenty of reason to question whether there is an arbitrary age limit on performance. Particularly in data just published there is a remarkable stability in people's own control of their performance up to their 70s and 80s in about 50% or even more compared with 25 year olds; half or more of the older people are performing as well as the younger ones, including speed of perception tests as well as several others. I wonder about the variability in your data—can we say whether there is an automatic change with aging or do these changes apply only to a certain group of older people and not to others? If so, we need to learn why.

Birren: There are several aspects of variability. One is the moment-to-moment variability within the organism and then there is a variability which loosely refers to individual differences which may be stable. I think our data will agree with what you have inferred from recent data, that the older fit subjects are more like the young subject than they are like the old unfit. You see the biggest difference in my distribution of the experimental results which show that it was the old unfit that were the slowest. With regard to the airline issue, I think that these data are laboratory measurements that have no direct translation into the cockpit of the aeroplane. I would proceed very carefully; I think that an experienced pilot at 60 is a much safer pilot to fly with than an inexperienced one at 35.

Robert: If I understood correctly your interpretation of the slowing down of the reaction, this is entirely limited to the central nervous system. In order to get a message from the brain through to the fingers, you must have not only a fast processing of the input of the information but also of the outgoing orders. This means that if your neuromuscular synapses are degraded, then, even if the processing is fast, the execution could be slow.

Birren: Yes, That's possible. Earlier in my career I investigated the nerve conduction velocity. There is a little bit of evidence that it changes slightly with age, but it's a trivial variable in the total picture. The next might be the synaptic delay at the model neuron and that would appear perhaps to be an increase by a thousandth of a second. Again it's a small factor in the total picture. Tentatively I think to this point that these changes are proportional. Anything mediated by the central nervous system is affected in a similar way, that's the general hypothesis, whether it is a model response or is dealing with a sensory input.

The Position of the Old in Tribal Society

Report from a field study in West Africa

Leopold Rosenmayr

Institute of Sociology, Vienna University and Ludwig Boltzmann Institute for Social Gerontology and Life Course Research, Austria

PURPOSE AND AIMS OF THE INVESTIGATION

Demographers and sociologists have furnished evidence that the ratio of young to old is changing quickly in developing countries, even in the poorest ones, and will change even more drastically in the coming century. So there will be considerably more old people in absolute and relative terms and the health needs of this group will increase. It should be noted that in 1975 slightly more than half (52%) of all persons aged 60 and over lived in the developing countries. By the year 2000 over 60% of all older persons are expected to live in those countries, and it is anticipated that the proportion will reach nearly 75% by 2025 (WAA 1982). Still more recent data show the greying of the Third World is approaching fast.

The vast majority of children in developing countries are integrated into and socially protected by clans and kinship. Due to rural-to-urban migration

Table 1
Population 65 and over in millions

	1980s	2000s	2020s
Developed countries	128	166	230
Developing countries	132	237	530
World	260	303	760

From Laslett (1989).

Challenges in Aging
ISBN 0-12-090163-3

25

and the severing of kinship ties, this is no longer generally the case for the old in many developing countries of the world, including the poorest ones.

The problem became of particular interest to me in connection with the Plan of Action for the UN Conference on Aging, held in Vienna in 1982. At that time, a growing consciousness of the percentage increase of old people in the so-called developing countries and particularly in Africa stimulated the interest, not only of African governments, but also of researchers in various parts of Europe and in the USA. I defined the aims of my own research in the following way:

1. To find out—as a structural analyst—what social integration meant in tribal society and what role the elderly played therein.

2. To study—participating as a concerned observer, eager also to learn from the traditional model of tribal society—whether this integration in tribal society was primarily due to the "wisdom" of the old or whether there were other principles at work that constitute the powerful and respected position of the old, particularly old men (Rosenmayr 1988a).

3. As an observing and often perplexed participant—to determine the particular health needs of old people in one specific ecological and cultural environment in the Third World and how they could be coped with.

In order to realize my research plans I made several decisions: one was to co-operate closely through friendship ties and with local healers and experts in folk medicine and to invite Western and African representatives of Western medicine to the area. From both groups I expected specialized knowledge of local diseases, of medical culture and an appropriate way of discussing health needs with village people.

For the first phase of the study I made the decision against random samples of individuals. First, it is not really possible to carry them through in rural areas, second the questionnaire method creates a bias in favour of men as women refrain from answering and third the subtle issues of power cannot be approached adequately. In order to better understand social structures and settings I proposed to carry out the research on entire villages and clans.

All methods imply limitations. However, the study of health within networks of social relations in one particular ethnic and ecological context permitted us to understand health, environment and culture as an internally interconnected network.

This way we elaborated a model of village studies which will hopefully permit in the future more of our type of integrated research of a multi-focused character, interconnecting studies on agro-econonmic, cultural, and sociostructural factors with health factors.

It proved to be enormously important to establish close co-operation with local healers. Through them we tried to understand the several cultural influences and traditions concerning health.

We could clearly see in tribal society that in several ways their meanings were not ours, and *vice versa*. We interpreted what was observed by us but we also interpreted the perspectives and interpretations of the healers and of the people of the village, perspectives which are part of their own cultural framework and thus part of how they understand their life.

In addition to our own first-hand attempts at interpretation we felt the necessity to understand the way in which village people interpreted themselves and health and sickness in their culture, drafting the meanings of their own lives from their culture. We attempted to look with them, with "their eyes" at what we saw. We came to the following conclusion.

In bicultural situations where traditional tribal symbols and practices mix with recent Western influences one ought to live and look with "two souls" and ought to live on two levels of consciousness. For a better understanding of the psychological and health needs of the old in the first phase we used medical examinations of various age groups.

ELEMENTS OF THE ECOLOGICAL SETTING OF THE STUDY

The central region of the Republic of Mali (Fig. 1) is characterized by extreme dryness and by regions where the forests show vast areas with millions of corpses of trees and bushes. Desertification is progressing. During the dry season violent winds blow sands and cause—to illustrate one aspect of the ecological situation—a large number of eye diseases, particularly among children but also among older people through chronic conjunctivitis. There is great danger that cataracts may develop; they become a particular handicap for the old and not unfrequently lead to blindness.

Millet raising is the main form of agriculture in the area. Whenever the harvest permits it, surplus production of millet is sold to voyaging traders. Millet pudding and millet soup form the nutritional basis. Treenuts complement the scarce animal fats. Sheep and goat meat are eaten on festive occasions only. Rarely are cattle slaughtered. Less than half of the 20 extended families (clans) of the village we studied own small herds of cattle. Only three families own 30 or more cattle. The meat of animals slaughtered is always distributed among the community and is never the sole property of individuals. The act of dividing the meat of the slaughtered animal takes place in public and is carried out by some village elders. This is already one of the functions of the old according to the seniority principle.

The nutritional distribution follows the general characteristic that the old

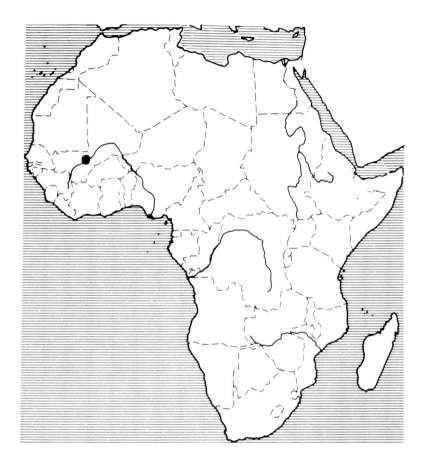

Fig. 1. Map of Africa indicating (●) the area of our research 1983–1987.

men associate in groups and become active in the village in this form and on many other levels. This is important for the social conditions of their health, as they are expected to remain active to solve village problems even if they are handicapped or blind. As concerns "leisure", participation in village dances of the old men and women is also quite common and is much appreciated by all the villagers. So the old remain integrated and actively participate through social recognition and encouragement.

Sonongo, the village we studied, located about 100 km west of the city of Ségou, with no roads leading to it, has approximately 400 inhabitants. A total of 20 extended Bambara families (clans) inhabit the village, each of which has between 7 and 30 members. Polygyny is the dominant Bambara marriage pattern; the males have a clearly dominant position in all external and "political" matters. Either the father or the eldest brother is the head of the several households of one clan or extended family. Half of all children born alive die before the age of 5 of unclear postnatal infections, or of diarrhoea, measles, pneumonia, meningitis or parasites.

Land is not owned privately but originally allocated by the village chief to the lineage chiefs (heads of families) and then remains apportioned on the basis of tradition. The quantity and quality of donkeys, carts and ploughs varies from one family to another. Activities are hectic during the rainy season, the farmers do not have much work to do in the dry season. During this period parents with their very young children go to the dried-out zones to cut wood from the dying bushes and trees. Approximately two-thirds of the male youth and one-third of the female youth leave temporarily for the city during the dry season each year to work as weavers, market helpers or maids and return to Sonongo thereafter, but some leave for good, without announcing it when they go.

Out of 15 hand-dug wells in Sonongo approximately eight provide water. Women go to the wells at approximately 4 a.m. and also sometimes late at night. Some wells completely dry out during the dry season, so that only two remain in use and yield water. In some years all food is consumed and hunger is spreading.

AN ANTHROPOLOGICAL CONCEPT OF AGING

Aging is a universal process of life yet its forms vary greatly all through the different species of the biological order. With evolution also the forms of aging evolve and take on different functions in individual and social animal life by generating higher life expectations and gradually increased fitness late in life. These improvements generate evolutionary changes which permit the development of extended protective roles for the offspring.

Also leadership and scouting capacities in the latter part of animal life develop which have no direct relation to procreation and rearing of the young but increase survival chances of the genes of the group.

All these crystallizations of leadership and scouting roles and thereby often also of power positions of older (mostly, but not exclusively male) individuals within social networks in animal groups required higher orders of neurobiological structures. On the other hand, cerebral growth was stimulated and thus evolved through more complex social organization and the stimuli emanating therefrom. Naturally, such evolutionary processes, based on individual and group selection, cannot be explained just on the basis of competition of the intrinsic capacities of the individuals and groups themselves, but must also be understood in view of the ways these individuals and groups interact with the various dimensions of environment.

As we turn from biological to human society this relationship to the environment begins to take on a very different significance. Not only the scope—the plasticity of human reactions to the environment excels by far any other animal species—but also the quality of the coping with environmental changes on account of the uses of complex tools, symbols and the communication by language. Human "relation" to environment follows purposeful and planned action based on defined co-operative networks with interactive codes. The latter crystallize with the genesis of types of pastoral and sedentary agricultural societies. Hunters and collectors have less definite structures; it is much more difficult for them to stabilize and elaborate incest taboos.

For our understanding of the seniority principle in pastoral and particularly in sedentary tribal society it is crucial to take into consideration the great dangers and obstacles menacing work and procreation, individual and social survival. In order to subsist and to endure these societies had to (and have to) wage a battle against a sometimes very hostile natural environment and are at the same time forced to defend themselves against intrusion, occupation, homicide and slavery from other (often neighbouring) groups which may have developed different styles and codes of social organization and behaviour.

My interest in the study of aging in Africa grew out of my fascination with encountering actually living tribal society. In this type of society I hoped to find early forms of human behaviour and social ties which, if I understood them well would improve—by means of comparison—my understanding of man, of human motivation, of life goals and values.

Can we learn something from "primitive society", even if we are self-critical enough and reject any suggestion to quickly transplant what we find in the tribal world to the enormously complex economic and social reality of so-called "highly developed" society?

Do forms of tribal society, their organization by age sets, their structures of clans ruled by the seniority principle, mark a certain type or stage in the development of the human race? Although it appears to be justifiable to look at man in the context of the evolution of life on this planet and to consider human life as a particular and unique form of life, human history (including tribal societies which change over time) is of an order different from biological evolution, and all hypothetical analogies ought to be handled with greatest care. I think that this is important also in view of the changes occurring in (up to now) traditional and often isolated tribal societies if and when "modernization" hits them through information, transportation and production technology, from the radio set to the plough and the motor scooter. Such processes are not just "evolution of society".

In human society change is induced through purposeful action which creates a network of economic and social structures. Purposeful action also changes needs and aspirations, and this action is characterized by the all-powerful information systems and value orders man has created. If people no longer accept certain rules and sanctions and they reject idols adored for a long time, then the moment of change has come. The steering of historicosocial development in human society takes place on a rail different from the genetic code and its manifestation in certain living populations. The distribution of the genetic code is not insignificant and its operation on the human individual is powerful; sociocultural change however is a second level of control for behaviour and its "selection". If I therefore discuss some aspects of the evolution of the phenomenon of aging it should not be overlooked that man, constituting a uniquely special kind of nature, has, in addition to the information within the genetic code, created the cultural supercode of a non-nature-bound information system.

To understand the variability of a significantly extended period of adult life in human history and culture, the study of old age in Africa, its value, power and vulnerability may help.

THE POSITION OF THE OLD IN TRIBAL SOCIETY (FEATURES FROM THE BAMBARA ETHNIC GROUP)

Seniority is a generally applied principle of power distribution. It is not based on the often quoted "experience" or "wisdom" of older individuals. Nor is it the accumulated individual knowledge of the old which is of primary importance. However, this accumulated individual knowledge is sometimes an argument used to legitimize the power which the old have and thereby can enforce norms and make decisions. In reality, it is the other way round: seniority gives power to privileged subgroups and individuals who affirm traditional rules as representatives of the collectivity.

Let me try to summarize: human behaviour to provide food, clothing and shelter, intentional and co-ordinated action to hunt or to farm was always bound to rules; also the control of procreative activities, of mating and mate selection, was organized by codes. These codes contained norms and were often institutionalized by means of rites and symbols. It is important to note that these codes were of an "intentional selective" character. To give an example: cross-cousin marriage (as we found it in Sonongo) brought two advantages: it avoided both sibling marriage and the marriage of complete strangers. Behaviour was organized by code, it may be mentioned, and assured calculated genetic risks. Complete strangers might have been felt as too dangerous and from a genetic point of view this "feeling" may have been justified. In this instance, the role of the old is clear: they see that these mate selection rules are inforced. No "wisdom" is necessary to perform such tasks, only executive rigour and power within the clan and the village to oppose the "whims" of individual desire and preference.

By defending the gene pool and operating as agents of selection the old might be called "wise" only in an "objective" sense, in as much as they perhaps unconsciously protect a fragile system.

The social power they had enabled them to defend their groups, clans, villages and tribes against the hostile environment. They had traditional rules to follow, into which they had been initiated when they were young. A relatively inflexible tribal society which Emile Durkheim characterized by the notion of "mechanical solidarity" (Durkheim 1969) must filter the social influences from outside because the impact of these influences might threaten or destroy the society if not screened through careful selective "mechanisms" and procedures.

The old, in order to perform their executive tasks, have accumulated a great deal of information about what should be done in their societies. Though perhaps to a limited extent, they have accumulated more "experience" in as much as they have had to react to more situations that needed decisions. Thereby a certain increase in competence occurred. If there are rules of the society, the individual's rise experience is not very important for the required decisions. Experience grows effectively if situations in which decisions are taken vary greatly and if the normative margin of the decisions is wide—which is not the case with the traditional seniority position in tribal society. It must always closely follow a strict code of rules.

We may say that the old, as executives of the system, are not required to produce individual decisions and therefore they are challenged to much less than wisdom. On the other hand they have achieved a position that goes far beyond wisdom in as much as they have the power to regulate their society.

Wisdom is a type of second level knowledge, a competence to judge and handle knowledge, to integrate different and even contradictory information and to apply all of this to some form of inner or outer action. Criteria for wisdom have recently been elaborated in various ways (Baltes and Smith 1990, Rosenmayr 1990), but in spite of differences in the definition of wisdom it becomes clear that wisdom requires a personal synthesis based on a certain amount of both social and individual freedom. The wise person must have flexibility and must have the capacity to reflect upon himself as the basis for finding a variety of solutions which he is then capable of offering or of suggesting to others.

In Bambara society the traditional healer or Marabou to some extent did perform such tasks and continues to do so wherever the traditional system

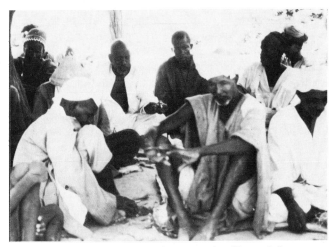

Fig. 2. Group of older Bambara men in village of Sonongo.

is still operating. Such people in tribal society were already "specialists". In early high culture, as reflected by classical Greek epic or dramatic poetry, there is much evidence of the wise old man as a consultant to the king or of the warning function which has been associated with the name of Kassandra.

It is my intention in this paper to state clearly that the often repeated assumption that old people in tribal society are respected because they are wise is misleading. We may even say that it is not old age as such that is respected, but that it is the seniority principle in tribal society which merits respect as the central model for survival and "filtered change". The traditional tribal society, for reasons of self-defence against other societies and against nature, has generally to be "closed" and opened only to the extent that its mechanisms could cope with influences from outside. It cannot be denied that the brutal opening of traditional tribal society caused by influences of technology and different non-traditional life styles due to "modernization" destroys many values of coherence and co-operation. On the other hand the principle of seniority has not proven capable of accepting more individual freedom and has, in general, not responded to the fundamental changes modernization has brought to Africa and its, up to now traditionally organized, more or less isolated, rural societies.

Let me examine another aspect which supports my view that it is the social structure which defines the position of the old and not *vice-versa* (Fig. 2). Seniority is closely related to the power of the word. In a culture with no written tradition, verbal power is decisive. It reinforces status. The young men may only listen, they are not yet allowed to speak in any formal public discussion. The old men do all the talking. The more responsibility a man acquires through his advancement in the seniority system, the more he is required to talk. And the more he talks, the more he affirms his status. Therefore, the quality and expressiveness of his rhetoric improves and his social and power expectations also grow. Mastering the word in response to, in many ways, submissive individual and group expectations enhances both power and influence.

Finally I have to look into the relation between power and potency of older men. Within the traditional tribal setting the old African man cannot be subjected to power limits from outside unless the tribe is conquered by another one and its members are drawn into slavery. Also, even now, a village chief who has lost his sight cannot be deposed; he is provided with helpers who "see" for him. Although the village chief cannot be deposed merely because of impotence, his deficiency becomes known and erodes his prestige from inside. When this occurs he is likely to resign, unlike the situation with blindness, which his society can accept.

POTENCY AND POWER OF OLDER MEN

In the system of polygyny, a man accumulates more wives the older he gets. This is a matter of social prestige with an economic function because the women work for him and thus add to his modest prosperity. Each day he visits a different one of his wives in her hut or (depending on the tribal rules) she comes to his hut. And as unlike as African eroticism may be from that of other world civilizations in many respects, in Africa also the woman expects the sexual act on this occasion.

Potency has a strong social significance. If a man is not potent *vis-à-vis* a woman he is also socially unfit for a ruling position according to the principles underlying tribal society. And therefore, as I learned from the jocular comments made by the old men (the initiation companions), potency plays a central role in the power structure of the family and of the village. With the help from a great variety of powders and magical practices, potency is strengthened, an example of this being the powder obtained from grinding the horn of a rhinoceros. There is no doubt that the aggressiveness of the rhinoceros is considered to be the model of the desired aggressiveness of one's own phallus. On account of the social significance of potency the powerful old man is the target of witchcraft. And because he is a dreaded rival, this powerful old man is bewitched with the help of various secret methods, so that he will lose his potency, and may therefore be deprived of his power. He, on the other hand, protects himself by making use of counterchant, of magical powders and anti-witchcraft.

As observers of Bambara, we must see sexuality, in analogy to Michel

Foucault's suggestion, within the framework of a "dispositif social", i.e. within the interdependences of functions and powers of the respective society and the way this society interprets nature and morals.

Seniority functions as a multi-level social instrument, and the more diversified its application becomes in the kinship network, in the village and in the tribe, the more reinforcement it receives.

The seniority principle unfolds its efficacy within the wider framework of ecological and supraregional determinants such as wars, famines, plagues of crickets and droughts. It structures and controls the tribe in order to make it resistant against violation and losses. The morally devastating effects on village and kinship caused by tribal wars and the kidnapping by slavers often fragmented tribal society. Under such conditions, seniority had a reorganizing effect. Long-lived elders imparted a selective advantage to their families and tribes—they prevented chaos as a clear "order of ruling" existed.

If the whole socio-economic system is also orientated toward stabilization then the principle of seniority can operate well as a mechanism for the distribution of power, but if the socio-economic system becomes change orientated, relative to super-regional and international market fluctuations and to competitive production—as is the case in the process of Westernization—then the system cannot fulfil this homeostatic task and adjust social life to these new conditions. The introduction or expansion of new forms of work and technology create severe difficulties for the application of the seniority principle.

THE SENIORITY PRINCIPLE AS ROOTED IN CHILDHOOD SOCIALIZATION

In Bambara culture, mothers have extremely close relations with their small children. For a long unbroken period of time, approximately 20 months, the mother literally and symbolically ties the infant to herself. The child often stays fixed to the mother by straps. On many occasions the mother carries the child on her back while crushing millet, dragging up buckets of water from a well, or working in the fields. Even during village dances when the women appear in their best clothes, the youngest child is carried on the back of the mother. The emotional root of the seniority principle lies in the adherence to the yielding mother.

Our research on early childhood socialization revealed that the child is never frustrated orally; it may drink or suck and play at the mother's breast as often as it wishes. The only restriction is that the child may not bite the breast, and mothers have gentle techniques to discourage them from doing so. Cleanliness training is also done with great patience. The child

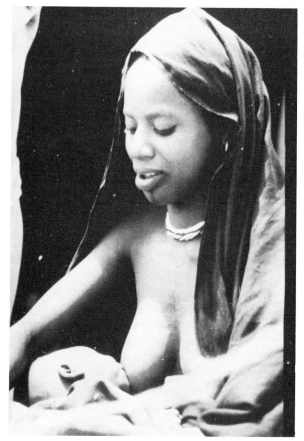

Fig. 3. Yielding motherhood; the basis of strong group identification.

learns in practically all areas of his needs that it may depend on the mother
(Fig. 3).

Immediately after weaning at the age of 2, boys and girls become part
of an informal children's group of their own and often a special homestead
located within the area of the clan. Children in this group range from 2 to
7 years of age. They are taken care of by older girls, yet mostly do not
stray too far away from their own mothers. Additionally, the girls who lead
the groups behave in a way very similar to the mother. The decisive
organizational root of the seniority principle lies in the group.

In early childhood socialization of the Bambara culture, the mother is
the child's only dominant reference figure. As a result of this structure,
there is no "classical" competition between the son and the father for the
mother. Identification with the male parent as it develops from rivalry with

the father (the Oedipus complex) does not take place in Bambara culture. Traditional African personality formation differs from the historical European model of growth. Cohesion within the children's group—and later within the initiation society for young adolescents—is emotionally based on unity with the mother, real or symbolic as is the case in Komo mythology, in which maternal imagery dominates.

The deep oral satisfaction achieved during the first 2 years, the shift of emotional need satisfaction from the dyadic mother–child relation to the children's group, and the continuous step-wise reinforcement of the collective orientation may be interpreted as the crucial psychosocial foundation for acceptance and internalization of the seniority principle.

Childhood socialization prepares the individual for the acceptance of the seniority principle and the social organization of initiation. The further developments of the life course reinforce the readiness of the group to accept authority, which means to "enthrone" the seniority principle. The group pressure to which the young children are exposed immediately after leaving their mothers paves the way for the acceptance of the old as leaders and of the ancestors as a spiritual reference group to identify with. The Ton organization for children and later the Komo initiation groups for the young engrain step by step this collective mentality. An orientation toward a strong solidarity with age-equal or age-similar peers supports the seniority principle.

Much of the practice of continued initiation is connected with the crucial symbols of "secret mothers" of the Bambara tradition. The Komo initiation society revolves around four "mothers" related to a life order in which participants mature by passing from one stage of knowledge to the next. To acquire the knowledge which is symbolized by the four mothers, an initiate must endure an internal journey. The gradual maturation of self-control and self-satisfaction expressed through the process of initiation is comparable to certain forms of meditation and asceticism found in Asiatic and, to some extent, European cultures. Mythology reinforces the mother influence.

INITIATION AND ANCESTORS AS REFERENCE TO CULTURAL STABILITY

The most harmonious aspect of reciprocal young–old relations occurs relative to initiation into the so-called secret societies. There, the young need the old initiation masters and the latter "need" young disciples to offer them respect and veneration. Initiation societies like the Komo are part of the large age set organization prevalent in traditional Bambara society.

Age sets in West Africa may be formally defined as linear or cyclical models (Rosenmayr 1978) or treated as simple informal age groups as was the case in the Bambara village Sonongo. Age sets vary greatly from one African society to another according to the "composition and internal organization of the local group" (Paulme 1971). Therefore opportunities for theory building are limited. Further, age sets are losing their structural meaning and power on the African continent maybe more quickly than their organization, ritual and myths can be preserved by written records.

Age sets represent a collective non-familial aspect of the seniority principle. They are founded as particular age cohorts and are formally defined by common circumcision ceremonies. Initiation is expressed through various educational and ritual practices based on myth. Traditional African society makes available this mythological, life-orientated knowledge to a cohort of its growing members, who then constitute an age set. This age set may receive a name from a standardized consecutive name pattern, or an individualized non-recurrent one, or none at all.

As has been observed by various anthropologists, these age sets or age classes follow a principle different from lineage organization and are clearly community orientated (Paulme 1971, p. 20). Where they are more formal institutions as in the case of the nomadic Masai, they serve to recruit cadets for their "armed forces". The relationship between the concrete age groups may be marked by differentiated access to and use of very different weapons: variation in size and type of spears characterizes traditional Masai age groups. These externally marked differences, however, occur mostly in societies where the age set system prevails over the kinship system as is indeed the case with the traditional Masai tribes (Rosenmayr 1978).

Initiation is re-enacted even in later life on an ever more complex level (Rosenmayr 1982). In some societies such as the Senufo of the Ivory Coast in West Africa, new physical and psychological tests are required for access to a new age grade in adulthood. Thus age sets fulfill an "enculturation function" that "lasts throughout the individual's life" (Bernardi 1985). Most crucially for our purposes, members of younger age groups treat the members of the older groups as their seniors.

In Sonongo a children's group continues to play an important role in socialization. After a period of informal yet close relationships in mixed groups, the young boys of Sonongo form a task-orientated organization, the "Ton", at around the age of 7. The Ton is headed by a somewhat senior boy. Co-operation and qualities of unbroken mutual support are learned in this group which forms a sort of help brigade and performs work needed for the organization of community feasts. "Tribal closeness" is the result of these socialization processes, not competitive behaviour. As there is little room for individual competition, there is little achievement motivation born and developed. In this way, age sets reinforce the seniority

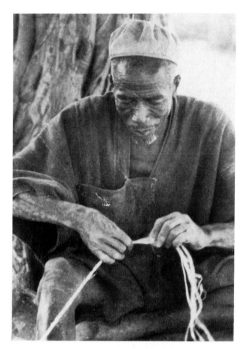

Fig. 4. Seri Sakko, initiation master of Sonongo still venerates the ancestors by sacrifices.

system not only through organizing society in terms of age cohorts but also by stressing communal solidarity over individual goals.

Much of the practice of continued initiation seems to have disappeared in Sonongo and its immediate region under the pressure of Islamization. Some of it still existed but was kept secret from us. However, the Komo initiation society still retains influence. Adult initiation in Sonongo transcends a mere power function and is concerned with the criteria of maturity. The content comes from Bambara mythology which is extremely rich and meaningful.

An equally significant buttress of the seniority system in Sonongo is the process of ancestor worship. "One is always in the power of the ancestors", said Seri Sakko (Fig. 4), one of my informants in Sonongo, "and one has to renew their forces in order to place oneself under their protection." He recommends killing a cock for the ancestors. It must be one which has already crowed, otherwise you risk having a child born mute. One may send special messages and requests to the ancestors by putting dried dates (which are rare delicacies to the inhabitants of Sonongo and the whole region) into the millet balls.

In explaining Bambara ancestor worship, Dominique Zahan (1974) says that when intoxicated—after having imbibed the millet beer sacrifices—the dead allow themselves to be directed and influenced. An even stronger effect can be expected from blood sacrifices because blood expresses the rhythms of the life span of the sacrificed creatures. Man's limited life span is (by means of the blood shed in the sacrifice) integrated into the realm in which his ancestors repose. When the ancestors accept the offering of blood poured out upon their altars, they cannot help but feel grateful to the living.

The ancestors may start to speak. They are capable of an articulation in language if—according to the seniority principle—the head of the clan concentrates very hard on hearing them on the day when they are venerated. They send teachings or messages applicable to the problems of life (Sow 1977). You can try to influence the ancestors but they never become partners in a contract. They do represent order and they are models for the living. In this way ancestors and older men resemble each other and both exemplify the seniority principle.

In relating to the ancestors, people have to acknowledge a collective unity which becomes part of their consciousness through socialization. The black African psychiatrist Sow, on the basis of his own childhood experiences, holds that the unity of the black African personality is founded upon a spiritual principle represented by the ancestors. This principle locates the self in the continuity of living and dead generations. Continuity is not based on biological reproduction but rather derives from the spiritual realm. This spirituality, according to Sow, represents an ancestral substance occurring in each member of the tribal society. This "substance" is seen as constituting the African self (Sow 1977). The life principle is mortal but the spiritual ancestral principle is immortal. It connotes communal solidarity. And the latter is supported by the seniority system.

Special attention has to be given to the forces of myth and ritual. Myth is the basic force to structure self-interpretation, which is necessary to give meaning to aging and age group relations. In a traditional, particularly in a non-literate society, age relations are the structural backbone of a "stable" and self-sufficient subsistence economy (Amoss and Harrell 1981, Holmes 1983, Kertzer and Keith 1984). Clearly, ancestor myth is regionally shaped and developed. There are few African societies where it does not exist or where it exists only marginally. Yet where it exists, it forms a stabilizing unity and is incorporated into socialization practices. Without understanding initiation and ancestor worship there is no understanding of the seniority system.

Under the pressure of an often brutal and economically dysfunctional "modernization" process, individual competition has become a social necessity. Attitudes and expectations based on the seniority principle therefore easily become obstacles to modernization. The spirit of individual achievement is being fostered in some of the most intelligent tribal rural youths who have come in contact with aspects of Western society, often first through radio emissions which they listen to on cheap small sets originating from Japan. Westernization means that, in one way or another, the young will have to reject the system from which they stem. Thus we arrive at one of the social and cultural contradictions in contemporary African society, a contradiction which is particularly painful because rejection of the old seniority-based tribal system also means rejection of African identity, a requisite for individual and political self-assertion of individuals. It is the collision of systems which produces generational conflict and cultural anomie.

TRADITIONAL SOCIOMORPH AND COSMOMORPH VIEWS OF HEALTH

Health and sickness are viewed and interpreted by the village people from both a *cosmomorph* and a *sociomorph* point of view according to the (Bambara) tribal doctrine. Health by the Bambara is looked upon as a state which can be restored through various forms of participation in the macro- and microcosmos of nature. Astrological constellations (macrocosmos) have to be observed and microcosmic elements of nature (herbs, baths in water of boiled herbs, burned roots, burned bones of animals, etc.) have to be taken. Such contacts with nature are looked upon as treatment. This health attitude corresponds to the general cultural attitudes prevailing in all other areas of life, including hunting. These attitudes reflect a faith in various forms of "soul" animating plants and deer. After killing an animal in the bush the soul "evaporating" from the dying animal has to be respected and measures have to be taken not to be damaged by it (Fig. 5).

Faith in the healing forces of nature is a correlate of a general belief attributing "soul" to all living creatures be they plants or animals. Thus it is ultimately the "great soul" in the realm of living nature which influences the soul of the sick person. In this particular sense it might be appropriate to speak of "animism".

Older people impressed me to be more convinced of this correspondence and interference with animistically interpreted nature than the younger ones, even if they—the old—during their earlier years had spent longer periods of time in town.

The diagnosis and treatment of sickness is sociomorph in a double sense. First, the expectation to be cured is *related* to a healer who is a person

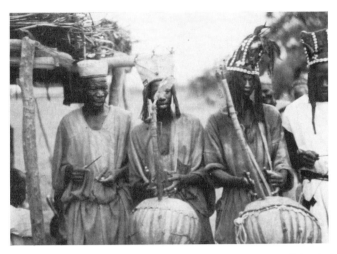

Fig. 5. Hunters are particularly sensitive to the "traffic of souls" in their natural environment.

with high social recognition. The traditional healer is the social reference person for any cure. He will prescribe the therapy, and it is nearly sacrilegious not to follow his prescriptions. The healer carries the weight of tradition and he is therefore highly respected. A second aspect of sociomorphism in the restoration of health is the very general behaviour of grouping around the injured, sick or in any way suffering person. The clan feels obliged to be present on the occasion of the medical examination, of the treatment and of various acts to help the patient. At first sight I found this burdening and irritating in case of first aid to seriously injured persons. Later I more and more understood that onlooking and standing around was not just curiosity but a form of social participation in a serious personal event of the sick person. The accumulation of people around a sick person I started to understand as an important expression of solidarity and support to this person.

Illness may be considered as corresponding to some evil constellation in the social network or as a result of a serious violation of the rules of the social network. It is often seen as the result of some malediction. Illness may spring from maledictions of offended opponents. Illness may be the consequence of the curses of a relative or of an authority figure. The old aunt who demands quiet at night several times and is not taken seriously by a group of youngsters who continue to be noisy finally curses one or several of them. The young then fall ill and suffer seriously for a long time unless the old person "lifts the ban", annuls the malediction.

We may interpret such sickness as the result of strong anxieties and as psychosomatic consequences. Many such cases occur. There are more latent neurotic dispositions in tribal society than its quick idealization on romantic grounds may suggest. Such disturbances reveal the sociomorphic character of at least an important set of sickness.

In the case of "spirits" seen—as balls of light in the dark bush, as flashes in the night courtyard—we rediscover the interaction with nature. It took a long time in Sonongo until the old permitted the use of torches during the night, because of anxieties in view of unexpected sudden flashes as different from the well-accustomed sight of burning wood in the fireplace. I rarely saw an old person "splitting" the night by using a torch in Sonongo. The young, however, made ample use of them.

One of the great surprises of our research on the health and care of the elderly in the tribal village of Sonongo was the following: many interpretations of the old concerning their own sickness or health were still strongly based on beliefs as just described. However, they willingly accepted Western drugs in cases of severe sickness, or aspirin against headache, drops to cure eye troubles, or pills to stop diarrhoea or constipation. We may speak of a cultural syncretism in matters of health. It appears important to me to point to this non-exclusive cultural attitude vis-à-vis health in the traditional society studied, which developed also among its older members, even if to a smaller extent.

The local hierarchy (following the seniority principle) becomes effective also in view of health resources. We could practically never deny priority of assistance to the old even if some other cases appeared to be more urgent. Also, some of the village dignitaries expected to receive drugs or vitamins particularly if they themselves came and asked for them. To some of them—personality variables did play a certain role in causing differences also between older people—the quantity of a medicament was looked upon as an expression of acknowledging their dignity. The more pills, the more drops, the more some of them felt respected. Here again we may discover the sociomorphic relationship to health. The higher the status, the more entitlement to be healed and be supplied generously with drugs. The drug is looked upon as a gift, as some form of tribute. All these aspects are important for designing and distributing medical aid and for medical education, including its most primitive forms.

SOME SOCIOMEDICAL FINDINGS OF OUR STUDY

Fifty-nine of 200 inhabitants of Sonongo were examined medically by Prof. Stemberger. For a better understanding of the health needs of the old in

Table 2

Average age and sex of persons who underwent medical
examinations

Sex	Average age (years)	Number
Male	40	30
Female	39	29

the first phase medical examinations of various age groups were compared
with each other. (Age data were self-ascribed estimates.)

The examination comprised the inspection of the skin, the examination
of the anterior eye sections, of the teeth and the throat as well as the
auditory canal and the eardrum. The heart and the lungs were examined
by way of auscultation and percussion, the liver, the spleen and lymph
nodes by way of palpation.

Let me give a brief survey of the major medical problems of the older
population in the area, noting that 10–12% of the people are 50 and over.
Only half of the children born reach the age of 5. Because of the high
infant mortality rate and—compared to Western standards—highly increased
forms of mortality in youth and early adulthood, old people are relatively
healthy. This is an effect of selective survival.

We found very low blood fats due to nutritional habits; good heart and
respiration functions, yet reports of rather frequent pneumonia; a relatively
good skin condition of the elderly in contrast to the high incidence of
dermatological problems with children; low schistosomiasis and malaria due
to the relative dryness of the area.

The outstanding problems of health of the old which we found in
Sonongo were cataracts, malaria and rheumatism. Fifteen to 20% of the
people of 50 and over suffer from cataracts. Malaria is particularly
burdensome for the elderly as the high fever consumes much of their energy
and there is little chance to effectively lower the fever without special
medication. Deaths due to such exhaustion are not infrequent.

The low rate of intestinal infestation in Sonongo can be attributed to the

Table 3

Age group distribution of the medical examination

Age group	Male	Female	Average age (years)
0–29 years	13	14	16.1
30–59 years	9	8	50.4
Over 60 years	8	7	69.1

Table 4
Age group distribution of *Ancylostoma* and *Schistosoma haematomium*

Age	*Ancylostoma*	*S. haematomium*
Under 30 years	1/27	3/38
30–60 years	3/17	0/17
Over 60 years	2/15	0/15

fact that human faeces in this area are never used as a fertilizer: thus faeco-oral infection is largely ruled out. This explains the complete absence of *Ascaris* and *Trichuris* eggs in the stool specimens. These data can be even better understood if we relate them to our observation that the inhabitants of Sonongo consistently used properly built latrines. This certainly explains the low rate of hookworm infestation and the absence of *Strongyloides* infestations. The low rate of infestation with *Schistosoma haematomium* can be undoubtedly explained by the geographical situation, the long distance from prominent infection areas and the low degree of mobility of the Bambara (above all of the older ones). Sonongo is situated about 100 km west of the River Niger; persons of 50 and over very rarely travel in the donkey-drawn carts such a long distance.

The nutritional habits of the village population of Sonongo are nearly exclusively based on millet consumption as everyday food. Therefore it was interesting to determinate cholesterol, triglycerides and apolipoproteins A1 and B values and to compare them with European averages. Particularly low values were found for apolipoprotein B. Resulting from these values the quotient apolipoprotein B/apolipoprotein A1 (which is a measure for cardiovascular risk) came out very low. If compared with data from Europe, only the values of European newborns are lower than this quotient found in adults in Sonongo. Already in babyhood, Europeans have a cardiovascular risk quotient higher than the average quotient in Sonongo.

The majority of the test persons in the group of those aged over 60 showed significant titres both in the Treponema-unspecific VDRL and in the Treponema-specific hemagglutination test. Positive serological findings were less frequent. In the age groups under 30 years there was not a single test person that would have to be classified as being in need of treatment on the basis of the respective serological finding. As those under 30 years were seronegative, we must assume that the transmission of syphilis was brought to a halt about 30 years ago within the framework of a mass treatment effort, which, however, was not effective in so far as the infected persons were not completely cured. Up to now this assumption cannot be supported by relevant literature.

Our antibody findings suggested that malaria is not highly endemic in this region, since only 72% showed significant antibody titres in the group aged 0–29 years. Antibody examinations in holoendemic malaria regions of West Africa have shown significant antibody levels among all inhabitants starting from the second year of life.

The differences between men and women in our study may be explained by the fact that the men travel much more and are therefore exposed to *Anopheles* to a greater extent than are the women, whose sphere of activity is rather within the village and the neighbouring fields.

A report on findings concerning health and sickness in an African village of a rural tribal society would be incomplete without some reference to the relation between traditional "folk medicine" and Western medical diagnosis and medicaments. One might expect that this relationship would be particularly conflictive if we look at the old people in the villages. Is it true that their rejection of Western medicine is more widespread than the doubts and reticence of other age groups?

As far as my observations go this is not the case. Particularly in the less accessible and therefore often more tradition-dominated regions practices of African folk medicine as described for the Bambara by P. J. Imperato prevail (Imperato 1977). However, elements of Western medicine were not rejected, but integrated, as we widely observed. We can speak of a cultural pluralism in view of health matters, even in very isolated regions. There remains a small percentage of older people who completely reject Western medicine; an estimated one out of six older persons reject Western medicine.

PROPOSAL OF MEASURES TO IMPROVE HEALTH CONDITIONS OF THE OLD IN RURAL AREAS IN AFRICA

What are some of the possible measures to improve health conditions of the old?

Local Dispensaries

The improvement of the accessibility of health care of the old heavily depends on a small stock of first-aid kits and a set of important medicaments. They will find their way to the most needy people in the very poor communities if this medical stock (village pharmacy) is controlled not by an individual dealer but by a village committee. In tribal society (and not only there) the traditional forms of village organization do permit such control. Village committees serve as instruments for socially balanced distributions. The processes of this distribution function relatively well if there are only three or four basic drugs, and if some first-aid kit is available. It is therefore worthwhile to institutionalize village committees for local health to satisfy basic community health needs and thereby the needs of the old. The question remains open where the initial input of medicaments and first-aid material will come from.

It may be suggested that international campaigns, particularly by WHO (or the UN directly), be started in view of the growing needs of older people in the Third World, primarily for the health outfit for village usage. In urban areas a certain success with district pharmacies administered by local committees has been achieved. When such pharmacies (aid posts) are started with a supply donated from outside, the refilling of stocks ought to be the responsibility of the local committees. The health administration of the government should be viewed as a potential network to assist in this process of distribution at least to regional centres from where the villages could obtain the medicaments.

Co-operation with Local Healers

The support of local healers appears as one of the important bridges to bring help to the elderly in the village. The older people relate themselves faithfully to the local healer and they will accept Western medicaments better if the local healer is in agreement with such a supply.

All possible health aid which can be brought to the villages in isolated regions should be given to the village as such. There should be a village development programme within which both health and social integration of the elderly are supported. Some African governments originally had thought that special social or health policy or special initiatives for the old would best be established in analogy to specialized First World health institutions of the welfare state. This is, according to our findings—obtained in co-operation with medical experts and government representatives of the Republic of Mali—the wrong way.

Health Education

Progress in the supply of medicaments, treatment and consultation can be made if it is possible to select a small number of villagers, and to bring them as a group for a period of at least 2 months to a small town where a local hospital operates. There the groups can be trained to administer first aid and to distribute such medicaments as are necessary for the basic health of the whole village population, including the elderly. It should be noted that dosage is often different for older people so that not only the know-how concerning the medicament but also concerning its specified dosage is required.

Stabilization and social integration of the elderly in the village is a prerequisite for the satisfaction of their health needs. The integration of the elderly under conditions of rural exodus necessitates the agricultural development and the socio-economic stabilization of the village. Naturally there have to be at least minimal ecological changes to permit the socio-economic continuity of the village on the soil. If agroproduction can continue or even expand, then the survival of the village ought to enable the integration of the old. It is within the economic and the social context and the process of this integration that the health problems of the old ought to be understood and tackled.

Mass Media Health Programmes

Radio programmes in African countries become a growing potential of influence and will possibly be an important factor in health education. They increasingly influence women who previously were completely cut off from non-local, extra-regional information. Radio now starts entering even the most isolated regions. This is important also in view of the health of older people. Up to now in most African tribal societies women were the affective centres of society. Their emotional support permitted the survival of the most vulnerable individuals and groups, e.g. children and frail elderly. As concerns information, they significantly lagged behind men. Women are the first to help, in social as well as in medical terms. Now women increasingly receive information through the mass media, particularly if and where regular programmes for the rural population are institutionalized, as is the case in the Republic of Mali. Health of the old thus might figure in a special health information programme. Such a programme could influence conditions for help. Knowledge, however, remains without power if a stabilization of the rural community on the basis of agrarian improvement does not take place.

Health support to the old in Africa is certainly not possible, has no real chances for success if it is conceived of or operated as an isolated activity without integrating it into the economic and social aspects of community development.

SUMMARY

Empirical findings from a 5-year field study project in Bambara villages in the Sahel region of the Republic of Mali (West Africa) are reported and interpreted. The traditional position of the old is placed in cultural and mythological context and described against the background of socio-economic changes. The seniority principle underlying traditional African society is explained. It encompasses also polarities other than parental and filial relations. It determines priorities, e.g. by ranking brothers according to the order of birth, and by ranking social units.

Age sets, ancestors' worship, child rearing, socialization practices and rituals are interpreted as elements of a sociocultural system in which the rules of seniority provide an organizing force.

The paper describes the ways in which breaks in the solidarity of the traditional community occur. Strategies are discussed in order to indicate how the health and care of the old could be improved. In its final evaluation of findings the paper argues for communal integration and community-centred health care. Social organizations are discussed in order to indicate how (on the basis of village committees) innovations could be integrated into slowly transforming traditional power structures.

ACKNOWLEDGEMENTS

I should like to express my gratitude to Prof. Heinz Stemberger who accompanied me on the first trip to Sonongo and to whom I owe valuable medical analyses some of which I am using here. Dir. Heide Reinisch, psychologist, helped me to understand mother–child relations and socializ-ation practices in groups as explanatory elements of the seniority principle. To Prof. Manfred Kremser I owe many insights into anthropology, particularly into witchcraft and healing; Dr. Erwin Ebermann through depth interviews and his mastery of the Bambara language enabled me to understand better the unfathomable depth of the African soul and the contradictions dwelling therein. Last but not least I should like to thank the Ludwig Boltzmann Society, Vienna, for supporting this study over the years.

REFERENCES

Amoss, P. and Harrell S. (eds) (1981). "Other ways of growing old: anthropological perspectives". Stanford University Press, Stanford, CA.
Baltes, P. B. and Smith, J. (1990). Weisheit und Weisheitsentwicklung. *Zeitschrift für Entwicklungspsychologie und Pädagogische Psychologie* (in press).
Bernardi, B. (1985). "Age and class systems". Cambridge University Press, Cambridge, MA.
Durkheim, E. (1969). "The division of labor in society". The Free Press, NY.
Ebermann, E. (1989). Gundofen. Die geheimen Dinge—Fetische und Geheimbünde

bei den Bambara. Gespräche mit Eingeweihten über die Fetische und die Geheimgesellschaften der Bambara in Mali. Afro-pub (Beiträge zur Afrikanistik 38), Vienna.

Foner, N. (1984). "Ages in conflict. A cross-cultural perspective on inequality between old and young". Columbia University Press, NY.

Holmes, L. (1983). "Other cultures, elder years: an introduction to cultural gerontology". Wichita State University Press, Wichita, KS.

Imperato, P. J. (1977). "African Folk Medicine", York Press Inc., Baltimore, NY.

Keith, J. (1985). Age in anthropological research. *In* "Handbook of aging and the social sciences" (R. H. Birren and E. Shanas, eds). Van Nostrand Reinhold, NY.

Kertzer, D. and Keith, J. (eds) (1984). "Age and anthropological theory". Cornell University Press, Ithaka, NY.

Koty, J. (1934). "Die Behandlung der Alten und Kranken bei den Naturvölkern". C. L. Hirschfeld, Stuttgart.

Kremser, M. (1984). Zur Geschichte des Bambara-Dorfes Sonongo in Mali. Vienna (mimeographed).

Kremser, M. (1986). Das Sandorakel "CEN" bei den Bambara. *Wiener Volkskundliche Mitteilungen* **28**, 5–31.

Laslett, P. (1989). The demographic scene—an overview. *In* "An aging world" (J. M. Eekelaar and D. Pearl, eds) p. 5. Clarendon Press, Oxford.

Paulme, D. (1971). Classes et associations d'âge en Afrique de l'Ouest". Plon, Paris.

Rosenmayr, L. (1978). Fragmente zu einer sozialwissenschaftlichen Theorie der Lebensalter. *In* Die menschlichen Lebensalter—Kontinuität und Krisen" (L. Rosenmayr, ed.) pp. 428–457. Piper, Munich.

Rosenmayr, L. (1982). Die gesellschaftliche Stellung der Älteren als Problem der Kultur. *In* "Aspekte des menschlichen Alterns" (Österreichische Akademie der Wissenschaften, ed.) pp. 31–47. Verlag der Österreichischen Akademie der Wissenschaften, Vienna.

Rosenmayr, L. (1988a). More than wisdom. A field study of the old in an African village. *Journal of Cross-Cultural Gerontology* **3**, 21–40.

Rosenmayr, L. (1988b). Die Schnüre vom Himmel. Über Alte und Ahnen bei den Bambara in der Region von Segou. *Psychosozial* **6**, 63–88.

Rosenmayr, L. (1990). "Die Kräfte des Alters" pp. 86–88. Edition Atelier, Vienna.

Simmons, L. W. (1970). "The role of the aged in primitive society". Archon Books (reprint from Yale University Press, 1945).

Simonton, D. K. (1990). Creativity and wisdom in aging. *In* "Handbook of the psychology of aging" (J. E. Birren and K. W. Schaie, eds) pp. 320–329. Academic Press, San Diego, CA.

Sokolovsky, J. (ed.) (1990). The cultural context of aging. Bergin and Garvey, New York.

Sow, I. (1977). "Psychiatrie dynamique Africaine". Payot, Paris.

Tout, K. (1989). "Aging in developing countries". Oxford University Press, NY.

WAA (1982). Vienna International Plan of Action on Aging, Paragraph 8, Final Report. Vienna (mimeographed).

Zahan, D. (1974). "The Bambara". K. J. Brill, Leiden.

Discussion

Williams: This was a marvellous presentation. A nursing anthropologist, who has been working in the black valleys of West Virginia, recently told me that when a person gets ill there she/he goes first to her/his mother. If there is no mother they go to the mother figure in the valley; beyond that it's anybody who has ever had any nursing training; beyond that it's the pharmacist; and finally, if absolutely necessary, it's the doctor. I wonder if there is any sequence like this or anything different about how a person proceeds in the village to get help.

Rosenmayr: The person in the village will first go to the local healer and will expect him to give some solution to his or her problems. The prescriptions that the local healer then gives are taken with the feeling that the healer is a great authority. So it would be completely wrong to leave the healer out of any institutionalization on a local basis of a pharmacy or a dispensary, but the local healer, if he is integrated, will permit ways of treatment that are not in his repertoire.

Age-associated Memory Impairment: Conceptual Background and Treatment Approaches

Jerome A. Yesavage

*Veterans Administration Medical Center, Palo Alto,
California and Department of Psychiatry and Behavioral
Sciences, Stanford University School of Medicine*

INTRODUCTION AND OVERVIEW

The general setting of this work is cognitive training for mildly memory-impaired elders (Poon *et al.* 1978, Cavanaugh *et al.* 1983). In the past, memory losses associated with normal aging were called "benign senescent forgetfulness" (Kahn *et al.* 1975, Craik 1977, Poon 1985). A National Institute of Mental Health (NIMH) Workgroup, however, has suggested that when such losses exceed one standard deviation from mean performance for young adults on standardized tests of recent memory, the diagnosis "age-associated memory impairment" (AAMI) should be applied (Crook *et al.* 1986). The reason for a formal diagnosis is that even this level of loss, averaging about 30% between age 20 and 70 on standardized tests, may be associated with dysphoria and excess disability. The AAMI diagnosis is currently under review by the Organic Subcommittee of the American Psychiatric Association's DSM-IV Workgroup for inclusion in the new version of their Diagnostic and Statistical Manual (DSM).

Below I'll describe our prior work which has centred on improving function in practical areas of memory impairment such as face–name recall, list learning and reading retention. I'll describe the "pretraining" concept

Challenges in Aging
ISBN 0-12-090163-3

list learning and reading retention. I'll describe the "pretraining" concept and explain how our group has used nonmnemonic "pretraining" to improve the effectiveness of classic mnemonic techniques in the elderly. I'll outline the gaps in our knowledge of the effectiveness of these techniques in the elderly, especially "Why is there so much variability of response to treatment?" and "What are the predictors of successful response to treatment?" I'll then describe our current large-scale studies which have shown that "old-old" subjects have much more difficulty learning complex mnemonics than do "young-old". I'll explain these results in terms of changes in information processing capacity and speed of information processing in the old-old. Finally, I'll present pilot work which takes these changes into consideration thereby attempting to address the problems the old-old have learning mnemonics.

PREVIOUS STUDIES OF MEMORY TRAINING AND KNOWLEDGE GAPS

Previous Training Studies and the "Pretraining" Concept

What are mnemonic devices?

Several mnemonic devices can facilitate recall of material such as name–face pairs and lists. A standard mnemonic for learning faces and names involves three steps for encoding: (1) choosing a prominent feature of the person's face, for example in my case, my bushy eyebrows; (2) developing a concrete, high-imagery transformation of the person's name, in my case, a SAVAGE Indian's feather head-dress; (3) forming a visual image associating the prominent feature and the transformed name, in my case, imagine the feathers growing out of my eyebrows. To recall the name, three steps are also required: (1) recognizing the prominent feature of the test face, the eyebrows; (2) utilizing that feature as a retrieval cue for the image association, seeing the feather head-dress; (3) deriving the actual name from the transformation. This mnemonic technique has been shown to provide young subjects a powerful strategy to recall names and faces they wish to remember (McCarty 1980). A more complex device, the method of loci, can be used for list learning. This device associates list items to a fixed list of places (or "loci"). Recall of the list is achieved by imagining each locus and then "seeing" the item associated to it (Bower 1970). Failure to use such organizational strategies appears to contribute to older subjects' poor memory performance (Craik 1977).

Pretraining and why elderly find mnemonic devices difficult to use

Unfortunately, we and others have found that the elderly have difficulty using mnemonic strategies for a number of reasons including anxiety, inability to form visual images, and relatively superficial encoding of associations (Poon *et al*. 1978, Yesavage 1985). Our research has attempted to deal with such age-related deficits that limit older persons' ability to learn mnemonics *before* trying to teach them the complex devices themselves. Our procedures thus involve supplemental non-mnemonic "pretraining" combined with a mnemonic strategy and have been found to improve performance more than the same mnemonic intervention given without pretraining (Hill *et al*. 1988). Several different non-mnemonic interventions have been studied.

The types of non-mnemonic pretraining

Relaxation pretraining for state anxiety

We have examined relaxation training to offset the negative effect of state anxiety on performance (Yesavage and Jacob 1984). The idea behind this intervention is that anxiety in the elderly reduces information processing capacity because much capacity is wasted on useless ruminations usually about expected performance. This is similar to treatment for test anxiety in college students. Although various relaxation procedures may be of use, we prefer to use progressive muscle relaxation because it is simple and follows an easily accepted physiologic model.

Visual imagery pretraining to enhance image associations

We have also used visual imagery training to enhance ability to utilize an imagery-based mnemonic (Yesavage 1983). This technique is based upon difficulties older people often have producing visual imagery. This and our other methods have been elaborated by our trainer in a procedures manual (Lapp 1987). In this case the therapist uses colour slides and other interesting visual materials to slowly train the older subject to "see in the mind's eye" what is presented on the screen. This pretraining in the ability to create visual images enables the older person to better create image associations used in mnemonics.

Semantic elaboration pretraining to enhance verbal encoding

Finally, we have developed semantic elaboration training in which subjects are instructed to make verbal judgments in relation to visual images to encourage elaboration during encoding (Yesavage *et al*. 1983). Thus not only visual, but verbal processing of associated images is enhanced. The better the encoding of image associations, the better the retrieval. In the example of the mnemonic for my name, one would ask the question, perhaps, does he really look savage?

Overall effects of pretraining

In the several studies cited above the overall effects of the pretraining interventions are superior to learning mnemonics without pretraining (Hill *et al.* 1987). Furthermore, the amount of improvement is at least of the magnitude, 30%, of the memory losses which have been associated with AAMI (Yesavage 1985). The effect of interventions is stable at 6 months follow-up (Sheikh *et al.* 1986).

Knowledge Gaps about the Elderly and Mnemonics

Why is there so much variability of response to treatment?

Despite progress in developing effective cognitive training strategies for elders, one finds enormous variability of response to treatment. For example, although average name–face recall improves 2.55 pairs after treatment in our current studies, improvement ranges from −4 to +11 with a standard deviation of 2.56. Thus a major knowledge gap in our understanding of non-pharmacologic treatment for AAMI is: why do some subjects show major improvement while others actually do worse after training?

There have been only a few attempts to define predictors of response to memory training. One study examined specific predictors (Schaffer and Poon 1982). This study confirms the large individual variability in response to training and found that subjects with high verbal intelligence benefit most from training.

Familiarity with the target task and locus of control are learner characteristics which also have been associated with improved performance in response to cognitive training (Willis 1985). It was suggested that the high variability of response to training may be due to other non-specific factors: how materials are organized, utilization of examples, redundancy of information, monetary and social reinforcement, and previous performance success.

Could personality be a predictor of response to treatment?

It is possible that the wide variability in response to training may depend upon the personality of the trainee. There is evidence of a relationship between locus of control and performance on tests of intellectual ability in elderly people (Lachman *et al.* 1982, Lachman 1986a).

Our current work examined the relation of personality traits to the older adults' ability to benefit from cognitive training. Three previously validated methods of cognitive training based upon three types of non-mnemonic pretraining described above were used in this study. Two personality measures were given: the NEO personality inventory (NEO) and the personality in intellectual-aging contexts scale (PIC). Results of this study described below suggest other predictors of response may be more relevant to our understanding of the sources of variability than personality. Below we will discuss findings suggesting that age itself is an extremely important factor. These analyses will use the contrast between the "young-old" (less than 70 years) and "old-old" (70 and more years) to explain a significant amount of variability of response to treatment.

CURRENT STUDIES OF PREDICTORS OF RESPONSE TO TREATMENT

The results reported here in summary form have been reported in detail in a number of our recent papers and represent the major findings of our NIMH grant in this area (see Gratzinger *et al.* 1990, Yesavage *et al.* 1989, 1990 for detailed reports).

Methods

Subjects

Subjects were community-dwelling elderly recruited by newspaper ads, personal contact and local senior citizen centres for a "memory improvement" study. The data reported in this section are for 218 subjects. In addition, another 61 subjects completed the pilot studies also reported. Thus, a total of 279 subjects were studied.

Seventy per cent of the sample of 218 subjects were female. Average age was 67.74 years (SD = 6.86, range 55–87). They were screened for major active health problems, clinical depression, and marked cognitive impairment. We included only those with an MMSE score of 27 or higher (Folstein *et al.* 1975). The short form of the Geriatric Depression Scale (Sheikh and Yesavage 1986) screened for depression. They also completed a seven-point rating of education. Subjects on average had completed some

Jerome A. Yesavage

Table 1
Demographics for the three main conditions and two pilot conditions

	N	Age (years)	MMSE	Vocab.	GDS
Main conditions					
1. Imagery	74	67.69 (6.83)	29.20 (0.79)	24.55 (4.58)	2.44 (2.46)
2. Relaxation	67	67.92 (6.50)	29.18 (0.89)	23.94 (5.43)	1.70 (1.86)
3. Imagery + judgment	77	67.64 (7.25)	29.10 (0.88)	22.59 (5.51)	1.84 (2.13)
Total sample	218	67.74 (6.86)	29.16 (0.85)	23.68 (5.23)	2.00 (2.19)
Pilot conditions					
4. Comprehensive pretraining	37	67.51 (7.05)	28.89 (1.05)	19.49 (5.25)	1.49 (1.68)
5. Lengthened mnemonic training	24	67.50 (6.42)	28.54 (1.41)	22.17 (5.81)	1.92 (2.34)

SD in parentheses.

college and rated themselves as being in excellent or good health. Demographic information is included in Table 1.

Treatment conditions

Regardless of type of non-mnemonic pretraining condition, all participants received 8 h training in a classroom-type setting (2 h day^{-1}) in one face–name (4 h) and one list-learning (4 h) mnemonic. We used the standard name–face-learning technique already described. In addition, a list-learning mnemonic called the "method of loci" was also taught (Bower 1970). Mnemonic training was given in the second week of the programme.

The treatment conditions differed as to the type of non-mnemonic pretraining subjects received in the first week of the programme. All subjects received 6 h of pretraining. The three conditions were the same as those we have used in the past and are described briefly below.

Condition 1 ($n = 74$) used "imagery" pretraining: subjects received 6 h of instruction (2 h a day for 3 days) in the formation and elaboration of visual images using slides, art works and other visual material. This skill was then applied to the elaboration of imagery used in the mnemonics. The procedure for this condition was adapted from Yesavage (1983).

Condition 2 ($n = 67$) used "relaxation" pretraining: subjects in this condition received 6 h of instruction in the use of progressive muscle relaxation. The procedure is similar to that of Yesavage and Jacob (1984).

Condition 3 ($n = 77$) used "imagery + judgment" pretraining: in this condition subjects received two types of non-mnemonic training. First, they were given 3 h of training in the formation of visual imagery as in Condition 1. Second, participants were given 3 h of instruction teaching them to develop and verbalize their impressions of image associations to be used in mnemonic techniques. The protocol for this group was the same as Yesavage *et al.* (1983).

Procedures

Participants were tested for face–name and list recall before and after mnemonic training. In addition, certain personality measures were used.

Description of the face and name test

The name–face recall test follows the same procedures as Yesavage *et al.* (1983) and thus uses unique sets of black and white slide photographs of faces. Each set contains six male and six female faces randomly selected from a larger pool of slides. Common last names were also randomly assigned to the faces of each set. Each face slide is projected onto a screen while the name is shown on a sheet of paper and read aloud. After the last name–face pair is presented, there is a 4-min delay and subjects are given the recall test. For both study and test presentations faces are presented in random order at the rate of one per minute. Scores are the number of correct last names and range from 0 to 12.

Description of list-learning tests

As with the tests of name recall, we use equivalent test forms. These test forms have been used in previous research. Each form represents an alternate list of 16 common words to be learned by subjects.

Personality measures

Each individual was administered the NEO-PI and the PIC. The NEO-PI yields scores on three major domains: neuroticism, extraversion and openness to experience, as well as agreeableness and conscientiousness (Costa and McCrae, 1985). Six subscales or "facets" are calculated for each of the three major domains. Thus there is a total of 23 ($5 + 3 \times 6$) potential measures on this scale.

An additional perspective on the question of personality predictors of performance is that of Lachman *et al.* (1982) who report that context-specific personality measures are significantly better correlated with cognitive performance than are transcontextual measures, which can be used in any situation. Context-specific measures integrate reference to a specific situation in which a cognitive function is used. The difference simply illustrated is that between questions such as "Are you generally anxious?" versus "Are you anxious when you try to play the piano?" Dr Lachman has successfully used this approach in a series of studies on the interaction of cognitive function and personality (1982, 1986a,b). We used her personality in intellectual-aging contexts (PIC) scales in the reported research. This allows comparison of a transcontextual measure of personality (the NEO-PI) versus her context-specific measure (the PIC).

Subjects were randomly assigned to one of three conditions which varied according to the non-mnemonic pretraining administered prior to training in the mnemonic devices. We did not include controls in this project because control groups with non-specific pretraining have already been used in our prior work and in the current work we were interested in between-subject differences (Yesavage *et al.* 1983, Yesavage 1983, Sheikh *et al.* 1986, Hill *et al.* 1988).

Results

No significant differences were found between the three conditions in percentage of males and females, age, MMSE, vocabulary scores, depression or subjective health. There was a significant difference in formal education with more subjects in Condition 2 (relaxation) having completed advanced degrees. However, there was no relationship between education and improvement on either face–name recall ($F(3,213) = 0.19$, n.s.) or list recall ($F(3,213) = 1.01$, n.s.).

Improvement in face–name and list recall

Table 1 presents for each condition the mean age, MMSE, vocabulary score, and geriatric depression scale (GDS) score. To examine the effects of training on improvement in recall, our data were subjected to a mixed-model repeated-measures analysis of variance with type of training as a between-subjects variable and time of testing and type of measure as within-subjects variables. Over all conditions subjects improved from 3.20 at pretest to 5.75 at post-test on face–name recall and from 6.80 at pretest to 8.73 at post-test on list recall. The overall effect of training was significant; $F(1,215) = 173.86$, P < 0.001. However, the difference in improvement between conditions was not significant; $F(2,215) = 1.77$, n.s., and there was no significant interaction among condition, improvement, and type of task $F(2,215) = 1.40$, n.s.. A more detailed discussion of these results is in press in *Psychology and Aging*.

Relation of personality variables to recall improvement

The effects of individual difference variables on improvement were examined by computing the partial correlations between each scale and post-test scores on the names–faces and list-learning tests, controlling for pretest scores. We found only small correlations between the NEO measures and improvement. With respect to the PIC, a context-specific personality measure, results were only slightly better. Overall, these results suggest that these personality scales are not likely to be clinically useful predictors of response to treatment in this population (Gratzinger *et al.* 1990).

Relation of age to recall improvement

Following our analysis of the effects of training, we examined the relationship between improvement in recall and age and MMSE. Because preliminary analyses revealed no interaction between type of training and age or MMSE with respect to improvement in recall, we combined data from all three types of training for this analysis. For both types of recall we entered age and MMSE into a multiple regression analysis and examined the relationship of each variable to post-test scores after adjusting for the effects of both pretest score and the other variable. Overall, age and MMSE accounted for 11% of the variance in gain in face–name recall and 22% of the variance in list recall. Using regression analyses we found that age was related to improvement in both face–name recall ($t(1,214) = 5.18$, P $<$ 0.001) and list recall ($t(1,214) = 6.64$, P $<$ 0.001) after controlling for the effects of MMSE. Despite the limited range of scores (27–30), MMSE was also related to improvement in list recall independent of the effects of age ($t(1, 214) = 2.78$, P $<$ 0.01). However, the relationship between MMSE and improvement in face–name recall was not significant ($t(1,214) = 0.46$, n.s.).

In descriptive terms, while face–name recall improved 2.8 and 2.2 items for those under 70 and those 70 years old and over, respectively, improvement in list recall averaged 2.9 for those under 70 ($n = 133$) but was only 0.3 for those 70 years old and over ($n = 85$). Analyses of covariance suggested that improvement on the list-learning task was more strongly related to both age ($F(1,216) = 11.05$, P $<$ 0.01) and MMSE ($F(1, 216) = 5.50$, P $<$ 0.01) than was improvement on the name–face task. The combined data for these subjects are described as Condition 1+2+3 in Fig. 1 as the white column.

To determine if these results might be due to other variables indirectly related to age and mental status, we repeated the regression equation

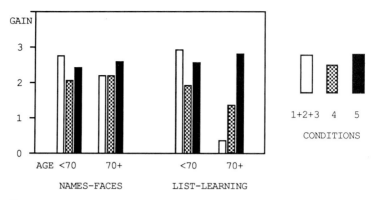

Fig. 1. Improvement in name–face and list recall by age and condition.

including education, subjective health, vocabulary scores and GDS scores
as additional variables. These variables did not change the relationship
between age, MMSE and improvement. See Yesavage *et al.* (1990) for a
full report.

Discussion and Implications of Pilot Work

General comments on task difficulty, age and AAMI

Although we have found that personality relates to successful memory
training, the amount of variance explained remains small at best. On the
other hand, we found that relatively crude cognitive measures such as the
mini-mental state exam (MMSE) also predict response to training even
using a restricted range of scores in the normal range (27–30). The strongest
predictor of response was age itself, and this effect cannot be accounted
for by MMSE score, anxiety, depression, education or subjective health.
Furthermore, age seems to affect the list-learning mnemonic more than the
face–name mnemonic. Thus we find that training techniques which have
been quite successful in improving the elderly's ability to use some
mnemonics may be inadequate for subjects older than 70 years. How can
one understand this effect of age on ability to learn certain mnemonic
devices?

A possible interpretation of the finding that subjects with lower MMSE
scores and higher ages benefit from one mnemonic and not from the other
is that their performance was negatively affected by the complexity of the
mnemonic taught. The face–name mnemonic is a relatively simple three-
step process: identify a prominent feature, construct a concrete name
transformation, and associate the two. The method for lists requires the

same three-step associative process, but also requires that subjects develop a list of loci or places to which they will link a set of visual images of the items to remember. If subjects cannot develop this list of loci, or find difficulty associating the list of items in sequence to the list of loci, or are unable to use the list in sequence to retrieve the items, the whole process fails. Thus the loci mnemonic is more demanding than the name–face technique.

If the old-old subjects could not benefit from one complex mnemonic, one wonders whether they would also fail in other training programmes using mnemonics with equivalent levels of complexity. Pilot data from 25 subjects on a reading retention study from our Teaching Nursing Home project supports this contention. In this unpublished data we found a negative correlation of −0.41 between age and gain scores for total recall after training. Although there may be different reasons why the old-old had problems learning reading techniques from the reasons they may have had for not benefiting from list-learning techniques, it is possible that a major factor was the complexity of the learned techniques.

The processing capacity model, the old-old and mnemonics

One way of interpreting our findings is the processing capacity model (Salthouse 1985b, Salthouse *et al*. 1989). Age differences in cognitive performance increase with the complexity of the task to be performed (Crowder 1980, Barr 1980). One could argue that information processing capacity declines with age and declines more in old-old individuals when compared with young-old individuals. This reduced processing capacity does not allow the concurrent use of multiple cognitive processes required by complex mnemonics thereby explaining why the old-old have difficulty with such complex tasks.

We have felt that one reason why our pretraining interventions work is that they increase the efficiency of processing. Because recent studies suggest continued decline of several cognitive functions in those over 70 (Crook *et al*. 1986, 1988), one should ask whether the deficits that are addressed by pretraining also become worse with advanced age, and whether a more comprehensive approach to remedy these deficits might be required in the old-old than might be required in the less impaired young-old. Thus old-old subjects might perhaps perform better with more comprehensive pretraining if such interventions allow for a more efficient use of their limited processing resources.

The speed of processing model, the old-old and mnemonics

There are other possible models to explain our results. It has been suggested that some deficits in cognitive performance on complex tasks are the consequence of the slowing of mental processing (Cerrella *et al.* 1980). Further, some data suggest that as task complexity increases cognitive slowing increases disproportionately (Welford 1977, Hale *et al.* 1987). A reduction in "psychological tempo" is seen as taking place across the range of information processing functions. Older people are slower both at basic levels of processing such as sensory registry and at levels of more complex functions such as reasoning ability (Salthouse 1985a). This phenomenon of cognitive slowing has been proposed as the overriding explanation for age-related memory decline (Waugh and Barr 1980).

While slowing as a universal decrement principle has been disputed (Kausler 1982), the concept leads one to suggest that additional instructional time and practice might be required for older subjects to learn a new cognitive process such as a mnemonic technique. In a review of intervention programmes, Poon *et al.* (1978) suggest that age-related differences in response to memory training could be reduced by providing more practice time for older subjects to master mnemonic techniques. Indeed, some studies show that when older subjects are given additional time to perform cognitive tasks they can compensate for their disadvantage in memory performance (Treat and Reese 1976) and in learning new skills (Elias *et al.* 1987). Furthermore, across cognitive tasks and age groups, performance improves with practice (Murrell 1970, Rabbit 1982, Baltes and Willis 1982, Poon 1985). Some argue that the likelihood of forming an accurate assessment of the potential benefit of mnemonic training will be increased if older subjects are given more time to become familiar with the task (Treat *et al.* 1981). Thus, increasing the time to learn (by providing additional practice time) for a complex mnemonic (method of loci) might be expected to improve performance for older subjects. Although there is extensive evidence that a number of mental processes slow with normal aging, no one to date has systematically examined the effect of increased time for the teaching of mnemonic devices.

Some pilot data presented below suggest that increased instructional time and enhanced pretraining may improve the ability of the old-old to benefit from training in a complicated mnemonic device.

PILOT STUDIES OF AGE AND BENEFIT FROM TRAINING

Because it appears that the deficits which are addressed by pretraining become worse with age, in the following study we ask the question of whether benefit can be maximized for the old-old by using a treatment which combines several applicable techniques. In addition we would like to know if age-related slowing of information processing could be attenuated by increased practice. In sum, can increased pretraining or increased practice enhance the ability of the old-old subjects to profit from complex mnemonic techniques?

Pilot Data on Pretraining and Age-related Effects

We completed a pilot "Condition 4" with 37 subjects. These subjects were given a comprehensive pretraining programme which combined our imagery and judgment pretraining with our relaxation training programmes. Our goal was to determine if this variation would help address the disadvantage that our old-old subjects appeared to have in benefiting from the memory retraining on the method of loci. This small pilot study was not designed to address questions about low-normal MMSE subjects.

Condition 4 had the same testing procedures and the same amount of time spent in pretraining and mnemonic training as did our first three groups of the main study. Subjects in this group first received 2 h of instruction in the use of the simple progressive muscle relaxation pretraining procedure from Condition 2. They were then given 2 h of pretraining in the formation of visual imagery as in Condition 1. Finally, participants were given 2 h of pretraining in developing and verbalizing their impressions of image associations as in Condition 3.

Pilot Data on Training Time and Age-related Effects

Another alternative to our current methods would be to increase training time to examine the possibility that the old-old require more time to learn mnemonic techniques. This strategy would be consistent with the large body of work documenting the slowing of information processing with normal aging cited above. For the 24 subjects in this "Condition 5" we added 2 more hours of mnemonic training for the method of loci (one additional class). In previous studies subjects had received 4 h of training. Thus we increased training time by 50%. In all other respects the treatment was equivalent to Condition 4, our other pilot study which had comprehensive pretraining.

Results of Analyses on Pilot Data

Recall performance in our two pilot conditions was compared to performance in our three main conditions by means of a $5 \times 2 \times 2$ (condition $\times$ time $\times$ mnemonic) ANCOVA with repeated measures on the last two variables and age as a covariate. We found a significant interaction among age, condition and time, $F(4,269) = 2.60$, P <0.05. In general, old-old subjects were more likely to benefit from the added features of our two pilot conditions than were young-old subjects. This effect appeared to be somewhat stronger for the more complex list-learning task; however, the four-way interaction was not significant ($F(4,269) = 0.85$, n.s.). Subjects in Condition 4 who were 70 years old and over ($n = 15$) scored 1.4 on list improvement and those in Condition 5 who were 70 years old and over ($n = 9$) scored 2.8 compared to an average of 0.3 for all old-old subjects in Conditions $1 + 2 + 3$ combined ($n = 85$). This pattern of results is presented in Fig. 1.

These pilot data suggest that comprehensive pretraining and lengthened mnemonic training may improve performance in memory tasks, and that these additional features will have a positive effect for the old-old learning a complex mnemonic technique.

LIMITS OF PILOT WORK AND NEED FOR FURTHER STUDY

Despite the encouraging results of these two pilot studies, our enthusiasm is tempered by several considerations. First of all, a direct comparison between Condition $1 + 2 + 3$ and the pilot conditions is strained because the pilot work was not run at the same time and subjects were not randomized across all five conditions. Although subjects in all conditions were found to be comparable on age, initial scores on name–face and list recall, depression scores and health status, significant differences existed between the pilot groups and Condition $1 + 2 + 3$ on vocabulary scores and MMSE scores (see Table 1). Furthermore, since Condition 5 combined both pretraining and learning time interventions, their relative impact could not be determined. Finally, the number of subjects in the pilot work over 70 years old was small and the issue of low-normal MMSE score subjects was not raised due to the small sample size. None the less, we are encouraged by these preliminary results. We currently have proposed research to further look at AAMI treatments in the old-old using samples carefully matched across conditions and of sufficient size to study issues of individual differences in response to treatment.

One should also note that although age accounted for a substantial amount of the interindividual variance in the current study even when controlling for MMSE score, it is possible that the relatively simple screening process failed to identify some subjects who may have been in the early stages of multi-infarct or senile dementia. Changes associated with these conditions might be difficult to document on simple tests such as the MMSE given our subjects' relatively high educational level and expected high level of premorbid functioning. *Post hoc* examination of the MMSE in our study showed that errors on the recall items were the errors most closely associated with poor performance on the memory course. This, however, is of little help in discriminating individuals because, although poor memory is often the initial complaint of the demented individuals, non-demented elderly also often complain of memory loss. Furthermore, such distinctions are clouded by Reisberg's finding that in following borderline cases (ratings of 2 on his global deterioration scale) similar to those with low-normal MMSE scores in our study, only 5% of these individuals progressed to diagnosable dementias (Reisberg *et al.* 1986). Although we found that both age and relatively low MMSE scores were independently associated with reduced performance on the complex mnemonic, we do not know how these two factors relate to a diagnosis of AAMI. This question cannot be answered with the current data or with the pilot results, but will be addressed in proposed studies.

Finally, future work should better characterize subjects on relevant cognitive measures such as measures of speed of processing and verbal ability. Such work might provide clues about specific deficits associated with impaired ability to benefit from treatment. At the very least, a means of screening out subjects unlikely to benefit would be created. Specific remediation strategies might be developed on the basis of such findings. These interventions would be analogous to the pretraining component of our memory retraining programmes for which, for example, we developed non-mnemonic training on verbal elaboration to compensate for age-related encoding deficits. Ultimately one could attempt to match type of training with type of cognitive deficit.

ACKNOWLEDGEMENTS

This research was supported in part by the Medical Research Service of the Veterans Administration, National Institutes of Mental Health grant MH 35182, National Institute on Aging Teaching Nursing Home project AG04458 and the Clinical Research Center for the Study of Senile Dementias MH-40041. The editorial and research assistance of Danielle C. Lapp and Leah Friedman is acknowledged.

REFERENCES

Baltes, P. and Willis, S. (1982). Aging and cognitive processes. *In* "Advances in the study of communication and affect" (F.I.M. Craik and S. Trehub, eds). Plenum Press, New York.
Barr, R. A. (1980). Some remarks on the time-course of aging. *In* "New directions

in memory and aging: proceedings of the George A. Talland Memorial Conference" (L. W. Poon, J. L. Fozard, L. S. Cermak, D. Arenberg and L. W. Thompson, eds). Lawrence Erlbaum Associates, New Jersey.

Bower, G. H. (1970). Analysis of a mnemonic device. *American Scientist* **58**, 497–510.

Cavanaugh, J. C., Grady, J. G., and Perlmutter, M. (1983). Forgetting and use of memory aids in 20 to 70 year olds in everyday life. *International Journal of Aging and Human Development* **17**, 113–122.

Cerrella, J., Poon, L. W. and Williams, D. M. (1980). Age and the complexity hypothesis. *In* "Aging in the 1980s: psychological issues" (L. W. Poon, ed.), American Psychological Association, Washington, DC.

Costa, P. T., Jr. and McCrae, R. R. (1985). "Manual: the NEO personality inventory". Psychological Assessment Resources Inc., Odessa, Florida.

Craik, F. (1977). Age differences in human memory. *In* "Handbook of the psychology of aging" 1st edn, (J. E. Birren and K. W. Schaie, eds). Van Nostrand Reinhold, New York.

Crook, T., Salama, M. and Gobert J. (1986). A computerized test battery for detecting and assessing memory disorders. *In* "Senile dementias: early detection" (A. Bes, ed.). John Libbey Eurotext.

Crook, T., Johnson, B., Youniss, E., Kelly A., Zadeik, A. and Bahar, H. (1988). Behavioral consequences of normal cerebral aging. *In* "L'vieillisement cerebral normal et pathologique" (S. A. Maloine, ed.). Foundation Nationale De Gerontologie, Paris.

Crowder, R. G. (1980). Echoic memory and the study of aging memory systems. *In* "New directions in memory and aging: proceedings of the George A. Talland Memorial Conference" (L. W. Poon, J. L. Fozard, L. S. Cermak, D. Arenberg and L. W. Thompson, eds). Lawrence Erlbaum Associates, New Jersey.

Elias, P., Elias, M., Robbins, M. and Gage, P. (1987). Acquisition of word-processing skills by younger, middle-age, and older adults. *Psychology and Aging* **2** (4), 340–348.

Folstein, M. F., Folstein, S. E. and McHugh, P. H. (1975). Mini-mental state: a practical method for grading the cognitive state of patients for the clinician. *Journal of Psychiatric Research* **12**, 189–198.

Gratzinger, P., Sheikh, J., Friedman, L. and Yesavage, J. (1990). Cognitive interventions to improve face–name recall: the role of personality trait differences. *Developmental Psychology*.

Hale, S., Myerson, J. and Wagstaff, D. (1987). General slowing of nonverbal information processing: evidence for a power law. *Journal of Gerontology* **42** (2), 131–136.

Hill, R.D., Sheikh, J. I. and Yesavage, J. A. (1987). Effects of mnemonic training on perceived recall confidence in the elderly. *Experimental Aging Research* **13**, 185–188.

Hill, R. D., Sheikh, J. I. and Yesavage, J. A. (1988). Pretraining enhances mnemonic training in elderly adults. *Experimental Aging Research* **14**, 207–211.

Kahn, R. L., Zarit, S. H., Hilbert, N. M. *et al.* (1975). Memory complaint and impairment in the aged. *Archives of General Psychiatry* **32**, 1569–1573.

Kausler, D. H. (1982). "Experimental psychology and human aging". Wiley, New York.

Lachman, M. E. (1986a). Locus of control in aging research. A case for multidimensional and domain-specific assessment. *Journal of Psychology and Aging* **1**, 34–40.

Lachman, M. E. (1986b). Personal control in later life. Stability, change, and cognitive correlates. *In* "The psychology of control and aging" (M. Baltes and P. Baltes, eds). Lawrence Erlbaum, Hillsdale, NJ.

Lachman, M. E., Baltes, B., Nesselroade, J. R. and Willis, S. (1982). Examination of personality–ability relationships in the elderly. The role of contextual (interface) assessment mode. *Journal of Research in Personality* **16**, 485–501.

Lapp, D. (1987). "Don't forget". McGraw-Hill, New York.

McCarty, D. L. (1980). Investigation of a visual imagery mnemonic device for acquiring face–name associations. *Journal of Experimental Psychology: Human Learning and Memory* **6**, 145–155.

Murrell, F. H. (1970). The effect of extensive practice on age differences in reaction time. *Journal of Gerontology* **25**, 268–274.

Poon, L. (1985). Differences in human memory with aging: nature, causes, and clinical implications. *In* "Handbook of the psychology of aging" 2nd edn. (J.E. Birren and K. W. Schaie, eds), Van Nostrand Reinhold, New York.

Rabbit, P. (1982). How do old people know what to do next? *In* "Advances in the study of communication and affect: aging and cognitive processes" (F. I. M. Craik and S. Trehub, eds). Plenum Press, New York.

Reisberg, B., Ferris, S. H., Borenstein, J., Sinaiko, E., de Leon, M. J. and Buttingher, C. (1986). Assessment of presenting symptoms. *In* "Handbook for clinical memory assessment of older adults" (L. W. Poon, T. Crook, K. L. Davis, C. Eisdorfer, B. J. Gurland, A. W. Kasalniak and L.W. Thompson, eds). American Psychological Association, Washington, DC.

Salthouse, T. A. (1985a). Speed of behavior and its implications for cognition. *In* "Handbook of the psychology of aging" 2nd edn. (J. E. Birren and K. W. Schaie, eds), Van Nostrand Reinhold, New York.

Salthouse, T. A. (1985b). "A theory of cognitive aging". Elsevier, New York.

Salthouse, T. A., Mitchell, D. R. D., Skovronek, E. and Babcock, R. L. (1989). *Journal of Experimental Psychology: Learning, Memory, and Cognition* **15** (3), 507–516.

Schaffer, G. and Poon, L. (1982). Individual variability in memory training with the elderly. *Educational Gerontology* **8**, 217–229.

Sheikh, J. I., and Yesavage, J. A. (1986). Geriatric depression scale (GDS): recent evidence and development of a shorter version. *Clinical Gerontologist* **5**,(1/2), 165–173.

Sheikh, J. I., Hill, R. D. and Yesavage, J. A. (1986). Long term efficacy of cognitive training for age-associated memory impairment: a six month follow-up study. *Developmental Neuropsychology* **2** (4), 413–421.

Treat, N. and Reese, H. (1976). Age, pacing, and imagery in paired-associate learning. *Developmental Psychology* **12** (2), 119–124.

Treat, N., Poon, L. and Fozard, J. (1981). Age, imagery, and practice in paired-associate learning. *Experimental Aging Research* **7** (3), 337–342.

Waugh, N. and Barr, R. (1980). Memory and mental tempo. *In* "New directions in memory and aging: proceedings of the George A. Talland and Memorial Conference" (L. W. Poon, J. L. Fozard, L. S. Cermak, D. Arenberg and L. W. Thompson, eds). Lawrence Erlbaum Associates, New Jersey.

Welford, A. T. (1977). Motor performance. *In* "Handbook of the psychology of aging" lst edn. (J. E. Birren and K. W. Schaie, eds). Van Nostrand Reinhold, New York.

Willis, S. L. (1985). Towards an educational psychology of the older adult learner: intellectual and cognitive bases. *In* "Handbook of the psychology of aging" 2nd edn. (J. E. Birren and K. W. Schaie, eds). Van Nostrand Reinhold, New York.

Yesavage, J.A. (1983). Imagery pretraining and memory training in the elderly. *Gerontology (Basel)* **29**, 271–275.

Yesavage, J. A. (1985). Nonpharmacologic treatments for memory losses with normal aging. *American Journal of Psychiatry* **142**, 600–605.

Yesavage, J. A. and Jacob, R. (1984). Effects of relaxation and mnemonics on memory, attention and anxiety in the elderly. *Experimental Aging Research* **10**(4), 211–214.

Yesavage, J. A., Brink, T. L., Rose, T. L., Adey, M. B., Lum, O., Huang, V. and Lierer, V. O. (1983). Development of a geriatric depression rating scale: a preliminary report. *Journal of Psychiatric Research* **17**, 37–49.

Yesavage, J. A., Sheikh, J. I., Friedman, L. F. and Tanke, E. (1990). Learning mnemonics: the roles of aging and subtle cognitive impairment. accepted for publication, *Psychology and Aging*.

DISCUSSION

Bergener: From our traditional point of view with our European classification system we have some problems with your term AAMI. Can you give a short definition?

Yesavage: The concept of AAMI (age-associated memory impairment) is that older people simply have more difficulty remembering things than younger people do, and probably the best analogy is with vision, i.e. as we get older we all develop a near-sightedness and the question comes up: is this a medical diagnosis or is it normal aging? What we try to do with this term is to put a tag on a phenomenon, whether that phenomenon is a disease or whether that's an age-related developed mental tag, it is not clear. We are trying to set up criteria. I understand from Dr. Gottfries that some more discussions are going on in Europe to set up criteria to define a population of people who seem to have experienced a decline from youth, and then to determine the biological, physiological and psychological aspects of these people, and then to look at treatment issues.

Nordin: It wasn't clear to me whether you taught the subjects a standard set of loci or whether you taught them each to develop their own set of loci. I think they will be more effective with their own set of loci than with the set that you impose on them.

Yesavage: They made their own loci.

Stähelin: How long would you think that the lag time between two training sessions should be?

Yesavage: The training time is 2 h a day for 2 weeks. We have set up the training like a course. I am a psychiatrist, but we do not use a psychiatric or a psychological model, we use an educational one. I think that this concept is well known in Switzerland. We have not really studied the best timing systematically, but I would say that we have a good experience with the above system. We have also tried to compress the time lag between the trainings, but I think that you do not want to give the older person too much too quickly.

Danon: Did you try to predict success by the state of health?

Yesavage: That's a very good question. We did so but we did not find any correlation with the state of health. But most of these people were rather healthy. The issue, I think, which was brought up very well by Dr. Birren earlier, is: there are healthy, and then there are very healthy. I would like to consult with some of my physically fit older statesmen to find out what is a quick test of physical fitness that one could do in this setting so that one could provide a more objective measure other than a questionnaire measure of fitness. Because it could be quite possible that the 60-year-old joggers are doing much better than 60-year-old sedentary people.

Sir Martin Roth: Was there a control of their health status?

Yesavage: Yes, but it was essentially a questionnaire measure, there was no performance measure.

Sir Martin Roth: Did you discover any correlation between performance and social class and educational status, or between performance in response to training against social class and educational status, because many epidemiological studies have found some correlation in respect of mental impairment of definable clinical kind?

Yesavage: The question is: is there a relationship between social class and education? What's interesting is that there was a baseline difference in performance. In other words, some of the better educated patients did better on baseline. But there was no difference in improvement. There was a parallel improvement regardless of social class or education. Well-educated persons might initially score 4 and less well-educated might score 2; after training the well-educated ones will score 6 and the less well-educated ones might score 4. So there is a parallel improvement, there is not a differential improvement with higher education.

Fries: Baltes found that he could equalize young and old by presenting performance lists and spacing the intervals. If the older people were given enough time between items, they could perform as well as the young. Is this the same phenomenon that you found on the training side or is it a different one?

Yesavage: It's the same thing on the training side. What we did with the testing is that we have given essentially an almost unlimited amount of time to do the testing, this is the same idea. What's interesting is that what you would think would be a tremendous amount of time for training, about 20 hours of training for these older people, if you take the same techniques to Stanford undergraduate students of psychology, you can train them in one afternoon. And what we are finding is that for the old-old, even the 20 hours or so were not enough.

Fejer: Your subjects were fortunate, so-called healthy elderly, and this may be an exception. Maybe there are between them young-elderly, young-old. Were these subjects absolutely free of any drug effect which would eventually influence the function of the CNS?

Yesavage: The patients were drug free. We have done analogous studies in a nursing home study funded by the NIA, with more impaired people and we found no drug effect.

Mrs Ermini: How did you measure the AAMI, what kind of test and what limitation criteria did you use in normal subjects vs AAMI?

Yesavage: The criteria we used were those developed by the NIMH work group, but they are not the ultimate ones, they are under debate now. You can use any standardized test which has norms for the different age groups. If the "old" group is one standard deviation below the "young" norm, then you have that group. We used essentially WAIS subscales and also rational memory scales. In addition, we have some standardized tests used in the past. I don't want to be ambiguous about the best tests.

Kanowski: How did you ensure that your probands did use a localization technique for learning a word list?

Yesavage: To verify the method of loci we developed two tests. First of all we get the persons to generate their set of loci before the examination and we collect that and test to see if they could generate the test. Then we give them a true and false test about the method of loci. What is interesting is that if you make one error on the true and false test your performance goes dramatically down and those errors are in the old-old group. So we have very good proof that the old-old just did not learn the technique.

Epidemiological Aspects of the Mental Disorders of Older Age

J. R. M. Copeland

*Department of Psychiatry, University of Liverpool,
P.O. Box 147, Liverpool L69 3BX, UK*

THE EPIDEMIOLOGICAL CHALLENGES OF THE DISEASES OF OLDER AGE

The two commonest causes of mental illness in old age are depression and dementia. This is particularly true in the community setting where the epidemiologist works.

The overall title of this course of lectures is, "Challenges in Aging". There are a number of challenges associated with investigations into these two diseases.

RECOGNIZING A CASE OF ILLNESS

First, there is the problem of recognizing a case of illness. Of course, such recognition is easy in hospital or primary care when patients present themselves or are brought by relatives who have already identified an illness. It is not so simple when the epidemiologist knocks on the door of someone's home. Where is the line to be drawn between normality and pathology? Community studies indicate that there is no clear point of demarcation. Within reasonable limits the point must be an arbitrary one. Doctors, who rarely see subjects in the early stages of an illness, may not be skilled at deciding where this point should be placed. Does accuracy matter? The answer is, we cannot be "accurate" where no external validating factor is

Challenges in Aging
ISBN 0-12-090163-3

available to guide us, we can only be consistent. It is important to be consistent if we are trying to compare the levels of illness between two localities or between two studies.

For some years medical doctors have assumed that their diagnosis of an illness was sufficient to identify "a case". Perhaps that was the situation when the results of a study were only of local interest to the planners of services or in everyday clinical practice. Now however, the scientific investigation of the cause of illness demands a more reliable method of case finding. Sadly, doctors like other human beings tend not to be consistent in their judgments. This has led to the introduction of standardized techniques for both examination and diagnosis.

Nor are the definitions of the illnesses themselves all that secure. With the elderly there is the added problem of normal aging. What is normal aging? We know comparatively little about it, so how do we recognize it from pathology? The safest policy is not to assume some symptoms are due to normal aging, but to record what is present and observe later what develops into recognizable pathology and what does not. Even when we are dealing with the more easily recognizable marked states there are problems, especially when making a diagnosis in the community where elaborate investigations are not immediately available. Dementia is one such example.

The two most important forms of dementia are senile and mutli-infarct dementia, but the distinction between them is probably not as clear cut as the names suggest. In our experience the stepwise course of multi-infarct dementia, so often referred to, is rare. Even the use of the term Alzheimer's disease, now so popular, brings its own dangers. It is easy to assume that because we give something a name we know what it is, yet Alzheimer's disease is a diagnosis made by exclusion when conditions of known cause are removed. In this paper we shall simply refer to senile dementia, not Alzheimer's disease. Nor is the pathology, so often referred to as the diagnostic gold standard, always quite what it seems. In most centres, standardized pathological methods for identifying illness are not used, so investigators must beware when drawing comparisons between studies.

The classical investigations of epidemiology have been those of prevalence (the amount of illness present at any one time) and incidence (the number of new cases occurring over a given time, usually 1 year). Henderson (1986) has reviewed the large number of prevalence studies and the few incidence studies of dementia undertaken over the last two decades. He draws attention to the disparity in the proportions of illness found by different investigations. Of course, if these differences were real they would be of considerable interest as they would prompt questions about the causation of dementia. However, he points out that such differences could easily be accounted for by different techniques of case finding, variable criteria of diagnosis, differences in sampling methods which select restricted age ranges or do not take into account the age structure of the base population. Some studies include only subjects living at home while others include those dwelling in institutions. Authors do not always describe how they distinguish mild from moderate from severe forms of illness.

If we are to make sensible comparisons between different studies then solutions must be found to these problems.

USING STANDARDIZED METHODS

In the 1960s a number of attempts were made to standardize the manner in which the psychiatric examination of the patient was carried out. Spitzer and Endicott (1969) in New York and Wing et al. (1974) in London developed their different methods for younger age groups.

In the 1970s we in the US/UK Diagnostic Cross-national Project were confronted by similar difficulties prior to starting our studies in older subjects. As a result we developed an interview method based partially on both the present state examination (Wing et al. 1974) and the mental status schedule (Spitzer and Endicott 1969), called the geriatric mental state (Copeland et al. 1976, Gurland et al. 1976). As neither of the preceding interviews dealt satisfactorily with organic symptoms, substantial modification, including the addition of many new items, was necessary. Since that time these standardized interviews have been further modified for community use, and have undergone updating in the light of the many studies which have used them. An informant interview, the history and aetiology schedule (HAS), has been added which seeks to collect information on the onset of the illness, a range of organic items thought to be associated with early dementia, family history and risk factors. Items for the Hachinski score (Hachinski et al. 1975) are asked and recorded in a standardized manner. The social status schedule allows the examination of expressed and judged need and the allocation to a social support network typology (Wenger 1984). The secondary dementia schedule records the findings of further investigations, if any, in order to allow the operation of the NINCDS-ADRDA criteria for dementia (McKhann et al. 1984). But while it is one thing to describe the illness and collect the symptoms in a standardized and reliable manner it is also necessary to determine "caseness", derive a differential diagnosis of the condition, and a level of syndrome severity in a way which will permit comparison with other studies.

WHAT IS A CASE OF ILLNESS? A CASE FOR WHAT?

The concept of caseness has caused much trouble to epidemiologists since the days of Snow's famous studies on the cause of cholera. Because this disease does not allow much difficulty in defining a case (cases of cholera are usually either obvious or dead) epidemiologists have tended to go on treating "cases" as things, to be identified rather like butterflies and then hunted. There have been endless discussions about how cases are to be defined for diseases with a variable clinical picture or where there is no clear distinction between illness and normality, as is the case with much mental illness (Copeland 1981). Such discussions miss the point, that cases like illnesses themselves are not things of independent existence, not like butterflies, but are concepts found only in the minds of the investigators. The tubercle bacillus as it goes about its ordinary life style, caseating a lung here and there, is not aware that it is supposed to be the agent of an illness. It is only the medical doctors, deeply prejudiced as they are against certain organisms in favour of human beings, who so choose to designate the things they dislike and feel the need to persecute them. Human concepts should only persist for as long as they are useful. Today's definitions of disease and today's cases may be completely superseded tomorrow. It follows then, that the concept of a case is to be defined by what it is useful for, and what is useful for one study may not be useful for another. Such an approach if it were followed fully might lead to an improvement in design, but would also lead to a lack of comparability between studies. It is necessary to find a compromise, to define the core of a case which will be useful for a range of studies and yet be capable of adaptation to other purposes.

Psychiatrists, like other doctors, seem able to recognize the point at which a collection of symptoms forms an identifiable group carrying with it implications for types of management and prognosis. It is probably also the point at which the clinician realizes intervention would be desirable in order to ameliorate unwanted symptoms. This point we designate in our studies as a "syndrome case". When a syndrome is chosen as the overall diagnosis, we define a "diagnostic case". When I use the term "case" in this paper I refer to "diagnostic cases".

Although levels of illness in a population assessed by two methods may be found to be similar, there is usually some disagreement on the actual individuals selected as cases. This often causes surprise and may be advanced as a demonstration of the failure of a particular method. In fact, given a condition whose symptoms are on a continuum with normality, it is not a surprising finding. I think the reason is something like this. There is a core of subjects on which everyone agrees they are cases of the condition. There is also a group in which all agree they are not cases. Then there is a small group which is very difficult to decide about. In fact, for one reason or another, it may be impossible to be sure, so that any decision for the group can be little more than a guess with more or less equal chances of choosing one way or the other. This means that selection is almost random with similar proportions designated cases and non-cases although they may not be the same persons.

This group of subjects with indeterminate states, who are to be found in all studies, makes it even more important in our view to have a consistent means of designating cases, with clear definitions which can be applied in the same way regardless of how difficult the clinical diagnosis may be.

STANDARDIZED DIAGNOSIS: THE AGECAT SYSTEM: SUPERSEDING THE TWO-STAGE DESIGN

How are we to translate these ideas into standardized methods of case finding and diagnosis? The answer came with computerized methods. Both Spitzer and Endicott (1969) with DIAGNO and Wing *et al.* (1974) with CATEGO had developed computer systems for diagnosis in younger age groups. For the elderly with their multiple pathology it was necessary to have a system which identified co-morbid states each with its own level of diagnostic confidence or severity. In addition, a large part of any diagnostic system in this age group was likely to concern the diagnosis of the different varieties of dementia, so a substantial history section depending on an informant interview was essential.

A computer system can be designed to replicate the clinician's diagnosis with surprising success. It has the great advantage of being consistent when faced with doubtful cases.

The automated geriatric examination computer-assisted taxonomy (AGECAT) was devised, not by an analysis of the data sets but on the basis of clinical principles. It is not an expert system but a branching decision tree program. Stage one of GMS-AGECAT varies according to the schedule from which the data have been derived. It condenses the various items of the interview into some 150 symptom components which are then further grouped during stage two, according to their importance for allotting subjects to levels of diagnostic confidence on each of eight diagnostic clusters. The diagnostic clusters are: organic, schizophrenia/paranoia, mania, depression, obsessional, hypochondriacal, phobic and anxious.

At this stage each subject is allotted to such a level on each of the clusters. Some clusters have five levels and some six. Psychiatrists tend to select levels three and above as representing syndrome case levels and one and two as subcase levels. In the rest of stage two the clusters are compared one with another according to the hierarchy of syndromes listed above, to provide a principal diagnosis, a subsidiary diagnosis if that is appropriate, the levels of confidence, profiles of symptom scores which are sensitive to change over time and various scores of organicity and depression.

A number of studies have now been completed which show good reliability between raters for individual items of the geriatric mental state (GMS) (Copeland *et al.* 1976, Henderson *et al.* 1983).

HAS-AGECAT draws on data from the HAS to allot subjects to the different subcategories of dementia and records a range of associated pathology.

The validity of the AGECAT diagnosis has now been assessed both by comparison with psychiatrist's diagnosis (agreement on organic states reaching kappa values 0.80–0.88, and for depression 0.76–0.80) and by outcome studies (see below) (Copeland *et al.* 1986, 1987a).

Computer algorithms for DSM 111R and draft ICD 10 have also been developed. Several versions of the interviews now exist in modular form for community use, designed to deal either with the whole range of mental illness or only with organic states (especially dementia) and depression. The most recent development has been the coming of lap top computers. The interviews are now available along with the AGECAT program adapted for computer application in the field. Interviewers take the computers into the subject's home and data are recorded directly on to disc. Older persons seem to enjoy the new technology. The saving in paper, storage, input time and expense is matched by the improved accuracy, the instant availability of results and the opportunity to keep a constant check on the quality of the data. We believe this is an important methodological advance.

ABANDONING THE TWO-STAGE SURVEY DESIGN

In practice, the computer method has also meant that the classical two-stage epidemiological study has been superseded. As the method has been developed for use by trained non-medical staff of the kind who would normally undertake screening, the AGECAT diagnosis can be applied to the full sample interviewed rather than a selected subsample, thus avoiding screening errors. We believe this is also methodologically important. A small subsample can always be followed up by a clinician as a check on the diagnosis although this is not strictly necessary.

RECENT EPIDEMIOLOGICAL STUDIES OF DEMENTIA AND DEPRESSION

In spite of the use of different assessment techniques, recent studies of the prevalence of dementia have tended to show roughly similar levels, with one or two surprising exceptions. In our London/New York community studies Gurland et al. 1983, Copeland et al. 1987b) we found twice the level of dementia in New York (8.4%) than in London (4.3%) when using the CARE interview which contained an early community version of the geriatric mental state. Kay et al. (1985) also using the GMS on a sample aged over 70, in Tasmania, found 7.7% dementia. Livingstone et al. (1990) using the short CARE in a London borough found 5.1% of dementia which rose to 7.3% when they added a sample of hospital-based subjects from the same area. Morgan et al. (1987) working in Nottingham and using the CAPE (Pattie and Gilleard 1976) found 4.3% dementia, rather higher than that found by Clarke et al. (1986) in Melton Mowbray using the same instrument. Shirayama et al. (1986) found 5.8% dementia in those aged 65 and over living in the Aichi Prefecture in Japan and Gavrilova et al. (1987) found 4.0% in a population aged over 60 in Moscow.

However, it is not possible to draw conclusions from the results of these studies because it is still not known whether the differences which are found are real, or artefacts of the different methods used.

Levels of depression in the various studies are even more disparate, with a wide range of levels which makes their interpretation almost impossible. Blazer et al. (1987) reported that 26% of their sample (part of the Epidemiological Catchment Area Study) had depressive symptoms, 19% mild dysphoria, 4% symptomatic depression, 2% dysthymia, 1.2% a mixed depression and anxiety syndrome, and 0.8% major depression. The last four figures, which probably represent varieties of depressive illness, total 8%. The authors suggest extending the DSM-111 diagnosis because of the apparent clinical relevance of cases lying outside this nomenclature. Kemp et al. (1987) reported that 26.7% of a sample in Los Angeles had depression or dysphoria and 0.7% major depression. Ben-Arie et al. (1987) however identified 13% of all kinds of depression in a small sample in Capetown. Murphy and Brown (1980) found 13.9% in a London-based sample and Kay et al. (1985) 13.9–14.8% in Hobart using the GMS. Again, it is difficult to compare these studies because of the different methods employed.

In our London/New York studies (Copeland et al. 1987b) we have shown that using the AGECAT diagnosis it is possible to make more reliable comparisons between different geographical areas. The levels of depression overall, including cases of bereavement, in London and New York were

19.5% and 16.2%, respectively (not a significant difference); this was against expectation.

THE GMS-AGECAT PACKAGE APPLIED IN RECENT STUDIES IN LIVERPOOL

A random sample of 1070 subjects aged 65 and over were interviewed using the GMS (community version) by trained non-medical raters whose reliability had been assessed against the project psychiatrists (Copeland *et al.* 1987a). At Year 3 the survivors were reinterviewed by psychiatrists in training using both the GMS and the HAS (the latter had not been available at Year 0) (Copeland *et al.* in press (a)). At Year 6 the survivors were interviewed again by trained non-medical interviewers. Diagnosis was made by the AGECAT computer method but psychiatrists' diagnoses were also available for Year 3.

The overall level of organic states at Year 0 was 5.1% (in the original paper this was cited as 5.2%; since then some amendments have been made to AGECAT which have produced small differences in percentages) (Copeland *et al.* 1987b). This finding is surprisingly close to the preliminary level in Zaragoza reported by Lobo *et al.* (1990) of 5.2% using the same methods.

What becomes of these organic cases of AGECAT levels of 3 and above? Table 1 shows that they have a poor prognosis, 83.3% are either dead or dementing in three years time. Even if we examine the subcases at Level 2, 41.7% of these are also dead or dementing by Year 3. This is a much higher figure than the 16%, 3-year death rate for the sample as a whole.

The organic diagnosis of AGECAT is associated with a poor prognosis and thus has some validation according to outcome.

BUT WHAT OF THE PREVALENCE LEVELS OF THE DIFFERENT DEMENTIAS?

Unfortunately the HAS was not available at the beginning of the study so it is not possible to say directly what proportion of organic disorders was dementing initially. However, as the HAS was given by the psychiatric interviewers at Year 3, it is now possible to make a reasonable estimate of the prevalence of dementia at Year 0 based on outcome. We obtain a figure of 4.3% when those organic cases which are known to have recovered are removed (they were almost certainly acute confusional states). Four point three per cent is also the figure for dementia in our London study after follow-up assessment.

Table 1

Dementia in Liverpool: random community sample including nursing and residential homes ($n = 1070$)

AGECAT diagnosis (01–5)			
Prevalence: clinically confirmed			
mild (01–2)			0.8%
estimate			
moderate to severe (03–5)			3.5%
total			4.3%
Year 3 ($n = 701$)			
Senile dementia Alzheimer type			3.3%
Vascular dementia			0.7%
Alcohol-related dementia			0.3%
Incidence			
All dementias			9.2/1000/year
Senile dementia Alzheimer type			6.3/1000/year
Vascular dementia			2.0/1000/year
Alcohol-related dementia			1.0/1000/year
Outcome of AGECAT organic disorders in 3 years			
Cases (03–5)	Demented	26.1%	83.3%
	Dead	57.1%	
	Other diagnosis	16.7%	
Subcases (01–2)	Demented	5.6%	41.7%
	Dead	36.1%	
	Other diagnosis	58.3%	

However, in addition to the information obtained at interview at Year 3 we also have information provided by the general practitioner on some of the subjects who died or refused interview because they felt too ill to be examined. This allows us to eliminate a further proportion known to have recovered, leaving 3.8%, identical to the proportion of dementia found in a rural population in the vicinity of Liverpool for whom it was possible to obtain similar information (Copeland et al., in press (b)).

If we assume that the subjects who refused interview or died before follow-up and for whom there is no information developed dementia in the same proportion as those for whom information is available, we arrive at an estimate based on clinical confirmed levels for mild dementia of 0.8%, for moderate to severe of 3.5%, making a total of 4.3% for dementias of all types of severity.

The proportion of dementia as a whole at Year 3 was very similar to that at Year 0. It may therefore be of interest to give the levels of the different types of dementia at Year 3 when the HAS was used as part of the assessment. Senile dementia of the Alzheimer type (SDAT) was 3.3%, vascular dementia (VSD) 0.7% (surprisingly low) and alcohol-related dementia (ARD) 0.3%. VSD was diagnosed using a standardized form of the Hachinski score (Hachinski *et al.* 1975). This score produced a good discrimination between those who scored hardly any points and those who scored relatively highly. The problem of overlapping scores on the Hachinski scale reported by others may be an artefact of hospital-based studies.

We may mention here the recent findings by Li *et al.* (1989) in Beijing and by Kua (in press) in Singapore. Both studies make an intuitive diagnosis based on the GMS used in Chinese populations. Surprisingly, both studies record levels of dementia of 1.8%, still rather below those reported from the West, even when adjustments are made for differences in the age structure of the base population. We hope to apply AGECAT to these data to see if the differences in diagnostic levels are confirmed.

It will be noted that recent figures for dementia tend to be below those often quoted. This has been an increasing tendency with the introduction of standardized techniques. It will also be noted how surprisingly similar the results from different studies are when such methods are used. This is a curious finding in a condition supposed to be causally associated with both genetic and environmental factors, and raises interesting questions.

WHAT ABOUT THE INCIDENCE OF THE DEMENTIAS?

The 3-year follow-up study allows us to assess the incidence of dementia and the 6-year study to check on the diagnosis of the 23 apparent incidence cases. In this way we were able to eliminate four cases who had recovered at Year 6. The overall figure for dementia is 9.2 per 1000 per year (6.3 for SDAT, 2.0 for VSD and 1.0 for ARD). As expected, the incidence of dementia as a whole rises with age: 65–74 years 3.8, 75–84 years 11.9 and 85+ years, 29.2 per 1000 per year. The overall figure is not dissimilar to that quoted by Mortimer *et al.* (1981). The figure for VSD is still low compared to other studies. We believe this is the first incidence study of dementia to follow up incidence cases for a further 3 years in order to confirm the diagnosis.

The levels of prevalence and incidence of dementia still indicate a major health problem in the future, extending well beyond the turn of the century for both the so-called developed and developing countries.

WHAT ABOUT THE LEVELS OF DEPRESSION?

Many studies in adults of all ages draw attention to the apparently large proportion of unresolved depression in the community. This study is no exception. The levels of depression in London and New York were almost identical, against expectation, as we were able to show that life in New York was more of a hardship for many elderly persons in terms of financial deprivation and contact with crime. The reason for this similarity may have something to do with the expectations of quality of life being lower in immigrant groups in New York (60% of the sample) who may accommodate to hardship more readily. However, the levels in both our northern rural community and Liverpool were almost half those in London, at 11.5%. We do not yet have a ready explanation for this difference either, except to suggest that family supports may be stronger in Liverpool and these may exercise a protective influence against adverse life events.

It is often stated that depression in the community is a comparatively trivial illness and one which if left alone will resolve without the need for intervention. We strongly contest this view. The case levels of AGECAT depression show a considerable increase of symptoms above those found in persons not designated as cases, furthermore these are levels of depression that psychiatrists judge should receive some type of intervention. They are not infrequently as severe as cases found in hospital settings.

However, we can now go one stage further and demonstrate the chronic nature of some of these illnesses. Table 2 shows the outcome of AGECAT depressive disorders 3 years after the initial interviews. A third or so of the cases are still cases 3 years later for both depressive neurosis and psychosis. Some 24% are dead. There is a significant tendency for the male depressives to die more frequently then the females, a finding already noted in some hospital-based follow-up studies (Murphy 1983). There has been a tendency for depression found in the community to be called the "common cold of general practice". It is not true. We also know from our studies that only 4.0% of the depressions receive any specific medication with antidepressants. This is not because they have never visited their doctors. Eighty per cent of the depressives in our sample were already on medication for a physical illness of some kind. Why then did they not receive treatment? MacDonald (1986) showed that in a London general practice depression tended to be over-diagnosed. What then is the explanation? It seems likely that doctors, like other health workers, tend to accept the popular stereotype of the elderly person as "understandably" miserable, and regard this as a social problem, or at best, as a consequence of normal aging. This is an error common to professionals who tend to see only the sick old. Those of us who have been privileged to meet a wide cross-section of older people in their own homes know that one of their endearing characteristics is the ability to remain cheerful in the face of considerable adversity. The need to change this stereotype remains one of the health problems for the future. It has implications for both undergraduate and postgraduate education as well as for the education of the general public.

Table 2
Depression in Liverpool: random community sample including nursing and
residential homes ($n = 1070$)

AGECAT diagnosis (D1–2, DN3–4, DP3–5)		
Prevalence	Subcase mild (D1–2)	10.7%	
	Depressive neurosis (DN3–4)	8.5%	11.5%
	Depressive psychosis (DP3–5)	3.0%	

Outcome of AGECAT depressive disorders in 3 years
Cases:

Depressive neurosis (DN3–4)	Still depressed	29.3%
	Subcase	12.2%
	Dead	23.2%
	Other	35.4%
Depressive psychosis (DP3–5)	Still depressed	36.0%
	Subcase	16.0%
	Dead	24.0%
	Other	24.0%
Subcases (D1–2)	Depressed case	17.9%
	Subcase	12.6%
	Dead	16.8%
	Other	52.6%

Proportion of community cases of depression receiving treatment with antidepressant medication	4.0%

WHAT NEXT?

A large number of studies are now beginning to examine these epidemiological issues in greater detail and to extend them to an assessment of risk factors for disease. The standardized methods which I have outlined are now in use in two multi-site studies organized by the World Health Organization and one by the Pan American Health Organization, in our own new longitudinal sample of 6000 subjects in Liverpool supported by the Medical Research Council of Great Britain and in their multi-site study in the UK, as part of the Eurodem studies and of studies in many other centres. For the first time it will be possible to make comparisons of prevalence and incidence between many centres and to analyse large data sets. The prospect is exciting.

Finally, one might ask, does the epidemiology of the mental diseases of older persons have a future in the age of molecular biology? Of course it does. Molecular biologists themselves rely on epidemiological methods for identifying samples of families for study, which have not been biased by hospital selection. Again, how else are early examples of illness to be recognized, so important for dementia where treatment would need to be applied at an early stage? There is the increasing realization that most treatment will be given outside hospital, where it will be important to recognize common diseases like depression, and medical audit will require to know why they are not being treated. The emphasis on community care has shifted the base of medicine away from the hospital, so it is the epidemiological method which will supply the data on which the principles of such care will be founded. Perhaps the most important general contribution of epidemiology to medicine has been in the move towards extending the medical model of illness from the simply biological, to encompass psychological and sociological elements, in keeping with the need to recognize the multi-causational nature of disease. The medical doctor can no longer expect to hold the dominant position in the care team, but by his or her training is nevertheless uniquely placed to co-ordinate the team and to understand the different contributions of its members as they seek to manage this extended concept of disease. The care of the elderly is one area where this approach will be most powerfully felt.

REFERENCES

Ben-Arie, O., Swartz, I. and Dickman, B. J. (1987). Depression in the elderly living in the community—its presentation and features. *British Journal of Psychiatry* **150**, 169–174.

Blazer, D., Hughes, D. C. and George, I. K. (1987). The epidemiology of depression in an elderly community population. *Gerontologist* **27**, 281–287.

Clarke, M., Lowry, R. and Clarke, S. (1986). Cognitive impairment in the elderly a community survey. *Age and Ageing* **15**, 2782–2784.

Copeland, J. R. M. (1981). What is a case, a case for what? *In* "What is a case, the problems of definition in psychiatric community surveys" (J. K. Wing, P. Bebbington and L. M. Robbins, eds). Grant McIntyre, London.

Copeland, J. R. M., Kelleher, M. J., Kellett, J. M., Gourlay, A. J., Gurland, B. J., Fleiss, J. L. and Sharpe, L. (1976). A semi-structured clinical interview for the assessment of diagnosis and mental state in the elderly. The Geriatric Mental State 1. Development and reliability. *Psychological Medicine* **6**, 439–449.

Copeland, J. R. M., Davidson, I. A., Dewey, M. E., Sharma, V. and McWilliam, C. Dementia, depression, pseudodementia and the neuroses: prevalence, incidence and three year outcome in the Liverpool community using the GMS-AGECAT package (In press).

Copeland, J. R. M., Dewey, M. E. and Griffiths-Jones, H. M. (1986). Computerised psychiatric diagnostic system and case nomenclature for elderly subjects: GMS and AGECAT. *Psychological Medicine* **16**, 89–99.

Copeland, J. R. M., Dewey, M. E., Wood, N., Searle, R., Davidson, I. A. and McWilliam, C. (1987a). The range of mental illness amongst the elderly in the community: prevalence in Liverpool. *British Journal of Psychiatry* **150**, 815–823.

Copeland, J. R. M., Gurland, B. J., Dewey, M. E., Kelleher, M. J., Smith, A.

M. R. and Davidson, I. A. (1987b). Is there more depression and neurosis in New York? A comparative study of the elderly in New York and London using the computer diagnosis AGECAT. *British Journal of Psychiatry* **151**, 466–473.

Copeland, J. R. M., Dewey, M. E., Henderson, A. S., Kay, D. W. K., Neal, C. D., Harrison, M., McWilliam, C., Forshaw, D. and Shiwach, R. (1988). The geriatric mental state used in the community replication studies of computerised diagnosis AGECAT. *Psychological Medicine* **18**, 219–223.

Copeland, J. R. M., Neal, C. D., Harrison, M. A. M., McWilliam, C. and Dewey, M. E. Is there more, or less dementia and other mental illness amongst rural communities of elderly people? A pilot study using the GMS-AGECAT package. (In press)

Gavrilova, S. I., Sudareva, L. O. and Kalyn, Y. B. (1987). Epidemiology of dementias in elderly and old age. *Zb Neuropatol Psikhiatr.* **87**, 1345–1351.

Gurland, B. J., Fleiss, J.L., Goldberg, K., Sharpe, L., Copeland, J. R. M., Kelleher, M. J. and Kellett, J. M. (1976). A semi-structured clinical interview for the assessment of diagnosis and mental state in the elderly. The Geriatric Mental State Schedule 2. A factor analysis. *Psychological Medicine* **6**, 451–459.

Gurland, B. J., Copeland, J. R. M., Kelleher, M. J., Kuriansky, J., Sharp, L. and Dean, L. (1983). "The mind and mood of ageing: the mental health problems of the community elderly in New York and London". Haworth Press, New York.

Hachinski, V. C., Illiff, L. D., Zihka, E., Du Boulay, G. H., McCallister, V. L., Marshall, J., Russell, R. W. R. and Symon, L. (1975). Cerebral flow in dementia. *Archives Neurology* **32**, 632–637.

Henderson, A. S. (1986). The epidemiology of Alzheimer's Disease. *British Medical Bulletin* **42.1**, 3–10.

Henderson, A. S., Duncan-Jones, P. and Finlay-Jones, R. A. (1983). The reliability of the Geriatric Mental State Examination. *Acta Psychiatrica Scandinavica* **87**, 1–9.

Kay, D. W. K., Henderson, A. S., Scott, R., Wilson, J., Rickwood, D. and Grayson, D. A. (1985). Dementia and depression among the elderly living in the Hobart community: the effect of the diagnostic criteria in the prevalence rates. *Psychological Medicine, 15, Psychiatry* **110**, 146–158.

Kemp, B. J., Staples, F. and Lopezaqueres, W. (1987). Epidemiology of depression and dysphoria in an elderly hispanic population—prevalence and correlates. *Journal of the American Geriatrics Society* **35**, 920–926.

Kua, E. H. The prevalence of dementia in elderly chinese. *British Journal of Psychiatry* (in press).

Li, G., Shen, Y. C., Chen, C. H., Zhao, Y. W., Li, S. R. and Lu, M. (1989). An epidemiological survey of age-related dementia in an urban area of Beijing. *Acta Psychiatrica Scandinavica* **79**, 557–563.

Livingston, G., Hawkins, A., Graham, N., Blizard, R. and Mann, A. H. (1990). The Gospel Oak Study: prevalence rates of dementia depression and activity limitation among elderly residents in inner London. *Psychological Medicine* 137–146.

Lobo, A., Saz, P., Dia, J.-L., Perez-Echeverria, M.A.J. and Ventura, T. (1990). The Liverpool–Zaragoza Study: background and preliminary data of case-finding method for a population study on dementias. *In* "Case finding for dementia in epidemiological studies" (M. E. Dewey, J. R. M. Copeland and A. Hofman, eds). Institute of Human Ageing, Liverpool.

MacDonald, A. J. (1986). Do general practitioners "miss" depression in elderly patients? *British Medical Journal* **292**, 1365–1368.

McKhann, G., Drachman, D., Folstein, M., Katzman, R., Price, D., and Stadlan, E. M. (1984). Clinical diagnosis of Alzheimer's disease: Report of the NINCDS-ADRDA Work Group under the auspices of Department of Health and Human Services Task Force on Alzheimer's Disease. *Neurology* **34**, 939–944.

Morgan, K., Dalloso, H. M., Arie, T., Bryne, E. J., Jones, R. and Waite, J. (1987). Mental health and psychological well-being among the old and very old living at home. *British Journal of Psychiatry* **150**, 808–814.

Mortimer, J. A., Schuman, L. M. and French, L. R. (1981). Epidemiology of dementing illness. *In* "The epidemiology of dementia" (J. A. Mortimer and L. M. Schuman, eds). Oxford University Press, New York.

Murphy, E. (1983). The prognosis of depression in old age. *British Journal of Psychiatry* **142**, 111–119.

Murphy, E. and Brown, G. W. (1980). Life events, psychiatric disturbance, and physical illness. *British Journal of Psychiatry* **136**, 326–328.

Pattie, A. H. and Gilleard, C. J. (1976). The Clifton Assessment Schedule: Further validation of a psychogeriatric assessment schedule. *British Journal of Psychiatry* **129**, 68–72.

Shirayama, H., Kasahara, Y., Kobayashi, H. *et al.* (1986). Prevalence of dementia in a Japanese elderly population. *Acta Psychiatrica Scandinavica* **74**, 144–151.

Spitzer, R. L. and Endicott, J. (1969). DIAGNO II: further developments in a computer program for psychiatric diagnosis. *American Journal of Psychiatry* **125**, 12–21.

Wenger G. C. (1984). "The supportive network: coping with old age". George Allen and Unwin, London.

Wing, J. K., Cooper, J. E. and Sartorius, N. (1974) "The description and classification of psychiatric symptoms". An Instruction Manual for the PSE and Catego System, Cambridge University Press, London.

Discussion

Bergener: What is your interpretation concerning the differences between the New York and the London dementia samples and what is the reason for the great variability in several investigations about the prevalence of depression, especially the percentage of subtypes and their classification?

Copeland: I don't think it's a sampling error, although you never can rule it out. Maybe there were more vascular disorders in New York. If that were true, we might expect a prevalence of stroke in New York. Prof. Gottfries would not agree because I think he believes that there might be two types of vascular disorder; but the prevalence of stroke was exactly the same in the two settings. We wondered about language and, tentatively, also about race, but we were able to exclude these possible factors as none of them seem to contribute. These studies should be repeated.

Williams: You may be aware of the recent report from Dennis Evans. The entire aged populated in East Boston was very carefully studied, and he finds approaching 12% of dementia in this population, almost 50% among those are aged 85 and older. Now, these figures are grossly larger than anyone else has yet reported and need to be further examined or confirmed. But we are seeing more data from various places that show great variability and challenges for methodology as well as for the studies. I do hope that your studies will collaborate with the World Health Organization special programme on research in aging which will be doing dementia comparative studies in seven different countries.

Reisberg: A number of studies have found that elderly depressed patients frequently develop dementia with 3-year follow-up, and I'm wondering if you found anything similar.

Copeland: We have looked into this problem and the short answer is "a few have". We looked also at the so-called pseudodementia to see if they had developed dementia and we found that about a third of them had. But, of course, the question was whether the diagnostic was correct at the beginning. We are looking very closely to the 6-year follow-up and shall be looking even closer in a much bigger sample we are getting now.

Twomey: Anecdotally one has the impression in treating depression in the elderly that there is a subgroup that seems to do very badly, no matter of what you do, maybe in 40, 50%. Is that anecdotal impression correct? Is there a method of identifying the potential responders from the potential non-responders to treatment and intervention on the basis that the one thing is to make a diagnosis but really the second thing is how you make the diagnosis useful to intervene therapeutically?

Copeland: This is a very important point. I ought to be careful when talking about treatment and the community because I think we do not yet know well whether the treatment would really improve these patients, although I think it's reasonable to assume that those who look as severe as those you see in hospital would probably improve. Maybe the others should be given the benefit of the doubt at this stage. I can't really comment on the system cases because we are in the middle of treatment studies. When we get very large samples, maybe we should pick up some of these cases and follow them through. It could be that the 6% of people who are depressed at all three occasions over 6 years will represent a resistant group.

Fejer (comment): We tried to make some epidemiological studies in Canada. In general we came to the conclusion that in both Canada and the USA the proportion of 65 year olds is about 10% now; in the coming 10 years it may increase to about 14%, and at the end of the baby boom in about 30 years it will increase tremendously. The study at Harvard University predicts an increase of even 50%. I am wondering about the proportion of 8–10% in those over 65.

Spiegel: What was actually your sample? Was it 65 and above, and was it only community people, so you did not include any institutionalized cases?

Copeland: That is an important point. They were 65 and above and were taken from GPs' lists. GPs continued to look after people in nursing homes and in residential accommodation, so we included all in the sample. We did not include, however, those who had gone to hospital and had been in hospital for at least 2 years. If they have been in hospital for less time than that we will have them on the lists. We did not include people who were in hospital chronically for more than 2 years.

Dekoninck: Could you differentiate already at the first interview between depressive people and SDAT?

Copeland: The AGECAT system gives you the differential diagnosis. When dementia and organic states overlap, the system itself will choose between the two. In a 3-year follow-up this choice is surprisingly acceptable: it differentiates between those who have become demented at year 3 and those who actually got better or remained depressed. One of the things we were surprised at was that this gnosis does not seem to be quite so difficult as one might have supposed.

Dekoninck: Do you have any autopsy controls for the difference between multi-infarct dementia, vascular dementia and SDAT?

Copeland: No, we don't have any autopsy at the moment.

Biological Markers in Dementia Disorders

C. G. Gottfries

*Department of Psychiatry and Neurochemistry, University
of Gotheburg, Sweden*

SUMMARY

As biopsies are not made in the diagnosis and in the study of the pathogenesis
of dementia disorders, the biological markers for the disorder must be
sought in the body fluids. The main source of information in the live
patient is the CSF. Neurotransmitters, their metabolites and enzyme
activities involved in the transmitter metabolism can be studied in CSF,
and data indicate that, to some extent, they reflect the metabolism in brain
tissue. It is obvious, however, that in spite of the reduced AChE activity
and lowered concentrations of HVA and 5-HIAA, there is such great
overlap when demented patients are compared with controls that these
markers have a limited diagnostic value. Further studies of CSF markers
are of interest, however. The concentrations of markers for amyloid and
paired helical filaments seem to be able to be recognized in CSF. A marker
for the ganglioside metabolism also seems possible to identify in CSF, and
this marker will then possibly constitute a marker for degeneration in grey
matter. Preliminary data also indicate that the identifying of sulphatides in
CSF may be a method for studying degenerative changes in white matter.

The finding of antibodies against neuron elements in CSF is also of
interest. The estimation of such antibodies will not only provide a diagnostic
method, but will also elucidate the pathogenesis of the dementia disorder.

Neuroendocrine disturbances in dementia disorders seem to be due to
overactivity of neuropeptides in the hypothalamus. This overactivity may
be due to reduced inhibitory tone from other centrally controlling systems
and possibly also to a disturbed feedback mechanism via the hippocampus,

Challenges in Aging
ISBN 0-12-090163-3

in which nucleus most of the cortisol receptors are found. The neuroendocrine disturbances found in AD/SDAT and VD are very similar to those found in melancholia.

Studies of blood, plasma and peripheral organs indicate that AD/SDAT is not only localized to the CNS. Muscarinic and nicotinic receptors are changed in the lymphocytes. Changes in the metabolism of fibroblastic cells also indicate general disturbances in patients with AD/SDAT.

In a subgroup of patients with SDAT, low vitamin B_{12} levels are found, which seem to be due to atrophic changes in the mucous membrane of the stomach. It is speculated whether age-caused changes in the mucous membrane of the stomach may cause deficiencies of essential nutrients causing the dysfunction of the brain.

INTRODUCTION

During the last two decades there has been very stimulating research concerning aging and dementia disorders. Neuropathological and neurochemical changes have been carefully described. As is obvious from this research, there are multiple changes in the neurotransmitter systems, in grey matter and in white matter. At the present level of knowledge, however, none of these changes can be singled out as of special significance for the aetiology of the dementia disorder. However, it is obvious that the changes are of importance in the pathophysiology of the disease, and sometimes the changes can also be directly correlated with the symptoms seen in the disorder.

Biopsies are not usually carried out in the diagnosis of dementia disorders. Biological markers for dementia must therefore be sought in the body fluids.

The aim of this paper is to discuss biological markers in the body fluids and their role for the diagnosis of the main groups of dementia disorders.

BIOLOGICAL MARKERS IN THE CEREBROSPINAL FLUID (CSF)

When interpreting the result of ante-mortem CSF studies it has been shown that several factors may influence the levels of neurotransmitters and their metabolites (Bertilsson and Åsberg 1984). Factors of importance are age, ventricular size, rostrocaudal gradients, height of the patient, circadian variation, physical activity, stress, neuroactive medication and intake of transmitter precursors. However, it has also been shown (Wester 1987) that there is a positive correlation of both monoamine and monoamine metabolite concentrations between ventricular cerebrospinal fluid and various brain regions. Thus, the biochemistry of CSF is useful to study as ante-mortem markers, at least of monoamine neurotransmission.

Cholinergic Markers in CSF

Acetylcholine (ACh) is found in the CSF in small amounts (3–479 pmol ml^{-1}) and cannot be used as a marker for the metabolism of acetylcholine in the brain (for a review see Giacobini and Elble 1990). Neither is cholineacetyl transferase (CAT) measurable in the CSF. The activity of acetylcholine esterase (AChE), however, and the levels of choline can be measured in the CSF. According to Elble et al. (1989) there is a significant reduction in AChE activity and an increase in choline (Ch) with advancing dementia of the Alzheimer type. The changes are not related to age. The authors interpreted the increase of Ch as being related to neuronal membrane breakdown and reduced uptake by cholinergic neurons. The reduction in CSF AChE activity is, of course, consistent with the depletion of cholinergic neurons in Alzheimer-type dementia (AD/SDAT).

As reported by McRae et al. (1990), the presence of cholinergic neuron-specific IgG in the CSF of a subgroup of AD/SDAT patients could be demonstrated by immunocytochemistry. In 1986, Singh and Fudenberg reported that the serum from AD patients contained antibodies which recognized neuronal elements in the rodent central nervous system, and Fillit et al. (1985) found that the serum from a subgroup of AD patients contained antibodies which recognize CAT molecules.

The importance of the cholinergic disturbed variables in CSF for the symptoms seen in the dementia syndrome was studied by Wester (1987). He could show that the degree of dementia, employing a global deterioration score and activity to daily life status, and also the Alzheimer-related symptoms dyspraxia and dysphasia were associated with low AChE in CSF. These findings, of course, support the already established finding of a cholinergic dysfunction as an important event in Alzheimer's disease.

CSF Markers for Monoamine Metabolism

Reduced concentrations of homovanillic acid (HVA) and 5-hydroxyindole-acetic acid (5-HIAA) in CSF of patients with SDAT have already been shown in 1969 by Gottfries et al. Although this finding has been debated, there are at present several reports confirming reduced HVA and 5-HIAA levels in CSF in patients with AD/SDAT (for a review see Hardy et al. 1985, Gottfries 1988). In a study by Parnetti et al. (1987), most of the monoamines and their metabolites were estimated in the CSF of patients with dementia disorders. This study showed that it was only the levels of

HVA and 5-HIAA in an AD/SDAT group that differed from a contrast group, while all other monoamines and monoamine metabolites did not decrease. In a study by Bråne et al. (1989), it was shown that the levels of HVA and 5-HIAA significantly correlated to rated symptoms of patients with AD/SDAT. Some differences were found between patients with early onset and late onset of the disease, but there is great overlap between these two groups and also between demented and non-demented patients, and therefore the acid monoamine metabolites have a limited value as diagnostic markers.

GANGLIOSIDES AND MYELIN COMPONENTS IN CSF

As previously shown (Gottfries et al. 1983), the concentration of gangliosides (GM1) is reduced in post-mortem human brain tissue (the caudate nucleus). It has also been shown that in white matter there are neuropathological as well as neurochemical changes, indicating degeneration of the myelin of white matter (Brun and Gustafson 1976, Gottfries et al. 1985, Svennerholm et al. 1988, Englund 1988). These findings have stimulated research concerning markers for ganglioside metabolism and white matter components in the CSF. As the gangliosides are accumulated in the synaptic cleft, they could be assumed to be markers for degeneration of grey matter, while sulphatides or cerebrosides could be assumed to be markers for white matter degeneration. Data at our institute indicate that there is significant increase of ganglioside GM1 in CSF from patients with early-onset AD (Blennow et al., 1990a). As this disorder is a parietotemporal lobe disorder, this finding is in agreement with the hypothesis that gangliosides are markers for grey matter degeneration. Preliminary data from our institute also show that sulphatides are significantly increased in patients with SDAT and non-MID vascular dementia. In these patients CT scan has shown white matter low attenuation. It thus could be speculated that concentration of sulphatides in CSF could be a sensitive marker for white matter degeneration.

Markers for Amyloid and Paired Helical Filaments in the CSF

The formation of paired helical filaments is an important factor in the pathophysiology of AD/SDAT. The neuropathology of AD/SDAT is also characterized by the presence of amyloid deposits. Using monoclonal antibodies to PHF, ubiquitin and synthetic beta-peptide by direct ELISA, Wisniewski et al. (1989) in preliminary studies found significantly increased concentrations of these markers for PHF and amyloid in CSF. These markers may be valuable tools in the diagnosis of AD/SDAT.

Neuropeptides in CSF

It is now well known that many peptides are found in the brain, and here the peptides are of importance for communication. Some peptides function as neurotransmitters or neuromodulators. They are released from nerve terminals and they influence other cells via receptors. Sometimes they coexist with other neurotransmitters, such as ACh and monoamines. Somatostatin-like immunoreactivity in brain tissue from patients with AD has shown a generalized decrease in many brain regions (for a review see Hardy *et al.* 1985). The levels of substance P are also reduced (Davies *et al.* 1982). As shown by Wallin et al. (1990a), increased concentrations of somatostatin, neurotensin, galanin and AVP can be found in the hypothalamus. In CSF from patients with AD/SDAT, the somatostatin concentration is decreased, as is the concentration of corticotropin-releasing factor (CRF).

BLOOD–BRAIN BARRIER DYSFUNCTION IN DEMENTIA DISORDERS

By measuring the serum and CSF albumin ratio, it is possible to get information about the function of the blood–brain barrier (BBB). In data from our institute, it was found that the BBB dysfunction, as marked by the albumin ratio, in patients with AD/SDAT could be related to vascular factors (Blennow *et al.*, 1990b). In a subgroup of AD/SDAT patients, mild vascular disturbances, such as heart dysrhythmia, hypertension and hypotensive crisis, were recorded, however, of such a low degree that they cannot be considered important for the dementia disorder. In the study it was shown that in patients with a diagnosis of AD/SDAT and with BBB dysfunction, the latter could be related to vascular factors.

In 53 patients with vascular dementia, who were compared with 50 healthy controls (Wallin *et al.* 1990b), the VD group showed higher mean albumin ratios compared with the controls. The albumin ratio was not significantly correlated to age. Neither was the albumin ratio related to individual clinical vascular factors. The altered BBB function was considered to be a consequence of a small vessel disorder which could also be of aetiological importance for the dementia disease.

NEUROENDOCRINE MARKERS IN DEMENTIA DISORDERS

In patients with dementia disorders, neurohormonal changes are described which are considered to be of pathophysiological importance for the

disorders. Post-mortem human brain investigations (Wallin *et al.* 1990a)
have shown that in the hypothalamus of patients with AD/SDAT and VD,
there are reduced concentrations of 5-HIAA and significant increased
concentrations of somatostatin, neurotensin, galanin and arginine vasopressin. According to Swaab *et al.* (1985) and Roozendaal *et al.* (1987),
increased activity of AVP is found in aged rats and in patients with SDAT.
As AVP is considered to be of importance for control of activity in the
hypothalamus–pituitary–adrenal (HPA) axis, these post-mortem findings
are of pathogenetic interest. The dexamethasone suppression test (DST) is
a laboratory test of patients with melancholia and increased activity in the
HPA axis is assumed in non-suppressors. In patients with AD/SDAT,
50–70% have pathological response to DST (Balldin *et al.* 1983, McAllister
and Hays 1987). The same pathological response to DST is found in VD.
Whether the increased activity in the HPA axis in these dementia disorders
is induced by an incapacity to turn off stress reactions or due to disturbed
higher controlling systems is at present not known.

As reported by Sapolsky and McEwen (1986), down-regulation of the
stress response is essential to health. The authors have studied neuronal
loss in the hippocampus of the aging rodent and the functional consequences
of such loss. They find that the capacity to terminate corticosterone secretion
when the stressor abates is impaired with age. Relative to young controls
corticosterone blood concentrations are elevated for prolonged periods
during habituation to mild stressors. In the old rat, there is decreased
sensitivity of the adrenal–cortical axis to feedback inhibition by circulating
corticoids. The hippocampus is the principal target tissue for glucocorticoids,
and a prolonged increase of the concentration of glucocorticoids causes
degeneration of the pyramidal cells of the hippocampus which are rich in
glucocorticoid receptors. In dementia disorders, the DST has shown that
several patients are non-suppressors, which means that these patients have
increased glucocorticoid levels in serum. This may be an exacerbating factor
in dementia after the disease has been established. Thus, prolonged stress
situations in the elderly may have aetiological/pathogenetic importance in
dementia.

As was shown in the post-mortem investigations by Wallin *et al.* (1990a),
there were reduced concentrations of 5-HIAA in the hypothalamus. It is
then of interest that treatment with citalopram, a 5-HT reuptake inhibitor,
seems to suppress the activity in the HPA axis (Balldin *et al.* 1988a, Nyth
and Gottfries 1990). Similar findings with tricyclic antidepressants have
been made in rats (Shimoda *et al.* 1988).

One method for assessing the postsynaptic NA sensitivity in patients is
to give the NA agonist clonidine, known to stimulate the secretion of the
growth hormone (GH) in animals as well as in humans (Lal *et al.* 1975,
Balldin *et al.* 1988b). The maximum GH response could be considered a

marker for the postsynaptic NA sensitivity. As shown by Balldin *et al.* (1988b), clonidine did not stimulate GH, yet depressed blood pressure levels were recorded in AD/SDAT patients. Thus, there seems to be a change in the alpha-2-receptor sensitivity involved in the GH secretion in AD/SDAT patients, while the receptors which regulate the blood pressure are unchanged. Another neuroendocrinal test is the challenge with a tyrotropin-releasing hormone (TRH). In normals, this test gives a TSH response. In a study performed at our institute, it was found that in 12 demented patients, four had a blunted response to TRH loading, as marked by a low TSH increase. However, in a study by Sobky (1986) a normal response to a TRH challenge was found in demented patients. A study by House and Jones (1990) investigated the serum prolactin changes in AD/SDAT patients loaded by meta-clopromide. The results showed data indicating increased sensitivity of the DA receptors in the tuberoinfundibular system, indicating a disturbance of the dopaminergic system in these patients.

Of interest are the considerable similarities between neuroendocrinal disturbances in melancholia and in AD/SDAT.

BIOLOGICAL MARKERS IN BLOOD

Several data indicate that AD/SDAT is a disorder not only restricted to the central nervous system (CNS).

As reported by Nordberg *et al.* (1990), there is a reduction of the nicotinic receptors in lymphocytes in AD/SDAT patients and in patients with Parkinson's disease, while this reduction is not found in vascular dementia. With regard to the muscarinic receptors, a decrease was found in the lymphocytes of the AD/SDAT patients, but not in other investigated groups.

Here it should also be stressed that studies from a number of laboratories indicate that the cellular processes involved in Alzheimer's disease occur in non-neural cells, including cultured skin fibroblasts. The Alzheimer amyloid precursor protein can also be studied in cultured skin fibroblasts. Among the abnormalities which can be linked by plausible hypotheses to the brain damage are those in cellular calcium homeostasis. Calcium has such a fundamental role in cell biology that abnormalities in its metabolism may be a critical "trigger point" in the cellular pathophysiology. According to Blass *et al.* (1990), the fibroblast culture system provides a convenient experimental tool for studying dynamic processes, such as cellular calcium homeostasis, which are less amenable to study in the autopsy brain.

Vitamin B_{12} (cobalamin) is one essential nutrient of well-known importance to the nervous system. Since the 1950s, vitamin B_{12} deficiency has been known to be more frequent in patients with senile dementia compared with normal elderly populations (Droller and Dossett 1959). At our institute, we have verified that low vitamin B_{12} levels in serum are frequent in patients with SDAT (Regland et al. 1988). Twenty-three per cent of the patients in the SDAT group and 50% (5 out of 10) of the patients in the group of confusional states were found to have serum vitamin B_{12} values below the lower reference limit (130 pmol l^{-1}). The SDAT group significantly differed from AD patients (6%) and VD patients (9%). According to Lindenbaum et al. (1988), patients with neuropsychiatric abnormalities due to vitamin B_{12} deficiency do not necessarily have anaemia or macrocytosis.

Monoamine oxidase (MAO) is found in the blood platelets, and, according to Adolfsson et al. (1980), there is an increase with age in the activity of this enzyme, and in patients with AD/SDAT there is a significant increase when compared with age-matched controls. Increased activity of MAO in platelets is also found in Huntington's chorea and Parkinson's disease (for a review see Regland 1990). Accordingly, MAO activity in platelets could be seen as a peripheral marker in primary degenerative dementia.

In 1980, Glover et al. reported on a highly significant increase in platelet MAO activity in patients with megaloblastic anaemia. Regland et al. (1988) found a significant relation between platelet MAO activity and vitamin B_{12} level in serum in patients with dementia disorders. In a follow-up study, Regland et al. (1990) verified that vitamin B_{12} directly influences platelet MAO activity. They also studied four patients with pernicious anaemia who all had extremely high activity of MAO in platelets. After adequate treatment with vitamin B_{12} platelet MAO activity was normalized. Also in SDAT patients, vitamin B_{12} substitution normalizes MAO activity in platelets.

Pepsinogen and gastrin are peptides secreted in the normal gastric mucosa. The blood levels of these peptides reflect the status of the gastric mucosa. From investigations of these peptides Regland (1990) concluded that low serum vitamin B_{12} levels in patients with dementia disorders are mostly due to atrophic gastritis with a subsequent malabsorption, probably caused by the combination of an insufficient production of intrinsic factors and acid in the gastric mucosa (for a review see Carmel et al. 1988).

Krasinski et al. (1986) calculated that 32% of all individuals above 60 years of age have mild to severe atrophic gastritis. Thus, it can be speculated that elderly people may have several deficiencies due to disturbed digestion and absorption of nutrients besides vitamin B_{12}. Vitamin B_6, calcium, zinc and selenium are trace elements that probably are dependent on acid secretion and pH in the gut. Amino acids, such as tryptophan and tyrosine, are dependent on an active transport over the mucous membrane, which may be disturbed in these patients.

It is obvious that vitamin B_{12} deficiency, and possibly other deficiencies, could be an important clue to our understanding of the pathogenesis of a subgroup of SDAT patients.

REFERENCES

Adolfsson, R., Gottfries, C. G., Oreland, L., Wiberg, Å. and Winblad, B. (1980). Increased activity of brain and platelet monoamine oxidase in dementia of Alzheimer type. *Life Sciences* **27**, 1029–1034.

Balldin, J., Gottfries, C. G., Karlsson, I., Lindstedt, G., Långström, G. and Wålinder, J. (1983). Dexamethasone suppression test and serum prolactin in dementia disorders. *British Journal of Psychiatry* **143**, 277–281.

Balldin, J., Gottfries, C. G., Karlsson, I., Lindstedt, G., Långström, G. and Svennerholm, L. (1988a), Relationship between DST and the serotonergic system. Results from treatments with two 5-HT reuptake blockers in dementia disorders. *International Journal of Geriatric Psychiatry* **3**, 17–26.

Balldin, J., Gottfries, C. G., Lindstedt, G., Långström, G. and Svennerholm, L. (1988b). The clonidine growth hormone test in patients with dementia disorders: relation to clinical status and cerebrospinal fluid metabolite levels. *International Journal of Geriatric Psychiatry* **3**, 115–123.

Bertilsson, L. and Åsberg, M. (1984). Amine metabolites in the cerebrospinal fluid as a measure of central neurotransmitter function: methodological aspects. *In* "Frontiers in biochemical and pharmacological research in depression" (E. Usdin *et al.*, eds) Advances in Biochemical Psychopharmacology vol. 39, pp. 27–34. Raven Press, New York.

Blass, J., Gibson, G. E., Black, R. S., Ko, L. and Sheu, K.-F. R. (1990). Cultured skin fibroblasts, "Alzheimer antigens", and cellular calcium homeostasis in Alzheimer's disease. *In* "Biological markers in dementia of Alzheimer type" (C. J. Fowler, L. A. Carlson, C. G. Gottfries and B. Winblad, eds) pp. 203–214. Smith-Gordon, Nishimura, Japan.

Blennow, K., Davidsson, P., Wallin, A., Fredman, P., Gottfries, C.G., Karlsson, I., Månsson, J.E. and Svennerholm, L. (1990a) Gangliosides in cerebrospinal fluid in subgroups of Alzheimer's disease. Submitted.

Blennow, K., Wallin, A., Fredman, P., Gottfries, C.G., Karlsson, I. and Svennerholm, L. (1990b) Blood–brain barrier disturbances in patients with Alzheimer's disease is related to vascular factors. *Acta Neurol. Scand.* **81**, 323–326.

Bråne, G., Gottfries, C. G., Blennow, K., Karlsson, I., Lekman, A., Parnetti, L., Svennerholm, L. and Wallin, A. (1989). Monoamine metabolites in cerebrospinal fluid and behavioral ratings in patients with early and late onset of Alzheimer's dementia. *Alzheimer's Disease Associated Disorders* **3**, 148–156.

Brun, A. and Gustafson, L. (1976). Distribution of cerebral degeneration in Alzheimer's disease. A clino-pathological study. *Archiv fuer Psychiatrie und Nervenkrankheiten* **223**, 15–33.

Carmel, R., Sinow, R. M., Siegel, M. E. and Samloff, I. M. (1988). Food cobalamin malabsorption occurs frequently in patients with unexplained low serum cobalamin levels. *Archives of Internal Medicine* **148**, 1715–1719.

Davies, P., Katz, D. A. and Crystal, H. A. (1982). Choline acetyl-transferase, somatostatin, and substance P in selected cases of Alzheimer's disease. *In*

"Alzheimer's disease: a report of progress in research" (S. Corkin, K. L. Davis, J. H. Growdon, E. Usdin and R. J. Wurtman, eds) Aging, vol. 19, pp. 9–14. Raven Press, New York.

Droller, H. and Dossett, J. A. (1959). Vitamin B-12 levels in senile dementia and confusional states. *Geriatrics* **14**, 367–373.

Elble, R., Giacobini, E. and Higgins, C. (1989). Choline levels are increased in cerebrospinal fluid of Alzheimer patients. *Neurobiology of Aging* **10**, 45–50.

Englund, E. (1988). "A white matter disease in dementia. A study with special reference to Alzheimer's disease". Academic dissertation, pp. 1–179. Wallin och Dalholm Boktryck, Lund, Sweden.

Fillit, H., Luine, B., Reisberg, B., Amador, R., McEwen, B. and Zabriskie, J. B. (1985). Studies of the specificity of antibrain antibodies in Alzheimer's disease. *In* "Senile dementia of the Alzheimer type" (J. T. Hutton and A. D. Kenny, eds) pp. 307–318. Allan R. Lince, New York.

Giacobini, E. and Elble R. (1990). Markers of cholinergic dysfunction in Alzheimer disease. *In* "Biological markers in dementia of Alzheimer type" (C. J. Fowler, L. A. Carlson, C. G. Gottfries and B. Winblad, eds) pp. 107–120. Smith-Gordon, Nishimura, Japan.

Glover, V., Sandler, M., Hughes, A. and Hoffbrand, A. B. (1980). Platelet monoamine oxidase activity in megaloblastic anaemia. *Journal of Clinical Pathology* **33**, 963–965.

Gottfries, C. G. (1988). Alzheimer's disease. A critical review. *Comprehensive Gerontology* **C2**, 47–62.

Gottfries, C. G., Gottfries, I. and Roos, B. E. (1969). The investigation of homovanillic acid in the human brain and its correlation to senile dementia. *British Journal of Psychiatry* **115**, 563–574.

Gottfries, C. G., Adolfsson, R., Aquilonius, S. M., Carlsson, A., Eckernäs, S. Å., Nordberg, A., Oreland, L., Svennerholm, L., Wiberg, Å. and Winblad, B. (1983). Biochemical changes in dementia disorders of Alzheimer type (AD/SDAT). *Neurobiology Aging* **4**, 261–271.

Gottfries, C. G., Karlsson, I. and Svennerholm, L. (1985). Senile dementia—a "white matter" disease? *In* "Normal aging. Alzheimer's disease and senile dementia. Aspects on etiology, pathogenesis, diagnosis and treatment". Proceedings of two symposia held at The CINP 14th Congress, 22–23 June 1984, Florence, Italy (C. G. Gottfries, ed.) pp. 111–118. L'Université de Bruxelles, Brussels.

Hardy, J., Adolfsson, R., Alafuzoff, I., Bucht, G., Marcusson, J., Nyberg, P., Perdahl, E., Wester, P. and Winblad, B. (1985). Review. Transmitter deficits in Alzheimer's disease. Critique: C. G. Gottfries, M. N. Rossor, C. M. Yates. *Neurochemistry International* **7**, 545–563.

House, A. and Jones, J. (1990). Increased response of serum prolactin to metoclopramide in senile dementia. *International Journal of Geriatric Psychiatry* (in press).

Krasinski, S. D., Russell, R. M., Samloff, M., Jacob, R. A., Dallal, G. E., McGandy, R.B. and Hartz, S.C. (1986). Fundic atrophic gastritis in an elderly population. *Journal of the American Geriatrics Society* **34**, 800–806.

Lal, S., Tolis, G., Martin, J. B., Brown, G. M. and Guyda, H. (1975). Effect of clonidine on growth hormone, prolactin, luteinizing hormone, follicle-stimulating hormone and thyroid stimulating hormone in the serum of normal men. *Journal of Clinical Endocrinology and Metabolism* **41**, 827–832.

Lindenbaum, J., Healton, E. B., Savage, D. G., Brust, J. M. C., Gartrett, T. J., Podell, E. R., Marcell, P. D., Stabler, S. P. and Allen, R. H. (1988). Neuropsychiatric disorders caused by cobalamin deficiency in the absence of anemia or macrocytosis. *New England Journal of Medicine* **318**, 1720–1728.

McAllister, T. W. and Hays, L. R. (1987). THR test, DST, and response to desipramine in primary degenerative dementia. *Biological Psychiatry* **22**, 189–193.

McRae, A., Blennow, K., Gottfries, C. G., Wallin, A. and Dahlström, A. (1990). Brain-specific antibodies in the CSF of patients with Alzheimer's disease and other types of dementias. In "Biological markers in dementia of Alzheimer type" (C. J. Fowler, L. A. Carlson, C. G. Gottfries and B. Winblad, eds) pp. 135–148. Smith-Gordon, Nishimura, Japan.

Nordberg, A., Adem, A., Bucht, G., Viitanen, M. and Winblad, B. (1990). Alterations in lymphocyte receptor densities in dementia of Alzheimer type: a possible diagnostic marker. *In* "Biological markers in dementia of Alzheimer type" (C. J. Fowler, L. A. Carlson, C. G. Gottfries and B. Winblad, eds) pp. 149–160. Smith-Gordon, Nishimura, Japan.

Nyth, A. L. and Gottfries, C. G. (1990). The clinical efficacy of citalopram in treatment of emotional distubances in dementia disorders. A Nordic multicentre study. *British Journal of Psychiatry* (in press).

Parnetti, L., Gottfries, J., Karlsson, I., Långström, G., Gottfries, C. G. and Svennerholm, L. (1987). Monoamines and their metabolites in cerebrospinal fluid of patients with senile dementia of Alzheimer type using high performance liquid chromatography–mass spectometry. *Acta Psychiatrica Scandinavica* **75**, 542–548.

Regland, B. (1990). Abnormalities of vitamin B-12 and other essential nutrients in dementia of Alzheimer type, and their clinical relevance. *In* "Biological markers in dementia of Alzheimer type" (C. J. Fowler, L. A. Carlson, C. G. Gottfries and B. Winblad, eds) pp. 215–219. Smith-Gordon, Nishimura, Japan.

Regland, B., Gottfries, C. G., Oreland, L. and Svennerholm, L. (1988). Low B-12 levels related to high activity of platelet MAO in patients with dementia disorders. A retrospective study. *Acta Psychiatrica Scandinavica* **78**, 451–457.

Regland, B., Gottfries, C. G. and Oreland, L. (1990). MAO activity in platelets is directly influenced by vitamin B-12 deficiency. Submitted.

Roozendaal, B., van Gool, W. A., Swaab, D. F., Hoogendijk, J. E. and Mirmiran, M. (1987). Changes in vasopressin cells of the rat suprachiasmatic nucleus with aging. *Brain Research* **409**, 259–264.

Sapolsky, R. M. and McEwen, B. S. (1986). Stress, glucocorticoids, and their role in degenerative changes in the aging hippocampus. *In* "Treatment development strategies for Alzheimer's disease" (T. Crook, R. Bartus, S. Ferris and S. Gershon, eds) pp. 151–171. Mark Powley, Connecticut.

Shimoda, K., Yamada, N., Ohi, K., Tsujimoto, T., Takahashi, K. and Takahashi, S. (1988). Chronic administration of tricyclic antidepressants suppresses hypothalamo-pituitary-adrenocortical activity in male rats. *Psychoendocrinology* **13**, 431–440.

Singh, V. K. and Fudenberg, H. H. (1986). *Immunology Letters* **12**, 277–280.

Sobky, A. (1986). Anterior pituitary response to tyrotropin-releasing hormone in senile dementia (Alzheimer type and elderly normals). *Acta Psychiatrica Scandinavica* **74**, 13–17.

Svennerholm, L., Gottfries, C. G. and Karlsson, I. (1988). Neurochemical changes in white matter of patients with Alzheimer's disease. *In* "A multidisciplinary approach to myelin disease" (G. Serlupi Crescenzi, ec.) pp. 319–328. Plenum, New York.

Swaab, D. F., Fliers, E. and Partiman, T. S. (1985). The suprachiasmatic nucleus of the human brain in the relation to sex, age and senile dementia. *Brain Research* **342**, 37–44.

Wallin, A., Carlsson, A., Ekman, R., Gottfries, C. G., Karlsson, I., Svennerholm, L. and Wilderlöv, E. (1990a). Hypothalamic monoamines and neuropeptides in dementia. *The European Journal of Neuropsycho-pharmacology* (in press).

Wallin, A., Blennow, K., Gottfries, C. G., Karlsson, I. and Svennerholm, L. (1990b). Blood–brain barrier function in vascular dementia. *Acta Neurologica Scandinavica* **81**, 318–322.

Wester, P. (1987). "Monoamine neurotransmitters in human brain and cerebrospinal fluid: methodological, functional and clinical studies". Medical dissertation New Series No. 185, ISSN 0346-6612, ISBN 91-7174-277-8, University of Umeå, Umeå, Sweden.

Wisniewski, H. M., Bancher, C., Barcikowska, M., Wen, G. Y. and Currie, J. (1989). Spectrum of morphological appearance of amyloid deposits in Alzheimer's disease. *Acta Neuropathologica* **78**, 337–347.

Discussion

Roth: It has been suggested that many of the neurochemical deficits associated with Alzheimer's disease may be secondary to neuronal loss. You have shown some muscarinic receptor changes in peripheral lymphocytes that are similar to those seen in some brain regions. I am wondering if there are any data to suggest that the number of receptors per surviving neuron are actually lower in the Alzheimer patients.

Gottfries: It's a very interesting question but I can't answer it and I wonder if there are any investigations that could answer it. But the reduction in the lymphocytes indicate that it would perhaps not only be a question of a loss of neurons.

Scuderi: It has been shown that the hippocampus has an inhibitory effect on hypothalamus pituitary adrenal axis secretion. I want to know, can't we think that hyperactivation of this axis in Alzheimer's dementia can be secondary to hippocampal damage?

Gottfries: Could damage to the hippocampus explain the neuroendocrine disturbances? It is, of course, an interesting question. A group from the United States suggests this. They say that in the hippocampus the receptors for the cortisol may be burned out by high levels; therefore the feedback loop initiated from the high cortisol levels in the serum will not function any longer, and therefore the hypothalamus is continuously active. So I think this damage to the hippocampus is a very interesting explanation.

Dolecek: I would like to suggest something else because the high levels of cortisol and of ACTH in old persons with and without dementia are well known, but if you use tests that show the integrity of the hypothalamo-pituitary-adrenal system, cortisol and ACTH are completely blocked, so probably the error is somewhere in the hypothalamus. Prolactin levels, especially in old males, are increasing significantly with increasing age and they have very significantly increased levels of oestrogens. And then another error of metabolism is in measuring very high levels of the cyclic adenosine monophosphate in practically all persons of old age, males and females. It means that the cells are under constant alarm or stress. So perhaps it works together with your ideology.

Gottfries: It's very interesting what you say. What you mean is that the disturbance is in the hypothalamus itself and it is not a question of a disturbed feedback loop only. I mean that one explanation does not exclude another one. I think they can be combined. If you ask the neuropathologists they say that you do not have very many senile plaques and fibrillary tangles in the hypothalamus. We have studied membrane components in the hypothalamus and they are quite normal. From a neuropathological point of view it seems that the hypothalamus is rather intact. However, what we know is that the hypothalamus is controlled by e.g. the cholinergic system, the dopaminergic system, the serotonin system, and a disturbance to these systems could explain that the inhibitory tone over the hypothalamus is lost.

Reisberg: I also think your findings are very comprehensive and very important. I wonder if you have observed any relationship between the neurochemical changes that you have been reporting, either the dopaminergic changes or the serotoninergic changes, or both, and the behaviour of disturbances which are so commonly seen in senile dementia?

Gottfries: Yes, there are several reports about that and we have also some reports. There is a group in Umeå in Sweden who studied the correlation between the reduced activity in the cholinergic system and behavioural changes and they have found correlations there. I can't explain to you in detail what they are. We have also investigated the cerebrospinal fluid content of homovanillic acid and 5-hydroxyindoleacetic acid and related that not only to cognitive but also to emotional disturbances, and we have correlations there. We are especially interested in the ratio between homovanillic acid and 5-hydroxyindoleacetic acid because we think these two systems balance each other in the brain. Therefore we have investigated the ratio between these and there you also find correlations. But they are rather weak correlations and, of course, you have correlations between homovanillic acid and motor functioning disturbances which you can expect.

Kanowksi: Isn't it a little bit premature or misleading to speak of biological markers of Alzheimer's disease because if there should be anything specific to AD the specificity should be expressed in terms of specificity and sensitivity compared to other types of dementia and normal controls. That is a methodological evaluation of specificity as psychologists use it if they are developing screening and discriminating tests between diseases and syndromes. I missed the evaluation of specificity and sensitivity of these biological measurements and I think before you have demonstrated specificity and sensitivity in statistical terms you can't speak of biological markers of AD.

Gottfries: I am glad that you brought up this issue because I agree with you, although I have said several times "markers for AD". But what I stressed was that these groups that we can delimit by these markers should be matched against the diagnosis. In fact I would like to study the specificity of these markers. But who should determine, who can take the patent of making diagnosis? Are neuropathologists the ones who should do that? Or clinicians? Or is it a neurochemist? What is most important in the brain: senile plaques? Cholinergic disturbances? Or a parietotemporal lesion diagnosed in the symptomatology? I don't think you can say that one of these makes the diagnosis. You have to check these, compare them and see if there are agreements. But I agree with you, it is premature to say that these are markers for a homogenous disease which may earn the name of AD.

M. Bergener

The contribution given by James Birren discussed findings that a wide range of behaviour slows down with age and that this slowing down is associated with other physiological and psychological changes. Results obtained in the laboratories of Dr. Birren's group suggest that older adults tend to be slow across all stages of information processing, especially if the stimuli are degraded and when the tasks imposed on the problems are unfamiliar for them. Cognitive capacities also seem to be limited with age. Current research shows that physical fitness and physical exercise serve in maintaining an appropriate level of performance and that cardiovascular disease for example on the other hand can be the course of a disproportionate slowness.

The social system in the West African tribal society relying heavily on the old persons in it was described in the next communication given by Leopold Rosenmayr from Vienna. The findings of a 5-year field study were discussed also in the context of a changing environment and society. The way in which the breaks and the solidarity of the traditional community occur was described as well as ways to adapt and to change the health attitude.

The third presentation marked the turning point from the discussion of many physiological topics to pathological conditions. Jerome Yesavage has given a description of a concept of age-associated memory impairment, sometimes also alluded to as benign senile forgetfulness. The description of training techniques, including a pretraining for the elderly to overcome the difficulties associated with degrading memory together with a presentation of the results, formed the core of his presentation.

Professor Copeland described epidemiological issues. First of all, the until now not fully solved problem of case definition in psychogeriatric research. A new concept of the term "case" was submitted for discussion, and the reliability of the diagnostic procedure which is the prerequisite for case finding and definition was addressed. The geriatric mental stage, AGECAT package, was presented together with reliability studies and preliminary results from studies in the UK and abroad.

The last contribution by Prof. Gottfries handled the biological and biochemical changes connected with dementing diseases. The intrathecal production of immunoglobulins found in dementia of Alzheimer's type and also in vascular dementias was described together with the already known changes in the metabolism of central monoamine neurotransmitters. Preliminary results have shown that concentration of the ganglioside GM1 was reduced in patients suffering from AD; the presence of antibodies against cholinergic neurone epitopes as well as a reduced glucose metabolism have been shown. These and other findings lend support to the hypothesis that the disturbances in AD are more general than suspected before.

Altogether, the contributions of the first block of the Sandoz Lectures showed that many results have now been collected, but that much research has yet to be done towards the understanding and correcting of pathological situations in elderly people.

Part II

Regulatory Factors of Cell Function during Aging

Neurohumoral Mechanisms of Aging

Vladimir V. Frolkis

Institute of Gerontology AMS USSR, Kiev, USSR

INTRODUCTION

One of the main tasks of gerontology is the establishment of general rules, the mechanisms of aging and development of age pathology. We have formulated the adaptation–regulatory theory, according to which age development is the result of the interaction of two processes: aging—the process of destruction, and vitauct (from Latin "vita"—life, and "auctum"—increase)—the process that stabilizes the viability, thus increasing the lifespan (Frolkis 1963, 1966, 1970, 1975, 1982). The mechanisms of aging are connected with the shifts in two systems of self-regulation: genoregulatory and neurohumoral. If we consider aging on the grounds of the system of self-regulation, then it is necessary, firstly, to make a general evaluation of the changes in its reliability and, secondly, to characterize the nature of shifts that take place in various chains of the self-regulating system. At aging there occur irregular changes in different chains of the system of neurohumoral regulation. When in some chains the symptoms of aging develop and in others, the processes of vitauct, then their interaction contributes to the prolonged preservation of homeostasis of an organism. All this takes place under the conditions of decreasing reliability of the regulatory system, of limitation of adaptation-regulatory mechanisms, which provoke the development of age pathology.

An important factor of changes in neurohumoral regulation is a genoregulatory shift in neurons, in the cells of endocrine glands. Once developed, these changes influence the regulation of the genome of other target cells. Genoregulatory changes taking place in the process of aging give rise to the changes in the correlation of syntheses of various proteins,

Challenges in Aging
ISBN 0-12-090163-3

to the possible development of earlier not synthesized proteins. These genoregulatory mechanisms of aging form the basis for the development of age pathology.

This paper presents data on the role of age-dependent changes of neurohumoral regulation in the formation of syndromes of aging; on the development of stress-age syndrome at aging; on the role of the limbic system and of the hypothalamus in age-dependent changes in neurohumoral regulation; and on the neurohumoral regulation of protein biosynthesis.

SYNDROMES OF AGING

The tendency to investigate the common mechanisms of aging often results in the situation when investigators focus their attention on general or universal aspects only and sometimes reject—be it consciously or instinctively—the individual or particular points of this subject, the species-specific and populational distinctions of aging.

In 1969/70 we proposed the concept of the existence of various syndromes of man's aging, of individual and populational specifics of this process (Frolkis 1970). The existence of common fundamental mechanisms of aging suggests that there are various qualitative and quantitative variants of development of this process, "the style of aging". All known aging syndromes can be classified by: (1) the rate of their development; (2) the sequence of aging of various systems in an organism. The rate of aging of individuals, of various human populations is different, which is confirmed by the different biological age of individuals without any expressed pathology (Ludwig and Smoke 1980, Ingram 1983, Voitenko and Tokar 1983).

The investigations run at the USSR AMS Institute of Gerontology have shown that the type of aging syndrome is defined mostly by the rate and nature of age changes in neurohumoral regulation. The syndrome of accelerated and premature aging is characterized by such a type of age changes, which leaves behind the aging of most individuals in the population. This syndrome has a number of donosologic symptoms related mostly to neurohumoral shifts—undue tiredness; lowered mental and physical efficiency; worsened memory; emotional instability; decreased reproductivity; retarded recovery of haemodynamic and respiratory shifts; increased sensitivity of heart and vessels to some humoral factors; delayed glycaemia curves; lowered levels of insulin, thyroxin, aldosterone and testosterone; changed correlation of various hormone concentrations etc. The comparison of changes in the concentration of ACTH and corticosterone; TSH and T_3, T_4; FSH, LH and testosterone, oestradiol provides evidence of the irregular nature of changes in excitability and in functional activity of various hypothalamic structures. All this complex of shifts determines the decrease in the adaptation abilities of an organism at aging and provokes the development of the age pathology.

Retarded aging is characterized by slower—in comparison to the whole population—rate of changes. The extreme display of this type of aging is the phenomenon of longevity (Dalakishvili 1987, Mankovsky *et al.* 1987). The extended clinicophysiologic investigations by the USSR AMS Institute of Gerontology have shown that the state of some functions of the nerve and endocrine systems (behavioural reactions, motor activity, bioelectrical activity of brain, speed of conduction through the peripheral nerves, concentration of some hormones in blood, etc.), certain characteristics of the cardiovascular system functioning and of the lipid metabolism in the long-livers correspond to those of the common group of people at the age of 65–75 years. The existence of this aging syndrome is also confirmed by the fact that the relatives of the long-livers have certain differences in the rate of age changes in comparison to the rest of the population (Glueck *et al.* 1976, Zdichynec 1978, Ho-Zhi-Chien 1982). Jamill and Milord (1981) and Nguen *et al.* (1981) have determined that the long-livers show relative stability in the values of humoral and cellular immunity. Mankovsky *et al.* (1987) have shown that relatives of the long-livers from Abkhazia are characterized by a higher mean frequency of α-rhythm in electroencephalogram, as well as by preservation of parameters of the induced potentials and by certain speed of psychomotor reactions. The optimal levels of androgens and oestrogens in the blood are maintained in this group for a longer time.

Dr. Kuznetsova of our group has shown that families with cerebral vascular pathology have an aging syndrome characterized by earlier age changes in electrogenesis of the brain (retardation of the frequency spectrum, decrease in reactivity and increase in the power of slow rhythms). They take place 10–15 years earlier than in the relatives of long-livers.

Figure 1 presents data on the changes in certain functions of the nervous system in the group of relatives of long-livers and in the group of practically healthy relatives of people suffering from cerebral ischaemia. The difference shown suggests that the aging syndromes differ in rate and expressiveness.

The clinicophysiologic study of aging people allows to single out some other syndromes of aging, which are characterized by more pronounced age-dependent shifts in some physiologic systems—nervous, endocrine, cardiovascular, locomotor and others. The distinction of aging syndrome by the rate of age-dependent shifts and by their expressiveness in the system is important, because it allows one to predict the possible development of one or another type of pathology.

The described aging syndromes can be observed not only in certain persons, but also in the population as a whole. The type of changes in neurohumoral regulation and in the state of the cardiovascular system determines the distribution of one or another syndrome in the population.

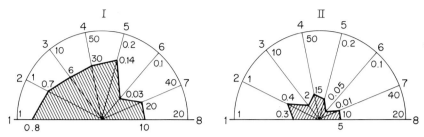

Fig. 1. "The profile of aging" of the central nervous system in the relatives of insult-sicks (I) and of long-livers (II): (1) the decrease in the frequency of θ-rhythm (Hz); (2) the decrease in the frequency of α-rhythm (Hz); (3) The decrease in the power of α-rhythm (%); (4) the decrease in reactivity (%); (5) the increase in the latent period (s); (6) the rise of tonus of the cerebral vessels (the time of the ascending part of the REG wave, s); (7) the rise of arterial pressure (mm Hg); (8) the decrease in the intensity of rRNA biosynthesis (%).

Figure 2 presents "the portraits of aging" of the population in three regions of the USSR—Ukraine, Abkhazia and Azerbaijan. These "portraits" are based on data of epidemiologic investigations run in the above regions by the workers of the USSR AMS Institute of Gerontology in Kiev. The population of the Ukrainian region is characterized by mixed types of aging syndromes, displayed by changes in both the central nervous and cardiovascular systems. The populations with high levels of longevity (Abkhazia, Azerbaijan) have peculiar regional aging syndromes. The Abkhazian aging syndrome is expressed by changes mainly in the cardiovascular system, while the Azerbaijanian "portrait of aging" is presented by changes in the central nervous system—neurogenous syndrome.

The shifts in the neurohumoral regulation system at different syndromes of aging correlate with each other differently. The natives of Azerbaijan are mainly Azerbaijanians, but there are many Russians as well. The life span of these two populations and their aging syndromes are not identical. The shifts in neurohumoral regulation are correlated differently in these two populations. The neurohumoral mechanisms of aging have their specific features. These shifts also define the type of age pathology and the life span of two populations living in the same region.

Well known are the species-specific distinctions of the life span. There are numorous data on the correlation between the species-specific characteristics of structure, metabolism and functions of an organism and the life span, which allow understanding of the basis of these distinctions (Sacher 1978, Economos 1980, Cutler 1984). Such an approach to the study of species-specific life span might be defined as phylogenetic. There is another approach which, however, is not used widely enough and which can be defined as phylo-ontogenetic. This is the study of peculiarities of aging of animals with different species-specific life span. This approach formed the basis for the complex study carried out by the investigators of the USSR AMS Institute of Gerontology in Kiev (Frolkis 1988). Age-dependent changes have been studied in more than 70 metabolic, structural and functional characteristics of mammals with different species-specific life span: mice, rats, rabbits, guinea-pigs, dogs and men. Age-dependent changes have been compared in adult and old individuals, taken at the age of 75–85% of their maximal species-specific life span.

The age dynamics of all characteristics might be classified into four groups. The first group contains the characteristics which do not change significantly with age. In the second group the longer the animal's life span or the longer he lives, the greater the characteristics change. We defined this group as chronobiologic. The third group includes the characteristics that change at aging identically for the animals with different species-specific life span. We defined it as ontobiologic. And the fourth group, the species-specific changes, contains characteristics expressed differently in animals with different species-specific life span. Figure 3 schematically presents all these changes. Certainly, the boundaries between them are arbitrary, since there could well be transition forms as well. What is important is that most age changes in neurohumoral regulation belong, according to our data, to the group of ontobiologic characteristics, that is, to the characteristics that correlate with the species-specific life span and that change with old age almost identically for the animals of different strains. This suggests that shifts in neurohumoral regulation take part in the formation of factors which influence the species-specific life span. Thus, for instance, the attenuation of the nerve control specifically, of vagus nerve influence on the heart—is an important mechanism of aging. It changes at aging identically for animals of different strains. The amount of testosterone in rats, rabbits, guinea-pigs and men decreases to approximately the same degree. The activity of adenylate cyclase, the contents of cAMP and cGMP in the heart and liver of animals of different strains do not change by old age; the activation of adenylate cyclase by adrenaline increases to the same extent.

So, age-dependent changes in neuhumoral regulation are in many respects decisive for the type of the aging syndrome, for the populational and species-specific characteristics of aging.

STRESS AND AGING

Numerous data on age changes in neurohumoral regulation and the general mechanisms of its shifts have been collected. The variety of changes developing in neurohumoral regulation at aging is so complex that it cannot be covered by a single notion. According to our investigations, as well as

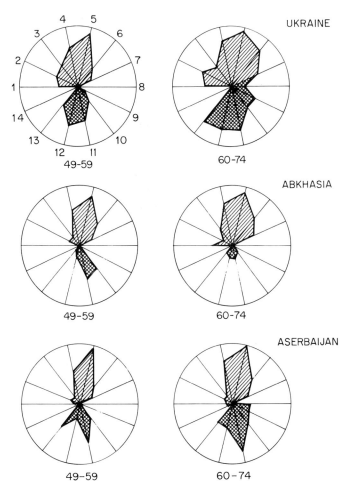

Fig. 2. Clinicophysiologic profile of age changes in men of different ages in three different regions of the USSR. Characteristics, describing the changes in the functional state of cardiovascular (1–7) and central nervous (8–14) systems: (1) the rate of arterial hypertension (%); (2) the rate of heart ischaemia (%); (3) the decrease of the ECG T-wave (mm); (4) the rise of tonus of the cerebral vessels (s); (5) the rise of arterial pressure (mm Hg); (6) the decrease of the vessels' elasticity (%); (7) the rate of heart pain (%); (8) the rate of extrapyramidal deficiency (%); (9) the rate of insult (%); (10) the decrease of ECG α-rhythm (Hz); (11) the growth of ECG latent period (s); (12) the frequency of ECG θ-rhythm (%); (13) the rate of headaches (%); (14) the rate of gerontal dementia (%).

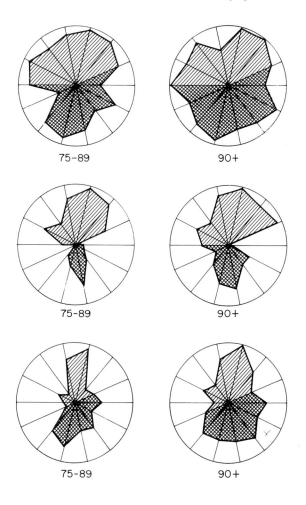

Fig. 2. Continued

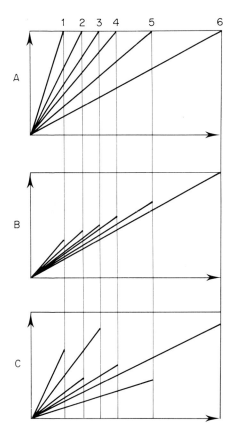

Fig. 3. Diagram of the species-specific distinctions of changes in certain character-istics in the process of aging: (A) ontobiological; (B) chronobiological; (C) species-specific; (1) mice; (2) rats; (3) guinea-pigs; (4) rabbits; (5) dogs; (6) men. Plotted on abscissa: the period of animal's life. Plotted on ordinate: the expressiveness of shifts in old age.

to the works of various other authors, there are many identical features in aging and stress effects. Their similarity gave origin to the concept of the "stress–age syndrome".

Selye (1976) defined stress as a common adaptation syndrome. The reaction of an organism to any strong exogenous or endogenous influence of the medium, to any disturbances in homeostasis is provided by, first, the specific response to a stimulator and, second, by unspecific response realized through sympathoadrenal, hypothalamo-hypophyseal, endocrine, and other tracts. The common adaptation syndrome observed in stress has, according to Selye, three stages: the stage of anxiety, when all the initial forces of an organism are mobilized; the stage of resistance; and the stage of exhaustion with increasing limitation of adaptation abilities of an organism. Selye distinguished the eustress—the syndrome which assists the preservation of health—and the distress—the syndrome, which is pathologic and leads to the development of diseases of adaptation. Selye states that the external development of the common adaptation syndrome with its three stages reminds us of the process of life with all its periods. In this sense the process of life can be compared to the adaptation syndrome extended in time.

What is the evidence for our concept of the "stress–age syndrome" developing at aging? First of all, the similarity of most symptoms of stress and aging. Apart from the known classical triad of Selye (activation of adrenal glands, atrophy of lymphatic system, haemorrhages in stomach and intestine), there exist numerous symptoms—neurohumoral, tissue, cellular, molecular—that characterize stress. Thus, typical stress reactions show increase in the amount of adrenaline, ACTH and corticosterone and vasopressin; decrease in the amount of insulin, TTH and T_3, T_4, aldosterone and androgens. In other words, activation of sympathoadrenal, vasopressin and hypothalamo-hypophyseal-glucocorticoid systems and decrease in activity of some other systems of an organism occurs. Figure 4 presents data of our group on age changes in the content of hormones in the blood of old and adult rats and in people of different age. Noteworthy is the pronounced activation of the stress hormonal systems: adrenaline, vasopressin, ACTH glucocorticoids; and the decrease in activity of some other hormonal mechanisms. At stress great significance is attached to decrease in thyroid activity and in the synthesis of sexual steroids. Many scientists note the activation of the ACTH-cortisol system, the increase in the blood content of vasopressin and adrenaline and the decrease in the blood content of thyroxin and testosterone (Malamed and Carsia 1983, Sonntag et al. 1987). According to the data of our group, the level of basal secretion of corticosterone by the adrenal glands, studied on old rats in vitro, increases. The rise in the content of vasopressin in the blood is accompanied by the drop of its content in the thalamus, hypothalamus, hippocampus, substantia nigra, and by its stable level in the hypophysis. Certain interest is presented by the data of Sato et al. (1987), who have shown that the increase in the content of catecholamines in the blood of old rats is accompanied by activation of electrical activity in the sympathetic nerve innervating the adrenal glands. According to many investigators, the content of insulin in the blood decreases at aging. Our group has shown that in old rats and elderly people with reduced tolerance to glucose, the content of insulin does not decrease, but increases. At the same time, the insulin activity, its physiologic effectiveness, become lower. In addition, the total content of insulin in the blood (serum and erythrocytes) decreases with age. Insulin plays an important role in the realization of stress, since

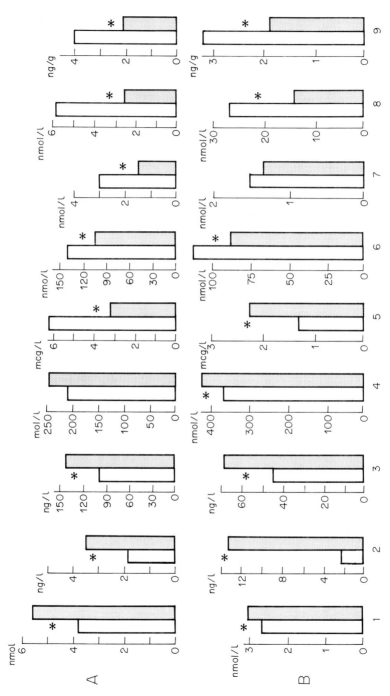

Fig. 4. Age-dependent changes in the concentration of various hormones in the blood of rats (A) and men (B): (1) adrenaline; (2) vasopressin; (3) corticotropin; (4) corticosterone, cortisol; (5) thyrotropin; (6) thyroxin; (7) triidothyronine; (8) testosterone; (9) insulin activity. Light columns: rats aged 8–10 months; men aged 25–30 years. Shaded columns: rats aged 26–28 months; men aged 60–75 years.

numerous counter-effects to a regulatory effect of catecholamines and glucocorticoids are realized through it.

As is known, the mechanism of stress development is greatly influenced by the hypothalamus, which via the corresponding liberins or direct nervous tracts, determines most stress shifts in an organism.

As can be seen from Fig. 5, the excitability of certain nuclei of hypothalamus changes at aging not only unevenly but also different directedly. Thus, the excitability of the anterohypothalamic, medial mamillary nucleus and of the rostral zone of the supraoptical nucleus increases; that of the caudal zone of the supraoptical nucleus and of the medial preoptical field does not change; and that of the lateral hypothalamic field decreases. Uneven changes in the excitability of the structures of the hypothalamus create the different-directed nature of neurohormonal shifts that develop at aging. The similar uneven changes in the excitability of hypothalamic structures take place at stress as well. The observed shifts in neurohumoral regulation at aging are influenced not only by the changes in the hypothalamus, but also in some structures of the limbic system.

Alongside the mechanisms leading to the development of stress, there exists an antistress system. This includes the changes in the central regulatory mechanisms, which inhibit the development of releasing factors, the activation of sympathoadrenal, vasopressin, and glucocorticoid systems. A certain role in realization of these influences is played by HAMC, glycine and opioid peptides. The content of enkephalins and β-endorphins in the hypothalamus decreases at aging (Tang et al. 1984), or does not change (Missale et al. 1983), or even increases (Steger et al. 1980). At the same time, the content of met-enkephalins and β-endorphins in the hypophysis increases (Missale et al. 1983, Tang et al. 1984). The number and affinity of opiate receptors in different cerebral structures change differently (Valueva et al. 1986). According to the data of our group, the content of neuropeptides in the blood does not change identically (Jensen et al. 1980, Piva et al. 1987) (Table 1).

When evaluating the development of "stress–age syndrome" it should be remembered that not all individuals necessarily have all the hormonal components, and that it is not a single characteristic only that should be evaluated, but a complex. There is data, for instance, according to which the content of glucocorticoids in blood does not change in old age (Verkhratsky et al. 1988). That is why it is so important to investigate the complex of neurohormonal shifts, to determine the stress–age syndrome, but not the characteristics of the state of dynamics of a single hormone, be it even a major one such as cortisol. Besides, in one person the neurohormonal "structure" might be changing and the stress–age syndrome would be registered at various stages of its development. An important role in the change of its development is played by progressing age pathology.

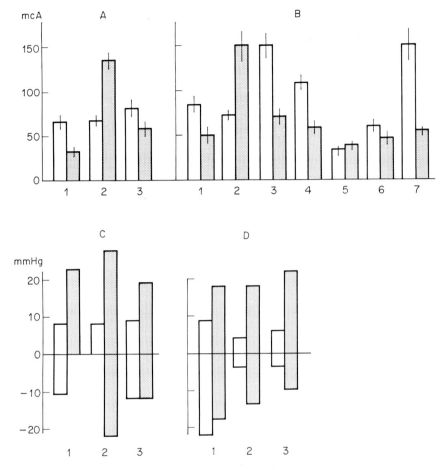

Fig. 5. Electrical thresholds of depressor (A) and pressor (B) reactions of arterial pressure and the magnitude of changes in arterial pressure at microinjection of acetylcholine (C) and adrenaline (D) in different zones of hypothalamus of adult (light columns) and old (shaded columns) rabbits. Zones of hypothalamus: (1) anteromedial; (2) mediolateral; (3) posteromedial, the part of supraoptical nucleus; (4) rostral; (5) caudal; (6) medial preoptical zone; (7) anterohypothalamic nucleus.

The development of stress reactions is characterized by definite behavioural and emotional shifts. Even during physiologic stress caused by direct influence on an organism, ignoring the emotional stress caused by psychogenic influences, first to develop are the emotional stressor reactions. The complex response to the emotional stressor situation is defined by both the nature of the provoking factor and the domination of involved neurophysiologic mechanisms and individual specifics of reaction (Waldman *et al.* 1979).

Table 1
Neuropeptide concentration in blood of rats of various age in pmol l^{-1}

Neuropeptide	Adult (6–8 months)		P	Old (28–32 months)	
Beta-endorphin	10.8	± 1.3		16.3	± 2.1
			0.05		
Metenkephalin	798.0	± 65.0		1400	± 110.0
			0.001		
Leuenkephalin	215.0	± 24.0		690.0	± 30.0
			0.001		
Neurotensin	29.0	± 3.1		24.0	± 2.5
			0.05		
Substance P	255.0	± 10		106.0	± 7.1
			0.001		
Vasopressin	3.1	± 0.7		7.3	± 1.1
			0.001		

From Valueva *et al.* (1986).

Prolonged emotional stress might form the basis for development of a variety of diseases. Positive emotional effects, however, in contrast to negative ones, do not result in the development of pathology. Moreover, as shown in experiments on animals, activation of the system of positive reinforcement might serve as an antistressor effect, which weakens the pathologic vegetative and morphologic effects in the cardiovascular system (Badikov 1982). At the same time, our experiments, run on rats, have shown that with age there develop signs of decrease in the functional abilities of the system of positive reinforcement (Fig. 6): the frequency of self-stimulation of the lateral hypothalamus and the range of currents capable of inducing the intensive self-stimulation become lower, and the motivating component of self-stimulation becomes weaker. At the same time, the chances of development of negative emotional symptoms become higher, which is expressed in decrease of electrical thresholds of defence reactions at stimulation of the ventromedial hypothalamus. So, it can be assumed that on the hypothalamic level of regulation favourable conditions develop for relieving the emotional stress reactions.

The data presented allow us to conclude that at aging of rats there develop, on various levels of the CNS, preconditions for shifting the emotional balance onto the side of negative effects. Really, it is more typical of old rats than of adult ones to have "the behaviour of distress", confirmed

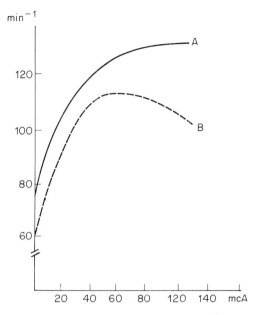

Fig. 6. Intensity of self-stimulation in adult (A) and old (B) rats at the gradual rise of the stimulating current from the threshold value: (1) threshold current. Plotted on ordinate: the frequency of self-stimulation (min^{-1}). Plotted on abscissa: the magnitude of the stimulating current (μA).

by the absence of swimming motions during a certain period; they have a sharp increase in stop periods in the first minutes.

The clinical investigations have shown that it is typical of old people to be emotionally inert, to have decreased variability of emotional states and increased significance of negative emotions (Schulz 1982). With age favourable conditions develop for negative emotional states; older people often experience anxiety, fear, perplexity, and finally, depression, which is the symptom of emotional disorder and which is diagnosed in 21–54% of patients of the geriatric clinic (Schulz 1982, Puccini 1986).

It is possible, without direct comparison of clinical and experimental data, to assume that there is a certain similarity in the shifts of emotional balance to the side of negative emotional effects. This phenomenon might speak of the chronic stress on the one hand, and might provoke the development of emotional stress reactions on the other.

The stress syndrome is characterized not only by neurohormonal shifts, but also by a complex of tissue and cellular changes. Similar shifts develop at aging as well. It means that at aging immunodepression develops; activation of lipid peroxidization increases; free-radical damage in the structures of cells, myocardium, stomach and intestine takes place; the sensitivity of some vascular zones to humoral factors increase; hypertensive reactions take place, and so on. Of course, one should not draw direct analogy between the shifts at stress–age syndrome and those at acute stress. They differ in expressiveness of neurohumoral changes and in duration of their effects. As is known, the long-lasting effect of many hormones might cause tachyphylaxis and might change the number and affinity of receptors.

Here, two basically significant questions arise: (1) why at a certain stage of aging does the age-dependent syndrome develop; (2) what influence has it on the rate of age-dependent changes and on the life span? The answers to these questions are assumptions rather than statements. It could be that the decrease in adaptation abilities of an organism, increasing at aging, results in a situation where the exogenous and endogenous stimulators cause the development of stress syndrome on this background. Also, the time factor in the influence of stimulators should not be overlooked. At aging it has a prolonged influence and might change from subthreshold factors into the threshold and over-threshold ones. As is pointed out by Dilman, time is a universal stressor. There is a concept of "chemical stress". Experiments with various chemicals show that their effect might cause, at a certain stage, the stereotype neurohumoral reaction, defined as stress. Then this stress reaction might be replaced by the stage of exhaustion, or by more pronounced local damages. Aging is characterized by growing changes in metabolism and in chemical reactions of the internal medium. These shifts, going through the chemoreceptive structures, might cause stressor reactions by direct influence on certain nerve centres. The role of the chemical stressor in the development of aging is proved by some of our data, showing that stressor reactions influenced by chemical factors are more pronounced in old animals than in adult ones. This fact was first proved as early as 1963 and was then confirmed by later work (Frolkis et al. 1963).

So, the age-dependent decrease in adaptation abilities of an organism, the increase in the chemical shifts, the prolonged influence of exogenous factors all these contribute to the development of stress–age syndrome. A more generalized approach allows us to assume that the disturbances in homeostasis influenced by aging are actually the signals for development of the stress–age syndrome.

The stress–age syndrome has a complicated influence on the rate of age-dependent changes and on the life span. It includes the destructive mechanisms—the symptoms of aging—and the protective mechanisms—the symptoms of vitauct. It is not that easy to make a boundary between them, since each component of the total reaction might have a different meaning for an organism in different life situations. Moreover, each hormonal shift might assist the adaptation of an organism by influencing one metabolic cycle, and its deadaptation by influencing another.

Finally, the stress–age syndrome itself changes in time; dependent on the

living conditions and current diseases, its components might change; its
stage of exhaustion might increase.

When evaluating the components of the stress–age syndrome, one should
take into account the literature data, showing that the geroprotective effect
is typical of glucocorticoids. They increase the life span of the culture of
diploid fibroblasts by 30–50%, increase the period of a single cycle of
growth and the level of proliferation and incorporation of ^{3}H-thymidine
into DNA (Cristofalo and Sharf 1975, Macieiro-Coelho 1975). Corticosteroids give an increase in the life span of cold-blooded short-living mice
(Bellamy 1968, Norris and Moor 1980). The increase in the life span
depends on the decrease in the concentration of TTH and thyroxin and on
the increase in the contents of vasopressin. The mice, fed with thyroxin,
have a shorter life span than the control animals (Ooka and Shinkai 1986).
Hypophysectomy, by itself, decreases the life span, while in combination
with substitution therapy by cortisone acetate increases it (Everitt *et al.*
1980). It is supposed that this increase in the life span is greatly influenced
by the drop in the level of thyroid hormones and, perhaps, of some other
thyroid hormones, which might affect not only the endocrine glands, but
other target tissues as well. The fact that development of the stress–age
syndrome might assist the prolongation of life is confirmed by experiments
with a calorie-poor diet. The diet-influenced prolongation of life is
accompanied by a neurohormonal shift, which Nikitin (1984) defined as the
"soft stress". The mass of adrenal glands and the width of zona glomerulosa
in experimental rats is doubled; the secretion of corticosteroids increases;
and the synthesizing ability of adrenal glands increases by almost 40%. At
the same time, these rats show lowered concentrations of thyroxin, insulin,
and testosterone during all their life.

It should be noted that the role of developing stress–age syndrome is
determined by other geroprotectors as well. We are well aware of the
geroprotective effect of many antioxidants, for instance of dibunol (2,6-di-
tert-butyl-4-methyl-phenol, BHT). Together with Dr Gorban we studied,
in the experiments on rats, the influence of dibunol on the hypothalamus–hypophysis–thyroid gland systems. As could be seen from Fig.
7, the administration of dibunol (in the dose of 100 mg kg^{-1}) results in
increased secretion of ACTH and corticosterone and in decrease of the
content of TTH and thyroxin. It can be assumed that it is not only—and
not as much the direct antioxidant influence of dibunol on the target tissue
that leads to the life prolongation, but its mediated effect via neurohumoral
mechanisms.

Selye (1976), in his time, believed that repeated stress would result in
exhaustion of the "adaptation energy" and would finally lead to the aging
of an organism. He saw ways for life prolongation in a peculiar fencing of
an organism from the medium factors. Later he slightly changed his opinion,

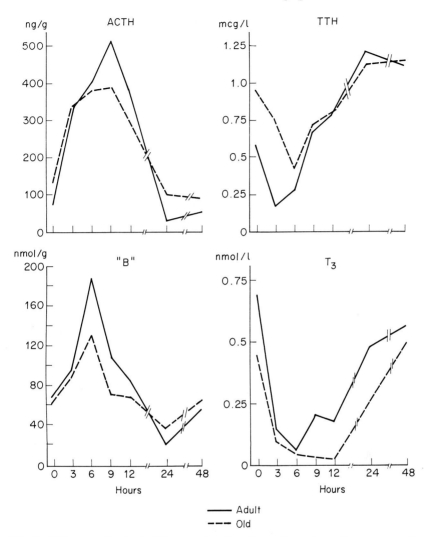

Fig. 7. Influence of a single injection of anti-oxidant, dibunol, on the concentration of ACTH, corticosterone(“B”), TTH and T_3 in the blood of rats of different age.

putting forward the concept of eustress and distress. In 1970 we worked out a somewhat different concept—various continuously repeating stressor effects of moderate power can "train" the protective mechanisms of an organism, the processes of vitauct, thus not only preserving but also prolonging the life. The experimental verification of this concept proved it to be true. Daily moderate stressor effects, including the cold, noise, electrical irritation, physical loads, and temporary limitation of the motor

activity, resulted in an increase of the mean life span by 18%, and of
maximal life span by 11%. At the same time, the extreme, "rude" stressor
effects shortened the life span.

Stress develops as a stereotype reaction and its neurohumoral component
does not necessarily correspond to the state of homeostasis of an organism,
with the state of its cells and tissues. This discrepancy increases with age.
Not only the hypothalamic centres, but other cerebral structures also take
part in the formation of neurohumoral mechanisms of stress. Their
excitability at aging does not change identically for all of them; moreover,
it might change different directedly. As a result, the neurohumoral
"structure" of stress might also change. Then, at a certain stage of aging,
at a certain rate of aging, the stress–age syndrome might cause not only the
adaptive, but also the destructive shifts, damaging the cells and tissues.

The described neurohumoral shifts at stress–age syndrome might provoke
the development of age pathology: atherosclerosis, arterial hypertension,
heart and cerebral ischaemia and diabetes. Thus, the rise in the concentration
of vasopressin, adrenaline, glucocorticoids, aldosterone and the drop in the
content of thyroxin and testosterone might provoke the development of
hypertensive reactions, spasm of coronary vessels and increase in the
thrombogenic potential of blood. The decrease in the insulin activity of
blood and the increase in glucocorticoids and catecholamines provoke the
development of diabetes, and the shifts in emotional zones contribute to
the development of depression, and so on.

So, in the process of aging there develops the stress–age syndrome. There
is also another side of the problem of stress and aging: how the neurohumoral
shifts develop at reproduction of stress in old animals. This problem was
investigated in our group by Verkhratsky et al. (1988). They reproduced
the emotion–pain stress in old and adult rats. In addition to the pain
stimulation they used noise and light effects. As can be seen from Fig. 8,
the regular repetition of the stress situation in old and adult rats
gives approximately identical dynamics of ACTH and corticosterone
concentrations in blood. At the same time, the secretion of aldosterone at
repeated stress suffers more in old rats than in adult, and the contents of
testosterone drops. According to our data the 5-min. emotion–pain stress
in adult and old rats leads to decrease in the content of vasopressin in the
hypothalamus and hypophysis, and to its increase in blood; its content in
blood increases in adult animals by 22, and in old ones by 6.

The data obtained were evaluated by the method of chief components—
one of the types of factor analysis. The evaluation included both the
concentration of hormones in blood and the shifts in the content of
norepinephrine, dopamine and serotonin in the anterior, middle and
posterior hypothalamus, and in the basal nuclei. The whole of the data file
was allocated on six chief components, one of which was in high correlation

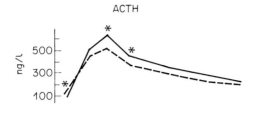

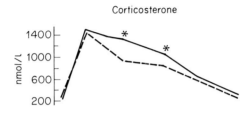

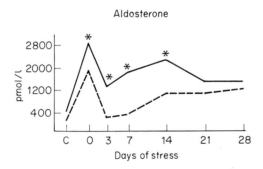

Fig. 8. Influence of chronic emotion–pain stress on the blood plasma ACTH and corticosteroids concentration in adult and old rats. Continuous line: adult rats; dashed line: old rats.

with the number of stress repetitions. The contents of this component in animals of both groups included norepinephrine from the hypothalamus zones and striatum, dopamine of striatum, which speaks of the leading role of catecholaminergic mechanisms in the development of stress. This component in old animals includes, in addition, the variables of serotonin of anterior and posterior hypothalamus. This suggests that the role of serotonin in the mechanisms of stress development becomes greater in old age. Consequently, the uniform hormonal reaction at stress in adult and old rats could be achieved through different neuromediatory shifts in the brain.

THE LIMBIC SYSTEM AND THE HYPOTHALAMUS

The neurohumoral regulation of homeostasis of an organism is to a great extent influenced by the limbic system and hypothalamus. Some investigators include the hypothalamus into the limbic system, while others exclude it from the limbic system. Still, all of them agree that numerous effects of the limbic system on the vegetative functions of an organism are realized through the hypothalamus. At the same time, an important role in the mechanism of most age-dependent changes in regulation, which are attributed to the hypothalamus, is played by the structures of the limbic system, realizing its influence through the hypothalamus.

There are numerous data on the morphological, neurochemical and electrophysiological changes in the structures of the limbic system at aging (Miller et al. 1984, Anderson et al. 1986, Krnjevic et al. 1988). Yet nobody has run the detailed analysis on the role of the limbic system in the mechanisms of changes in neurohumoral regulation of homeostasis or in the regulation of vegetative systems at aging.

The structures of the limbic system co-ordinate the cardiovascular shifts and various emotion-behavioural actions (digestion, sexual behaviour, rage, fury, fear, pleasure), providing the latter with corresponding energetic, vegetative shifts.

In our experiments, run together with Dr. Bezrukov, the stimulation of the dorsal hippocampus, and the central and medial nuclei of amygdaloid complex has shown the different age changes in electroexcitability of these structures of the limbic system: vasoactive elements of the corticomedial nuclei of amygdala in old animals were becoming less excitable; those of the central nucleus and anterior zone of amygdala more excitable; while the excitability of hippocampus in old and adult animals was identical for both groups (Fig. 9).

Our experiments have shown not only the different nature of changes in the thresholds of influences of the limbic system on the activity of cardiovascular system, but also the increased sensitivity of these formations to the influence of adrenaline and acetylcholine. As shown in Fig. 9, the AP shifts at microinjection of minimal doses of adrenaline and acetylcholine are significantly greater in old rabbits. However, these experiments have shown interstructural differences in the age-dependent characteristics of circulation reactions. The adrenaline injection gives more pronounced age-dependent difference in reactions from the central nucleus of amygdala; acetylcholine microinjection—from the hippocampus and medial nucleus of

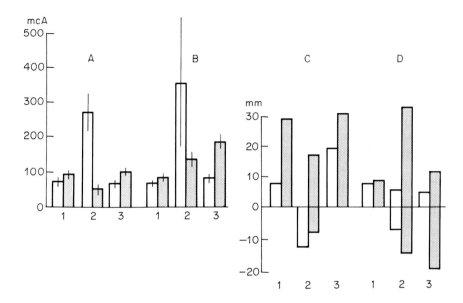

Fig. 9. Electrical thresholds of depressor (A) and pressor (B) reactions of arterial pressure, and the magnitude of changes in arterial pressure at microinjection of acetylcholine (C) and adrenaline (D) into the hippocampus (1), central (2), and medial (3) nuclei of amygdaloid complex in adult (light columns) and old (shaded columns) rabbits. Above the zero line: the magnitude of pressor reactions; below the zero line: depressor reactions.

amygdala. It can be admitted that the increase in the sensitivity of the haemodynamically active elements of the limbic system to certain hormones and mediators plays an adaptive role in the conditions of relative deafferentation of the central neurons, providing the corresponding level of influences on the blood circulation. At the same time, such an increase might be a significant factor of changes in the vegetative reactions at realization of the integral actions, actuated from the limbic system or realized through its participation.

The data obtained suggest that even in the range of a single, morphologically limited complex of nuclear aggregation of neurons, the functional changes and the influence of certain nuclei on the blood circulation are not identical in old age.

The noted peculiarities of influence of the limbic system could be connected, to a certain extent, with morphologically, metabolically and functionally irregular changes that take place in these structures in old age.

There are data, though contradictory, on the influence of the limbic system structures on the hypothalamo-hypophyseal-adrenal and hypothalamo-

hypophyseal-gonadal systems. Some authors believe that the limbic system
has a stimulating effect on the synthesis of corticosterone and testosterone
(Redgate and Fahringer 1973, Dunn 1987); others think that the limbic
system suppresses it (Dupont *et al*. 1972). There are no data in the literature
on how these influences change in old age. Verkhratsky *et al*. (1988) of our
group destroyed the structures of the limbic system of old and adult rats
and studied the change in the concentration of hormones in their blood.
They found that there were significant age-dependent differences. Thus,
the damage of the ventral hippocampus gave, 2 weeks later, an increase in
the concentration of ACTH in the blood of adult animals in comparison to
the initial value by 12.8 times; of corticosterone by 5.1 times; of aldosterone
by 3.3 times; and of testosterone by 2.5 times. In old animals with a
damaged hippocampus the concentration of the above hormones remained
without change 2 weeks after the damage. Damage to the dorsal hippocampus
gave a rise in the concentration of ACTH of 5.6 times in adult rats and
only 1.8 times in old ones; the rise in the concentration of corticosterone
was approximately the same, while for aldosterone and testosterone it was
higher in adult rats compared to old ones. The bilateral coagulation of
basolateral zone of amygdaloid complex induced, after 2 weeks, a more
pronounced increase in ACTH and corticosterone in old rats, while the
damage to the medial zone of the septum in adults. These data allow us to
draw the conclusion that under certain physiologic conditions they inhibit
the function of corresponding hormonal systems. For some structures these
inhibitory effects are less pronounced in old age, which might be considered
as one of the reasons for activation of certain hormonal systems and
development of stress–age syndrome. It was also found that not only
damaging, but also electrical stimulation of certain structures of the limbic
system gives a rise in the concentration of hormones in the blood. It looks
as if these two facts contradict each other. If a certain mechanism is activated
at the damage of the structure, then it means that this structure has an
inhibitory, not stimulating effect. Probably, each structure can have both
activating and inhibiting effects realized through various mediatory systems.
Twenty-four days after the damage of some structures of the hypothalamus
the level of hormones is recovered. However, on the background of the
damaged dorsal and ventral hippocampus, of the damaged basolateral zone
of the amygdaloid complex, the stress causes a more pronounced increase
in the content of ACTH.

Most vegetative shifts at stimulation of the limbic structures are realized
through the nuclei of the hypothalamus. Let us take, for instance, the
chain: hippocampus–fornix–mamillary body–anterior nucleus of hypothalamus–cortex of callosal convolution–presubiculum-hippocampus. The
nuclei of the amygdaloid complex are connected with the hypothalamus via
the terminal stria (with the medial preoptical zone, ventromedial and

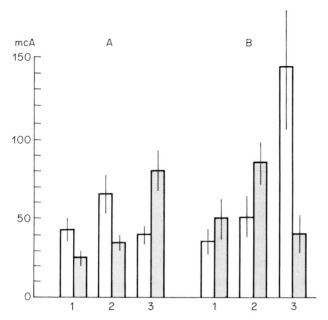

Fig. 10. Age specifics of interdependence between hypothalamic and limbic structures: (A) the thresholds of electrical changes in limbic structures at stimulation of: (1) supraoptical nucleus; (2) medial mamillary nucleus; (3) lateral hypothalamic zone; (B) the threshold of electrographic changes in the nuclei of hypothalamus at stimulation of: (1) dorsal hippocampus; (2) medial nucleus of amygdala; (3) central nucleus of amygdala.

paraventricular nuclei of the hypothalamus) and the lateral corticohypothalamic tract (with the lateral hypothalamic zone, lateral preoptical zone). The corticomedial group of nuclei of the amygdala has a great influence on the sympathetic zone of the hypothalamus, while the basolateral affects parasympathetic zone.

In our laboratory we have studied the age-dependent specifics of the influence of the hippocampus and some zones of the amygdala on the hypothalamic nuclei. The acute experiments, run on rats of different ages, have shown that in old rats the thresholds of the electrographic changes in the nuclei of hypothalamus at stimulation of the medial nucleus of the amygdala are higher, and of the central nucleus are lower than in adult animals, while at stimulation of the dorsal hippocampus they are practically the same for both the adult and old animals (Fig. 10). The thresholds of appearance of electrographic shifts in the limbic structures at stimulation of supraoptical and medial mamillary nuclei are higher in adult animals, while of lateral hypothalamic zone they are higher in old ones.

These changes in the structures of the limbic system and hypothalamus play an important role in the dynamics of the age-dependent changes in neurohumoral regulation. The hypothalamic and limbic formations take part in the regulation of different types of metabolism and of different activities of an organism. The attenuation of modulating influences of the medial nuclei of the amygdala on anterior and posterior zones of the hypothalamus might become an important factor contributing to the worsened regulation of the reproductive function and its vegetative provision. The strengthening of influence (at least, the decrease in the threshold of influence) of the central nucleus of the amygdala on the hypothalamic mechanisms of regulation of the vegetative homeostasis might play a significant role in easily developing affective behavioural reactions accompanied by substantial shifts in the activity of the cardiovascular system. Stability of the hippocampus excitability at the decrease of the post-effects of hypothalamic stimulation might form the basis for the impairment of the vegetative provision of the muscle responses, and the attenuation of the hypothalamic influence on the hippocampus might become a significant factor for worsening of some types of memory.

The age-dependent changes in the hypothalamus seem to be so important that this is where most investigators place "the biological clock" of aging of an organism (Everitt 1970, Samorajski and Ordy 1972, Dilman 1976, 1987). Some investigators connect the developing at aging changes with attenuation of the hypothalamus function, others with its activation.

In our investigations we have found a new approach—the systematic evaluation of age changes in the hypothalamus. The hypothalamus is a functionally and structurally non-uniform system. That is why the conclusion on the direction of changes in the "whole" hypothalamus should be made with great care.

In old age the activity and excitability of haemodynamically active elements of the hypothalamus, and the nature of the haemodynamic reaction change (Fig. 5). In old animals the excitability of the nuclei of anterior and posterior hypothalamus, of supraoptical nucleus increases, and the excitability of the lateral hypothalamic zone decreases. The difference in the thresholds of excitability between the most excitable and less excitable haemodynamically active points is less in old rabbits compared with the adult ones. Thus, the difference in the thresholds of the pressor reactions was half as large in old rabbits (51 μA) as in adult animals (100 μA). The state of isoexcitability creates the conditions for easier involvement in reactions of hypothalamic nuclei, for inadequate vegetative shifts in various situations. Along with the change in the electroexcitability in old age the sensitivity of some hypothalamic structures to mediators and hormones increases. Thus, the intrastructural injection of adrenaline and acetylcholine into the lateral, anterior and posterior zones of the hypothalamus results in more pronounced shifts in old animals (Frolkis and Bezrukov 1979). More

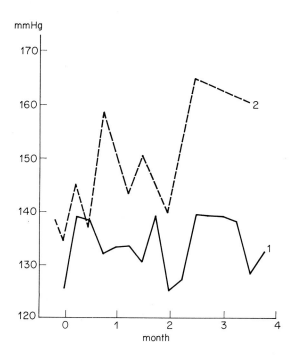

Fig. 11. Influence of the long-term stimulation of hypothalamus on the arterial pressure in adult (1) and old (2) rabbits.

pronounced differences are observed in the pressor reactions, but not in the depressor ones. Aging brings changes in the haemodynamic structure of reactions in response to stimulation of the hypothalamus. As found, change in arterial pressure, accompanied by increase in the ventricular ejection, occurs more often in old animals than in adult ones. In old age the range of haemodynamic reactions becomes smaller and the correlation between the intensity of stimulation and the power of response changes. The reflex bradycardia in old animals is less pronounced. The thresholds of excitability of the pressor responses change to a lesser extent than those of the depressor. The whole of this complex of shifts contributes to the development of arterial hypertension (Fig. 11).

The non-uniform functional changes in some structures of the hypothalamus can also be observed when studying the electrical activity of its nuclei. Thus, Bezrukov (1982) has run chronic experiments on rats with implanted electrodes, where he has shown the different retardation of frequency and indefinitive change in the power of some rhythms in the electrogram of various zones of hypothalamus of animals at aging. Old rabbits showed retardation of the θ-rhythm in ventromedial and mamillary nuclei, and of the β-rhythm in supraoptical and mamillary nuclei. The total power of electrograms substantially drops in the mamillary nuclei, slightly drops in the lateral hypothalamic zone, increases in ventromedial nuclei and does not change in supraoptical. If in young animals the total power of various nuclei substantially differs, then in old age there occurs, as a result of non-uniform shifts, the levelling of values of the total power of electrograms of different nuclei.

There are data on differently expressed morphological shifts in the nuclei of the hypothalamus (Hsu and Peng 1978, Sartin and Lamperti 1985). The whole of this complex of age changes in the hypothalamus we have defined as dysregulation of the hypothalamus (Frolkis 1975, 1982). We think that this dysregulation of the hypothalamus is the main cause for changes in its function, for decrease in its reliability, since regulation of any function of an organism is realized through participation of several hypothalamic structures. Thus, for instance, digestive behaviour is determined by interaction of "the appetite centre", located in the lateral hypothalamic zone, and of "the satiation centre", located in the ventromedial zone of the hypothalamus; thermoregulation—by interaction of the structures of anterior and posterior hypothalamus; reproductive function—by interaction of the preoptical zone and the nuclei of the median eminence, etc. That is why the dysregulation of the hypothalamus, the different-directed change of its nuclei results in the disturbance of some functions, in the regulation of which the complex of hypothalamic nuclei takes part. The different-directed change of excitability and of sensitivity of the hypothalamic structures to humoral factors distorts the integrative function of the hypothalamus and its ability to control the complicated adaptive processes. The dysregulation favours the phenomenon of "hypothalamic misinformation". This means that at aging the sensitivity of hypothalamic structures to nervous impulse and to various hormones and mediators changes unevenly and different direct-edly. At aging the sensitivity of different nuclei to the same humoral factor, or of one nucleus to different factors change differently.

An important role in the change of reactivity in any structure of the brain, including the hypothalamus, at neurohumoral shifts is played by feedback systems, by the influence of hormones on the structures of the brain. At aging irregular changes occur in the receptory binding of glucocorticoids in the cerebral cortex, hippocampus and hypothalamus. Magdich and Didenko (1988) of our group studied the age changes in the binding of corticosteroids by different structures of the limbic system, by hypothalamus and by hypophysis. In old animals irregular, different-directed changes in the binding of corticosteroids in various zones of the brain develop. Increase in the binding of corticosteroids by the receptors of the cells of hypophysis, and decrease in the binding by the cells of the hypothalamus, and increase in the binding by the cells of the hippocampus are noteworthy. All this might play a significant role in the intensity of influence of the feedback signals on the central formation of regulatory systems controlling the function of the adrenal cortex. Probably, the role of the feedbacks realized through the hypophysis increases in old age; the correlation of hypothalamus and hypophysis in the mechanism of regulation of most hormonal reactions changes. That is why, when evaluating age changes in hormonal feedbacks, it is important to differentiate reactions of the structures of the limbic system, of the hypothalamus and of the hypophysis.

It should be remembered that feedbacks from effectors to hypothalamus are realized not only through the hormones of the blood, but also due to the reflectory influences of receptors. In this respect, it would be reasonable to remember that at aging the reflexes from some mechanoreceptors of vessels, from internal organs, become weaker, and the sensitivity of chemoreceptors increases (Frolkis 1982). At aging redistribution of information coming via the canals of nervous and humoral link occurs. This results in "errors" in information on the state of internal medium of an organism, in realization of the hypothalamic programme, and of regulation of homeostasis.

The irregular nature of changes in the excitability of hypothalamic structures is one of the reasons for the shifts in the behavioural–emotional sphere. Stimulation of the medial hypothalamus in animals is usually followed by negative emotions; and of lateral hypothalamus by the development of reactions of self-stimulation. Experiments, run by Dr. Rushkevich, have shown that the negative emotion reaction at stimulation of the ventromedial nucleus takes place at the current of 126 ± 8 μA for adult rats, and 95 ± 4 μA for old ones. In other words, the excitability of the negative emotion zone increases with age. The intensity of self-stimulation at stimulation of the lateral hypothalamic zone is higher for adult animals. Dysregulation of the function of hypothalamus, hypothalamic misinformation, leads to the decrease of its reliability.

As shown by our group, prolonged stimulation of the hypothalamus for many days results in a more pronounced rise of arterial pressure, and in the development of disturbances in structure and function of the heart, and in the death of old animals. Morphological investigation of the heart of rabbits which died at old age has shown homogenization of cytoplasm, the disappearance of the cross striation throughout the myocardium of the left ventricle. Extensive areas of necrobiosis are found in the posterior wall of the left ventricle.

So, at aging the excitability, electrical activity, sensitivity to humoral factors of some structures of the limbic system and of hypothalamus change unevenly, and the correlation between them changes. As a result, the central programme of various complicated neurohumoral reactions and their reliability changes. In the long run, this results in limitation of adaptation–regulatory abilities of an organism, of its reliability, and contributes to the development of age pathology.

NEUROHUMORAL CONTROL OF PROTEIN BIOSYNTHESIS

Great significance for mechanisms of aging is attached to the changes in neurohumoral regulation, to the attenuation of the nervous control over the genome of cells, and the protein biosynthesis. Eventually, the genome regulation, its adaptation to the demands of a cell, is realized due to the intragenome mechanisms and to the influences of supracellular, neurohumoral mechanisms. The age changes in neurohumoral regulation result in shifts of the basal level of protein biosynthesis and, what is more important, in the limitation of adaptation reactions of the system. In the end, these neurohumoral influences are realized through hypothalamo-hypophyseal-hormonal tracts and the tracts of direct nervous influences. There are numerous works on the peculiarities of hormonal regulation of the genome. However, only a few of them are devoted to investigations on the influences from the nervous system (Gutmann 1976, Shimazu et al. 1978, Frolkis and Bezrukov 1979, Frolkis et al. 1979, Shimazu 1980). It would not be enough to know how the introduced hormone influences the protein biosynthesis in cells of animals of different ages. One should also know how it develops under natural conditions, under the conditions of "nervous" activation of hormone secretion from hypothalamus.

A series of works carried out by our group suggest that at aging the neurohumoral and hypothalamo-hypophyseal control over the processes of protein biosynthesis and over the state of the genome change. This limits the participation of biosynthetic processes in complex adaptive reactions of an organism, regulated and controlled by the hypothalamus.

The genetic induction of enzymes is considered to be an important adaptation–regulatory mechanism of a cell. The following enzymes of protein and carbohydrate metabolism are noteworthy: tyrosine aminotransferase (TAT), tryptophan pyrolase (TP), glucose-6-phosphatase (G6P) and fructose-1,6-diphosphatase (FDP). The activity of these enzymes increases under the influence of specific and unspecific substrates, of some hormones of glucocorticoids, and ACTH. Despite numerous literature data on the age specifics of basal activity of inductive enzymes, of substrate and hormonal induction (Kanungo 1980), the number of works devoted to the

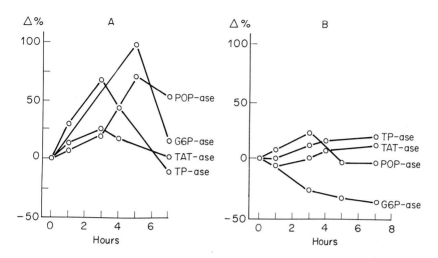

Fig. 12. Influence of a single stimulation of the hypothalamus on the enzymic activity in adult (A) and old (B) rats. Enzymic activity in sham-operated animals is taken as the basis. The time after stimulation (h) is indicated horizontally.

study of the central—hypothalamic in particular—mechanisms of regulation of inductive synthesis of enzymes is very scanty.

In experiments run on adult and old male rats the stimulation of the ventromedial nucleus of the hypothalamus resulted in the pronounced increase in the activity of TAT, TP, G6P and FDP in adult animals (Fig. 12). The preliminary administration of inhibitors of protein biosynthesis— actinomycin D or olivomycin—prevented the stimulating effect of hypothalamus stimulation on the activity of enzymes. The increase in the activity of enzymes at stimulation of the hypothalamus was not observed at preliminary adrenalectomy either. The increase in the activity of TAT, TP, G6P and FDP at electrostimulation of the ventromedial nucleus was less pronounced in old rats compared with adult ones. Together with decrease in the power of response, its latent period was increasing, and the shifts in the activity of some enzymes (TAT, TP) were delayed. The activity of G6P was decreasing in old rats. In adult animals "the exhaustion" of the inducing effect of hypothalamus stimulation was observed 3 days after the daily stimulation, whereas in old animals it was observed on the first day.

The possible influence of the hypothalamic zone on the processes of protein biosynthesis, realized by different tracts and in different ways in animals of different ages, is confirmed by data on determination of labelled orotic acid inclusion into nuclear and cytoplasmic fractions of RNA, and into the total RNA, obtained in collaboration with Dr. Muradian. The short-term stimulation of the ventromedial nucleus results in increased renovation of the total RNA, equal for both adult and old animals. However, the inclusion of the labelled precursor into various fractions of RNA was changing differently. Similar to the experiments with determination of enzyme induction, the activation of biosynthesis of RNA fractions in old animals was taking place later in time, and the stimulation effect of hypothalamus stimulation on the synthesis of RNA fractions was weakened.

So, aging brings about the situation when target organs can still respond to the adequate stimulation by activation of apparatus of protein biosynthesis, but the central—hypothalamic in particular—mechanisms are not able to maintain this level of adaptation reactions. In old age the range of regulatory influences of hypothalamus on biosynthesis of various classes of RNA and on genetic induction of some key enzymes becomes narrower.

When studying changes in the hypothalamic regulation of protein biosynthesis, data on the shifts of the level of chromatin might be especially useful, since with age a decrease in the portion of active chromatin occurs, and in the transcription activity, and also an increase in the amount of tightly bound protein. In collaboration with Khilobok, Moshzukhina, Goldstein and Muradian, we have studied the influence of electrostimulation of the hypothalamus on the state of chromatin in the liver of adult and old rats. The results of experiments have shown that 3 weeks after implanting the electrodes, the state of chromatin in old animals is actually the same as in intact animals. Electrostimulation causes the redistribution of chromatin fractions: the amount of low-active fractions decreases and, correspondingly, the amount of active fractions increases, in comparison with the control animals (Fig. 13). The specific activity of RNA increases in both chromatin fractions, and the size of the pool of labelled precursors remains the same. The ratio of protein/RNA remains without change in both the low-active and active chromatins. Electrostimulation causes a significant rise in the melting temperature of active chromatin.

The implanting of electrodes into old rats gives a decrease in the amount of low-active chromatin and an increase in the amount of the active chromatin. The ratio of protein/RNA remains without change in the low-active chromatin and decreases in the active chromatin. The growth of transcription in low-active chromatin at an invariable pool of labelled precursors increases. The melting temperature decreases in both fractions. The electrostimulation in old rats, in contrast to adult ones, does not cause any significant change in the contents of chromatin fractions, when compared to the control animals with implanted electrodes. Electrostimulation gives a significant decrease in the inclusion of labelled precursors into RNA of both fractions and a rise in the melting temperature of both fractions.

The data obtained suggest that the hypothalamus exerts a regulatory influence on the state of chromatin in the liver, and this influence changes

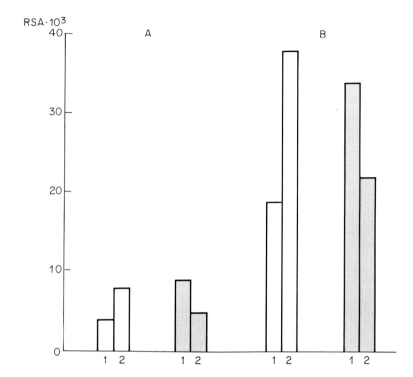

Fig. 13. Influence of electrostimulation of the hypothalamus on RNA synthesis in low-active (A) and active (B) chromatin: (1) control rats with implanted electrodes; (2) after electrostimulation. Light columns: adult rats; shaded columns: old rats.

in the process of aging. The fact that implanting of electrodes into the hypothalamus causes, by itself, the shifts in the state of chromatin over a long enough time, suggests the decreased reliability and the fragility of hypothalamic mechanisms of regulation in old age. It can be assumed that the change in the state of chromatin at stimulation of the hypothalamus is connected with both the nervous tracts of effect realization and the influence of hormonal regulatory factors, of hydrocortisone in particular.

All the obtained data confirm the existence of age differences in the influence of the hypothalamic zone on the systems of protein biosynthesis and genetic apparatus, and the possible dependence of these differences on age-dependent shifts in the ways of realization of the hypothalamus influence on the peripheral organs and tissues. The attenuation of potential abilities of hypothalamic regulation of the process of protein biosynthesis and of control over the activity of genetic apparatus is an important factor of reduction of adaptive abilities of an organism, a significant mechanism of aging.

So, the aging of a cell or of a cellular population should be considered in the boundaries of age changes in a definite system of self-regulation. Quite often, the primary changes in supracellular mechanisms—especially hypothalamic provoke the secondary shifts in genome and in protein biosynthesis of cells in the subject of regulation.

There are also some direct nervous regulatory influences on the protein biosynthesis, on the genome of a cell. These are realized via the tracts of vegetative nervous system, via somatic nerves. We have shown in an extensive series of works that at aging the nervous control over some cells and organs becomes weaker (Frolkis 1975, 1982, Frolkis et al. 1984). Such weakening of nervous control is connected with the destruction of neurons, of nerve endings; with change in the neuronal transport of substances; and with shifts in the synthesis and isolation of mediators. As is known, the age changes in nervous control are expressed differently in relation to different cellular populations and different organs. The work of our group has shown that at aging, changes in the nervous control of protein biosynthesis occur. This was shown on various subjects with the use of models of denervation. In some cases it was the surgical denervation—radicotomy—in other cases it was chemical—incorporation of selective adrenoblockers and cholinoblockers. The extent of changes in particular parameters of genome, of protein biosynthesis after denervation was the measure of the extent of changes in the nervous control.

In the experiments, run in collaboration with Dr. Bezrukov and Dr. Muradian, the denervation of liver was made by subdiaphragmatic dissection of the vagus nerves; by dissection of hepatoduodenal, hepatolienal, hepatogastric and suspending ligaments of the liver; and by denudation and phenolization of the area of solar plexus. The developing changes in transcription and translation were evaluated by shifts in the relative specific activity (RSA) of RNA and protein after incorporation of ^{3}H-leucine into animals. In old animals the denervation after 2 weeks resulted in significant increase of RSA of protein and RNA in the liver. This is confirmed by corresponding regressive equations (pseudo-operated adult rats—RSA of protein = $260 \pm 7.2t$; denervated—RSA of protein = $268 \pm 10.5t$; pseudo-operated—RSA of RNA = $250 \pm 3.3t$; denervated—RSA of RNA = $290 \pm 5.9t$). In old "denervated" rats, compared to pseudo-operated control animals, there were no shifts in the size of the relative specific radioactivity of RNA and protein. The weakening of influence of denervation on the intensity of RNA and protein biosynthesis in the liver of old animals is confirmed by the data of the disperse analysis. Thus, while in adult rats the influence of denervation on RSA of RNA was statistically significant ($F = 23.9$, $P < 0.001$), in old rats the corresponding F factor suggested the absence of denervation influence. Similar results were obtained in disperse analysis of data on protein RSA. It should be noted that more pronounced shifts in RNA and protein renovation in old animals took place under the influence of adrenoblockers (dihydroergotoxin, inderal) and of M- and N-cholinolytics (atropine, hexony).

This type of nerve influence on the protein biosynthesis might be defined as neurotrophic, determining the trophicity of a cell. Neurotrophic influences determine the adaptation of a cell to the conditions of life, and regulate the level of the function. That is why the specifics of neurotrophic influences, of nervous influences on the protein biosynthesis, depend on its initial level, on the peculiarities of the biosynthetic system.

An important role in an organism is played by the system of enzymes of microsomal oxidation. This defines the most significant mechanisms of detoxication. The enzymes of microsomal oxidation, cytochrome P_{450}, are induceable, which is decisive for adaptation of this system to the demands of an organism. At aging the inductive synthesis of these enzymes decreases, which might become a significant factor of disturbances in homeostasis of ´an organism in old age. Dr. Paramonova of our laboratory studied the influence of surgical denervation on the initial level and genetic induction of enzymes of microsomal oxidation (Fig. 14). The genetic induction of enzymes of microsomal oxidation was provoked in rats by a 3-day injection of phenobarbital at a dose of 80 mg kg^{-1}. As shown, the surgical vagotomy decreased the inductive growth in the contents of cytochrome P_{450} in adult animals and left it without change in old ones. The sympathectomy had no influence on the induction of enzymes in both adult and old animals. So, the system of microsomal oxidation of a liver is under neurotrophic control, which changes in old age. This control over various biosynthetic systems changes differently.

In experiments on skeletal muscles, run in collaboration with Dr. Yasechko, we determined age changes in the nervous control of protein biosynthesis. It was shown that by 30 min after denervation activation of protein biosynthesis occurred, the increase in the relative specific radioactivity by 56% in old animals. In adult rats similar shifts were not observed. The intensity of protein biosynthesis 5 weeks after denervation increased to approximately the same degree in the musculus gastrocnemius of old and adult animals (49% and 41%). There were only slight shifts in protein biosynthesis in the M. flexor digitorum longus of adult animals, while in old ones it increased substantially 30 min after denervation, as well as 5 weeks later (49% and 91%). The activation of protein biosynthesis at denervation is accompanied by progressive destruction of metabolism and of functions of skeletal muscles. It can be assumed that this activation results from the change in genoregulatory shifts. Such chaotic activation does not assist the preservation of the cell function. According to Gutmann (1976) and Parkhotik (1964), most metabolic shifts (intensity of tissue respiration, excitability, the contents of intracellular water, the concentration

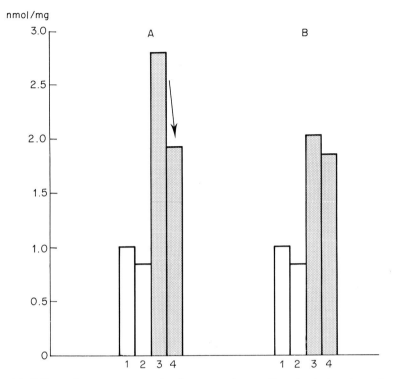

Fig. 14. Effect of vagotomy on the liver cytochrome P_{450} level (nmol mg^{-1} of microsomal protein) in adult and old rats: (A) adult rats; (B) old rats; (1) control; (2) vagotomy; (3) phenobarbital; (4) vagotomy + phenobarbital.

of potassium and sodium etc.) after denervation are less pronounced in old animals than adult ones. This fact confirms the concept that activation of protein biosynthesis, strongly expressed in old animals after denervation, is not followed by stabilization of the cell structure and function. There is a basic difference in the post-effects of denervation in the tissues of liver and skeletal muscles. The denervated liver continues to function actively. The denervated muscle—apart from changes connected with exclusion of neurotrophic influences—has shifts determined by exclusion of muscles from activity. Well known are the facts of muscle atrophy, resulting from inactivity.

Age changes in the intensity of protein biosynthesis in the skeletal muscles on the thirtieth minute after denervation provoke some interest. At that moment pronounced hyperpolarization of the cell membrane in adult rats occurs, the size of membrane potential increases by 4–5 mV. Old rats do not experience a similar hyperpolarization. Such hyperpolarization of muscular fibres is prevented by preliminary administration of an inhibitor of protein biosynthesis, actinomycin S or cycloheximide. This is explained by the fact that in the course of activation of protein biosynthesis a special peptide hyperpolarizing factor is synthesized (Frolkis 1981). In old animals the synthesis of this factor is weakened, which prevents the development of hyperpolarization. In our laboratory we have shown that the developing hyperpolarization on a feedback basis supresses the protein biosynthesis. The absence of such a mechanism in old animals becomes one of the factors of activation of protein biosynthesis at earlier stages after denervation.

So, neurohumoral and nervous control over the genome, and over the protein biosynthesis in the cell changes at aging. It is absolutely evident that such influences are realized through intracellular mechanisms of regulation, through regulatory system of genome itself. The age-dependent shifts in neurohumoral regulation are by themselves the reasons for the secondary age changes in the system of biosynthesis of regulated cells; and then they change and sometimes limit the inclusion of the cellular systems into the common adaptation–regulatory systems of an organism.

Gutmann (1976) noted the similarity of changes in protein metabolism in muscles at denervation and at aging. He believed that the decrease in the trophic function of a neuron was an important factor of aging. At the same time, the neurohumoral mechanisms of changes in the regulation of the genome and protein biosynthesis at aging might be much more extensive. The changes in concentration of even one hormone, the change in reception of it, might substantially influence the protein biosynthesis. At stress–age syndrome there actually develops a new "hormonal situation". This causes complex changes in the genome regulation, in the synthesis of various proteins. Really, the decrease in the concentration of sexual steroids, thyroxin, in the insulin activity of blood and the increase in the contents of glucocorticoids at stress–age syndrome, that is, the change in the correlation of anabolic and catabolic hormones, all lead to the shifts in the intensity of protein biosynthesis, in the correlation of synthesis of various proteins at aging. The attenuation of direct nervous control under such conditions changes the reactivity of protein-synthesizing systems to the whole complex of these shifts, and influences its state. Certainly, these shifts, taking place in cells, cannot be considered only as a result of age changes in neurohumoral regulation. The matter in question is different. The age changes in the genome regulation are superimposed by the shifts in neurohumoral regulation. The correlation of these two mechanisms is different in different cells. It depends on the function of a cell, its mitotic activity, and on the extent of nervous control. At the same time, these shifts in neurons in cells of endocrine glands result from the genoregulatory changes in themselves. All this determines the integrity of age changes in two circuits of the mechanism of aging of an organism.

CONCLUSION

For more than 25 years the author has been collecting data suggesting that age development is determined not only by aging of an organism, but also by vitauct—the process that stabilizes the viability of an organism. An important role in the formation of correlation between these two processes is played by shifts in neurohumoral regulation. They determine such important changes in an organism as shifts in behaviour, emotions, memory, mental and physical efficiency, reproductive ability, regulation of internal organs, preservation and damage of homeostasis and development of age pathology. Age-dependent changes in two circuits of self-regulation, two circuits of information transfer and treatment—genoregulatory and neurohumoral—are decisive for the basic mechanisms of aging connected with the shifts in the cell genome, in the protein biosynthesis.

By this paper the author tries to prove that apart from the basic mechanisms of aging there exist some individual, populational and species-specific distinctions in aging. They define the existence of different syndromes of aging, the formation of which is greatly influenced by the shifts in neurohumoral regulation. The type of aging syndrome defines the type of age pathology developing in an individual. At aging the stress–age syndrome develops, which means not only the activation of the hypothalamo-hypophyseal-adrenal system, of this most frequently described mechanism of stress. This is a whole complex of shifts—activation of some hormonal mechanisms and supression of others, weakening of the nervous control and metabolic changes in cells. The development of this complex has its own specifics. Its formation is connected with numerous manifestations of vitauct and aging, with development of age pathology. The development of the stress–age syndrome is connected with irregular, different-directed changes in different structures of the limbic system, in different nuclei of the hypothalamus. Its development is connected with changes in the intracellular bonds between these structures of the brain.

The changes in nervous control are considered as one of the reasons for the age-dependent shifts in protein biosynthesis. Being imposed on the genoregulatory changes in cells, they influence the age dynamics of the genome, and the protein biosynthesis. The developing genoregulatory mechanisms of aging form the basis for the development of age pathology. The genoregulatory mechanisms lead to the age changes in the correlation with synthesis of different proteins, to the decrease in the potential abilities of protein-synthesizing systems, and to the expression of earlier inactive genes. Dependent on the nature of genoregulatory changes in a person, atherosclerosis, diabetes, tumour, parkinsonism, Alzheimer's disease, or the combination of different types of pathology might develop. The development of genoregulatory shifts in neurons and in the cells of endocrine glands results in the changes in neurohumoral regulation, contributing to the development of age pathology.

REFERENCES

Anderson, K. J., Scheff, S. W. and De Kosky, S. T. (1986). Reactive synaptogenesis in hippocampal area CA 1 of aged and young adult rats. *Journal of Comparative Neurology* **252**, 374–384.

Badikov, V. I. (1982) Regulation of self-stimulation in animals as antistress factor. *Vestnik Akademii Meditsinskikh Nauk SSSR* **2**, 69–75 (in Russian).

Bellamy, D. (1968). Long-term action of prednisolone phosphate on short-lived mice. *Experimental Gerontology* **3**, 327–333.

Bezrukov, V. V. (1982). Hypothalamus during aging. *In* "Physiologic mechanisms of aging" (V. V. Frolkis, ed.) pp. 94–107. Nauka, Leningrad (in Russian).

Cristofalo, V. J. and Sharf, B. (1975). Stimulation of DNA synthesis by hydrocortisone during aging of human diploid cells in culture. "Proceedings of the 10th International Congress in Gerontology", Jerusalem, 1975, Abstracts, vol. 2, p. 11.

Cutler, R. G. (1984). Evolutionary biology of aging and longevity in mammalian species. *In* "Aging and cell function" (J. Johnson, ed.) pp. 1–47. Plenum Press, New York.

Dalakishvili, S. M. (1987). Complex characterization of some homeo-static indices. *In* "Abkhazian longevity" (V. Kozlov, ed.) pp. 227–242. Nauka, Moscow.

Dilman, V. M. (1976). The hypothalamic control of aging and age-associated pathology: the elevation mechanism of aging. *In* "Hypothalamus, pituitary and aging" (A. Everitt, ed.) pp. 634–667. C. C. Thomas, Springfield.

Dilman, V. M. (1987). "Four models of medicine" p. 280. Meditsina, Leningrad (in Russian).

Dunn, J. D. (1987). Differential plasma corticosterone responses to electrical stimulation of the medial and septal muscle. *Neuroendocrinology* **46**, 406–411.

Dupont, A., Basferache, E., Endroczi, E. and Fortier, C. (1972). Effect of hippocampal stimulation of the plasma thyrotropin and cortisone responses to acute cold exposure in the rat. *Canadian Journal of Physiological Pharmacology* **40**, 364–367.

Economos, A. C. (1980). Brain-lifespan conjecture: a reevaluation of the evidence. *Gerontology* **26**, 82–89.

Everitt, A. V. (1970). Food intake, endocrines and aging. *Proceedings of the Australian Association of Gerontology* **1**, 65–78.

Everitt, A. V., Seedsman, N. J. and Jones, F. (1980). The effects of hypophysectomy and continuous food restriction begun at ages 70 and 400 days on collagen aging, proteinuria, incidence of pathology and longevity in the male rat. *Mechanisms of Ageing and Development* **12**, 161–172.

Frolkis, V. V. (1963). Self-regulation of function during organism's aging. *Fiziologicheskii Zhurnal SSSR* **49**, 1221–1229 (in Russian).

Frolkis, V. V. (1966). Neuro-humoral regulations in the aging organism. *Journal of Gerontology* **21**, 161–167.

Frolkis, V. V. (1970). "Regulation, adaptation and aging" p. 480. Nauka, Leningrad (in Russian).

Frolkis, V. V. (1975). "Mechanismen des alterns" p. 380. Academie Press, Berlin.
Frolkis, V. V. (1981). "Aging: neurohumoral mechanisms" p. 320. Naukova Dumka, Kiev (in Russian).
Frolkis, V. V. (1982) "Aging and life-prolonging processes" p. 375. Karger, Wien, New York.
Frolkis, V. V. (1988). "Aging and life prolongation" p. 1985. Nauka, Leningrad (in Russian).
Frolkis, V. V. (1989). "Longevity: reality and potential" p. 215. Naukova Dumka, Kiev (in Russian).
Frolkis, V. V. and Bezrukov, V. V. (1979). "Aging of the central nervous system" p. 131. Karger, Basel.
Frolkis, V. V., Svechnikova, N.V., Verkhratsky, N.S. and Verzhikovskaya N.V. (1963). Stress, aged and adaptation. In "Mechanisms of aging" (D. F. Chebotarev, ed.) pp. 194–206. Zdorobje, Kiev (in Russian).
Frolkis, V. V., Bezrukov, V. V. and Muradian Kh. K. (1979). Hypothalamic-pituitary-adrenocortical regulation of induction of some enzymes of carbohydrate and amino acid metabolism in aging. Experimental Gerontology 14, 63–76.
Frolkis, V. V., Bezrukov, V. V. and Shevchuk, V. G. (1984). "Blood circulation and aging" p. 240. Nauka, Leningrad (in Russian).
Glueck, C. J., Gartside, P., Fallat, R. W., Sielski, J. and Steiner P. (1976). Longevity syndromes: familial hypobeta and familial hyperalpha lipoproteinemia. Journal of Laboratory and Clinical Medicine 88(6), 941–957.
Gutmann, E. (1976). Neurotrophic relations. Annual Review of Physiology 38, 177–216.
Ho-Zhi-Chien (1982). A study of longevity and protein requirements of individuals 90 to 112 years old in southern China. Journal of Applied Nutrition 34 (1), 12–23.
Hsu, H. K., Peng, M. T. (1978). Hypothalamic neuron number of old female rats. Gerontology 24, 434–440.
Ingram, D. K. (1983). Toward the behavioral assessment of biological aging in the laboratory mouse. Experimental Aging Research 9 (4), 225–238.
Jamil, N. A. K. and Millard, R. E. (1981). Studies of T, B, and "null" blood lymphocytes in normal persons of different age groups. Gerontology 27 (1–2), 79–94.
Jensen, R. A., Messing, R. B., Spiehler, V. R. et al. (1980). Memory, opiate receptors and aging. Peptides 1, 197–201.
Kanungo, M. S. (1980). "Biochemistry of aging" p. 294. Academic Press, London.
Krnjevic, K., Ropert, N. and Casullo, J. (1988). Septohippocampal disinhibition. Brain Research 438, 182–192.
Kulchitsky, O. K. and Orlov, P. A. (1977). Carbohydrate tolerance and functional activity of insular apparatus during aging. In "Insulin provision of an organism in old age" (V. V. Frolkis, ed.) pp. 34–45. Kiev (in Russian).
Ludwig, F. C. and Smoke, M. E. (1980). The measurement of biological age. Experimental Aging Research 6, 497–522.
Macieira-Coelho, A. (1975). The decline of RNA synthesis during the lifespan of fibroblasts in vitro. "Proceedings of the 10th International Congress on Gerontology", 1975, Jerusalem, Vol. 1, pp. 60–61.
Magdich, L. V. and Didenko, S. O. (1988). Receptor binding of corticosteroids in various parts of brain in adult and old rats. In "Endocrine mechanisms of aging and age-related pathology" pp. 21–25. Kiev (in Russian).

Malamed, S. and Carsia, R. (1983). Aging of the rat adrenocortical cell. Response to ACTH and cAMP in vitro. *Journal of Gerontology* **38**, 130–138.

Mankovsky, N. B., Mints, A. Ya., Kuznetsova, S. M. and Belonog, R. P. (1987). Neural system and psychic types. *In* "Abkhazian longevity" (V. Kozlov, ed.) pp. 216–227. Nauka, Moscow (in Russian).

Miller, A. K. H., Alston, R., Mountjoy, C. Q. *et al.* (1984). Automated differential cell counting on a sector of the normal human hippocampus: the influence of age. *Neuropathology and Applied Neurobiology* **10**, 123–141.

Missale, C., Govoni, S., Croce, L. *et al.* (1983). Changes of beta-endorphin and met-enkephalin content in the hypothalamus-pituitary axis induced by aging. *Journal of Neurochemistry* **40**, 20–24.

Nguen, Phuoc Du Ch., Dauwerchain, J., Mandin, A., *et al.* (1981). Vieillissement et immunologie: sous-populations lymphocytares sanguines et auto-anticorps seriques. *Medicine Actuelle* **8** (6), 15–18.

Nikitin, V. N. (1984). Experimental approaches to life prolongation. In "Progress of science and technology: general problems of biology" (M. Emanuel, ed.) pp. 6–43. Moscow (in Russian).

Norris, D. M. and Moore, C. L. (1980). Lack of dietary 7-sterol markedly shortens the periods of locomotor vigor, reproduction and longevity of adult female *Xyleborus ferrugineus* (Coleoptera, Scolytidae). *Experimental Gerontology* **15**, 359–364.

Ooka, H. and Shinkai, T. (1986). Effect of chronic hyperthyroidism in the lifespan of the rat. *Mechanisms of Ageing and Development* **33**, 274–282.

Parkhotik, J. J. (1964). Some indices of age pecularities of the course of denervation processes in the muscle. *Fiziologicheskii Zhurnal SSSR* **10**, 803–805 (in Ukrainian).

Piva, F., Maggi, R., Limonta, P. *et al.* (1987). Decrease of opioid receptors in the brain and in the hypothalamus of the aged male rat. *Life Sciences* **40**, 391–398.

Puccini, A. (1986). Ansia e depressione, alla ricerca delle cause vere: alcune storie per capire. *Medicina Geriatrica* **18**, 365–374.

Redgate, E. and Fahringer, E. (1973). A comparison of the pituitary-adrenal activity elicited by electrical stimulation of preoptic, amygdaloid and hypothalamic sites in the rat brain. *Neuroendocrinology* **12**, 334–343.

Sacher, G. A. (1978). Longevity and aging in vertebrate evolution. *Bioscience* **28**, 497–501.

Samorajski, T. and Ordy, J. M. (1972). Neurochemistry of aging. *In* "Aging and the brain" pp. 41–61. Plenum Press, New York.

Sartin, F. L. and Lamperti, A. (1985). Neuron numbers in hypothalamic nuclei of young, middle-aged and aged male rats. *Experientia* **41**, 109–111.

Sato, A., Sato, Y. and Suzuki, H. (1987). Changes in sympatho-adrenal medullary functions during aging. *In* "Organization of the autonomic nervous system: central and peripheral mechanisms" (C. Polosa and F. R. Calaresu, eds) pp. 27–36. Alan R. Liss, New York.

Schulz, R. V. (1982). Emotionality and aging: a theoretical and empirical analysis. *Journal of Gerontology* **37** (1), 42–51.

Selye, H. (1976). "Stress in health and disease" p. 180. Butterworths, Boston.

Shimazu, T. (1980). "Neuronal regulation mechanisms during aging" p. 185. New York.

Shimazu, T., Matsushita, H. and Ishikawa, K. (1978). Hypothalamic control of liver glycogen metabolism in adult and aged rats. *Brain Research* **144**, 343–352.

Sonntag, W., Gonszek, A. and Brodish, A. (1987) Diminished diurnal secretion of adrenocorticotropin (ACTH) but not corticosterone, in old age rats: possible relation to increased adrenal sensitivity to ACTH in vivo. *Endocrinology* **120**, 2308–2316.

Steger, R. W., Sonntag, W. E., Van Vugt, D. A. *et al.* (1980). Reduced ability of naloxone to stimulate LH and testosterone release in aging male rats; possible relation to increase in hypothalamic met⁵-enkephalin. *Life Sciences* **27**, 747–753.

Tang, F., Tang, J., Chou, J. and Costa E. (1984). Age-related and diurnal changes in Met⁵-Enk-Arg⁶-Phe⁷- and Met⁵-Enkephalin contents of pituitary and rat brain structures. *Life Sciences* **25**(9), 1005–1014.

Valueva, G. V., Frolkis, M. V. and Luchitsky, E. V. (1986). Age-related changes of blood neuropeptides in rats. *Fiziologicheskii Zhurnal SSSR* **32**, 604–608 (in Russian).

Verkhratsky, N. S., Moroz, E. V., Magdich, L. V., Didenko, S. O. and Kharazi, L. I. (1988). Steroid-hormone-secretion-regulating system under effect of stress in old age. *Gerontology* **34**, 41–47.

Voitenko, V.P. and Tokar, A.V. (1983). The assessment of biological age and sex differences of human aging. *Experimental Aging Research* **9**, 239–244.

Waldman, A. V., Kozlovskaya, M. M. and Medvedev, O. S. (1979). "Pharmacologic regulation of emotional stress" p. 359. Meditsina, Moscow (in Russian).

Zdichynec, B. (1978). Genealogic incidence of certain civilization diseases in a geriatric population versus pregeriatric group. *Journal of the American Geriatric Society* **26** (12), 534–539.

Discussion

Danon: Dr. Frolkis, you have mentioned that you found also cellular reactions to stress, which are similar to those that occur in aging, e.g. the decline of the immune system. Can you give us more details on changes in lymphocyte subsections, in granulocytes, in blood platelets, or in erythrocytes? I know that a lot of work has been done at your Institute about this.

Frolkis: We are studying only the levels of hormones in man, the contractile activity of the myocard, the structural changes in the myocard, the intensity of protein biosynthesis and RNA synthesis in the myocard and in liver and the system of microsomal oxidation cytochrome reactions, and behavioural reactions.

Danon: What about the circulation of blood cells?

Frolkis: We did not study blood cells.

Angelucci: Regarding the question about the situation of immune-competent cells in older rats, it is certain that mitogenic response of splenocytes is strongly reduced. I would like to make a comment on the first part of Dr. Frolkis's presentation, and also on Dr. Gottfries's presentation. The inhibition of the hypothalamo-pituitary-adrenocortical axis, which occurs both in the aging rat—which is a good experimental model in this direction—and in dementia, is very important. In some way it can really be used as a biological marker of dementia because this inhibition is mainly due to the fact that the special function of the hippocampus is being lost in the demented. The main function of the hippocampus is to compare previous experience and notions with the actual experience, and this is very difficult in the demented patient, as it is very difficult also in the old rat. There is a good example of this situation: the total or partial temporal and spatial disorientation, which is the inability to compare the past with the actual. There is also the important stimulation of the stress-activated hypothalamo-pituitary-adrenocortical axis. So, in view of these facts, maybe we have not a very specific, but a very regular biological marker of the hippocampal dysfunction, as also seen in conditions of dementia.

Scuderi: We have much evidence that hypersecretion of cortisol is secondary to an alteration of central control. I want to know from Prof. Frolkis if he thinks that the alteration of the hypothalamus-pituitary-thyroid axis is secondary to a thyroid failure or to a central control mechanism failure.

Frolkis: It would be secondary to thyroid function but primary to central failure. If one takes rats of 18 months, the level of thyreotropine is high, and only decreases at very old ages of 28 to 30 months.

Hofecker: We submitted rats to severe stress, from the sixth month onward to the end of their lives. As stressor we used overcrowding and noise. In old age the stressed rats showed better results in maze learning, higher spontaneous motor activity, and had a better survival characteristic than unstressed controls. Are these results compatible with the stress–age theory?

Frolkis: In our studies, the groups under stress remained identical and the stress lasted for 3 weeks only. Stress can also be good.

Hofecker: So you think that stress could prevent aging?

Frolkis: Yes.

Ermini: What would you call a good stress, and what would be a bad stress?

Frolkis: Pain, overexposure to light and noise is bad stress.

Angelucci: You asked about good and bad stress. Bad stress derives from unsurmountable situations, whereas good stress comes from situations which can be surmounted. In the Vienna experiment you have to exclude that your rats become easily accustomed to the sound stimulation or to the crowding situation. Maybe they organized it, they knew a hierarchy so that there was a full habituation and there was no more stress.

Ermini: So you would say the difference in the Vienna model was that they develop some kind of habituation to the stress and can turn it rather into a stimulus, and that in Prof. Frolkis's model there is the unused stress situation which is worse.

Angelucci: Yes, but the demonstrated damaging type of stressing procedure is to continuously change the stressor, not to use always the same stressor.

Neuroendocrine Factors in Aging Processes

Arthur V. Everitt

*Ageing and Alzheimer Disease Research Institute,
Repatriation General Hospital, Concord, University of
Sydney, New South Wales, Australia*

INTRODUCTION

The neuroendocrine system secretes hormones which have been shown to modulate many different aging processes (Everitt and Meites 1989). The concept of hormones as factors in aging had its beginnings 100 years ago in Paris, when Brown-Séquard (1889) announced that at age 72 he had been rejuvenated by an extract of testis. While the male sex hormone testosterone has since fallen into disfavour as a rejuvenative agent, the female sex hormone oestrogen is now widely used to counter the many ills of postmenopausal women (Doren and Schneider 1989).

The neuroendocrine system (Fig. 1) is very complex and involves interactions between several centres in the brain, the pituitary and the peripheral endocrine glands (thyroid, adrenal cortex, ovary and testis). Communication between components is achieved by means of neurotransmitters, hormones and other factors such as metabolites, nutrients and immune bodies. The major function of this system is to produce hormones which regulate the activities of almost every cell in the body.

The classical techniques of endocrinology have been used with considerable success to study the role of hormones in aging. Ablation of the pituitary (Jones and Krohn 1961, Everitt and Cavanagh 1965, Bilder and Denckla 1977), thyroid (Giles and Everitt 1967), adrenal (Landfield *et al.* 1978), ovary (Aschheim 1976, Schipper *et al.* 1981) and testis (Robertson and Wexler 1962) have all been shown to slow, delay or prevent the development of many age-associated processes. Conversely the administration of hormones

Challenges in Aging
ISBN 0-12-090163-3

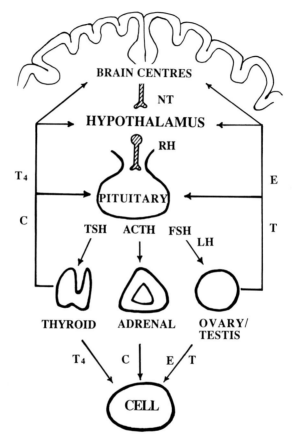

Fig. 1. The neuroendocrine system consists of centres in the brain (pineal, amygdala, hippocampus), the hypothalamus, the pituitary (or hypophysis) and its target glands (thyroid, adrenal cortex, ovary and testis). Centres in the brain secrete neurotransmitters (NT), while the pituitary and its target glands secrete hormones which regulate the actions of specific cells in almost all tissues of the body. The hypothalamus secretes releasing hormones (RH) which promote secretion of specific anterior pituitary hormones (TSH, ACTH, FSH/LH), which in turn control secretion of hormones by the corresponding target glands (thyroid, adrenal cortex, ovary/testis, respectively). Hormone secretion by the hypothalamic-pituitary-endocrine axis is tightly regulated by the feedback of the peripheral hormones thyroxine (T4), cortisol (C), oestrogen (E) or testosterone (T) on the hypothalamic-pituitary unit and other brain centres.

to endocrinectomized or intact animals is known to promote the development of certain age-related processes (Everitt and Meites 1989).

PITUITARY HORMONES

The pituitary gland (or hypophysis) located at the base of the brain occupies a central position in the control of the endocrine system (Fig. 1). It secretes at least ten hormones which regulate its target glands (thyroid, adrenal cortex, ovary, testis) and processes such as metabolism, growth and reproduction. Hypophysectomy, the surgical removal of the pituitary from young or middle-aged rats, inhibits the development of many aging processes (Everitt 1973, 1988). The absence of tissue stimulation by pituitary hormones and reduced stimulation by hormones of the thyroid, adrenal cortex and gonads after hypophysectomy diminishes tissue aging. Reduced hormone secretion also causes large decreases in metabolic rate (Denckla 1974), food intake and growth (Everitt *et al.* 1980) and cardiovascular function (Beznák 1963). A life-long lowering of body function levels might be expected to reduce the "wear and tear" aging of tissues. Reduction of metabolic rate diminishes the formation of metabolites such as free radicals and crosslinkers, thereby decreasing age-related damage in susceptible tissues.

A dietary hypophysectomy (Mulinos and Pomerantz 1940) is achieved by long-term food restriction, which decreases the secretion of most pituitary hormones (Campbell *et al.* 1977, Meites 1989) and retards the progress of many age-related processes (Masoro 1988, Snyder 1989).

These two anti-aging procedures of hypophysectomy and food restriction have been directly compared in a number of studies (Everitt *et al.* 1980, 1983, 1985, Wyndham *et al.* 1987).

The age-related inrease in the tensile strength of collagen fibres in tail tendon of male Wistar rats (Fig. 2) is halved by hypophysectomy and reduced by 30% in food restriction when both groups consume the same amount of food (Everitt *et al.* 1983). Tail tendons are removed from the rat under anaesthesia and tested *in vitro* by measuring the time a 2 g load takes to break an individual fibre immersed in 7 M urea at 40°C (Boros-Farkas and Everitt 1967). In *ad libitum* fed control rats the breaking time increases from 1 min at age 60 days (when rats are hypophysectomized and food restriction begun) to 100 min at 400 days and 200 min at 800 days. Clearly pituitary and other hormones are involved in collagen aging, as well as contributions from dietary factors and metabolites. Both thyroxine (Giles and Everitt 1967) and cortisone (Everitt 1973) have been shown to increase collagen aging.

Kidney aging is likewise inhibited by hypophysectomy and the effect is

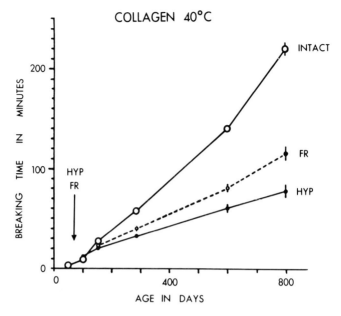

Fig. 2. The effect of age on the tensile strength of collagen fibres in rat tail tendon of control *ad libitum* fed rats (INTACT) as measured by the breaking time in minutes of an isolated fibre under a load of 2 g when immersed in 7 M urea at 40°C. Hypophysectomy (HYP) at age 60 days halves the rate of aging, while food restriction (FR) begun at the same age produces a 30% reduction. Reprinted with permission from Everitt and Wyndham (1982).

greater than that of food restriction (Wyndham *et al.* 1987). The thickness of the glomerular basement membrane (GBM) in the capillary tuft (Fig. 3) increases with age from 100 nm at 60 days at 200 nm at 400 days and 400 nm at 800 days. Like collagen aging, hypophysectomy halves the rate of thickening of the GBM and food restriction reduces it by 30% (Wyndham *et al.* 1987). Pituitary hormones, particularly growth hormone, are factors in GBM thickening (Oikawa *et al.* 1985), and age-related proteinuria (Everitt 1973). Age-related renal enlargement and proteinuria are also markedly inhibited by hypophysectomy (Wyndham *et al.* 1987).

Hind limb muscle age changes such as atrophy, histological changes and the development of hind leg paralysis in very old rats are all inhibited by hypophysectomy and long-term food restriction (Everitt *et al.* 1985). Hind leg paralysis is seen in about one-third of very old male rats aged 1000 days or more, but is completely absent in rats hypophysectomized early in life (Everitt *et al.* 1985).

Gross pathology in old age (Table 1) is greatly reduced in both hypophysectomized and food-restricted rats (Everitt *et al.* 1980). At autopsy

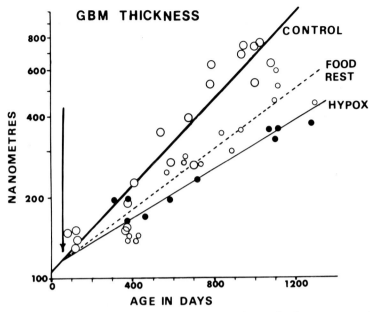

Fig. 3. The effect of age on the thickness of the glomerular basement membrane (GBM) of a capillary tuft in the kidney of the control *ad libitum* fed rat. Hypophysectomy (HYPOX) at age 60 days halves the rate of thickening, while food restriction (FOOD REST) begun at the same age produces a 30% reduction. Reproduced from Wyndham *et al.* (1987) with permission of Elsevier Biomedical Press, Amsterdam.

Table 1

Percentage of conventional male Wistar rats with gross pathology when dying at ages of 800 days or more

	Controls	Hypophysectomized	Food restricted
Number of rats	146	102	56
Any gross lesion	100%	58%	72%
Lung disease	75%	50%	57%
Any tumour	67%	12%	24%
Endocrine tumours	42%	5%	9%
Other tumours	26%	7%	14%
Internal haemorrhage	15%	17%	19%
Adrenal enlargement	75%	0%	7%
Heart enlargement	18%	0%	0%
Kidney enlargement	9%	0%	0%
Hind leg paralysis	29%	0%	6%

Data on smaller numbers of rats are reported elsewhere (Everitt *et al.* 1980; Everitt and Wynham 1982.

all old male control rats aged 800 days or more have one or more gross
disease (lung disease, tumours, hind leg paralysis, internal haemorrhage,
enlarged adrenal, heart or kidney). In hypophysectomized rats gross
pathology is seen in only 58% and in food-restricted rats 72%. Tumour
development appears to be particularly sensitive to pituitary hormones and
nutrition since the incidence is 67% in controls, 24% in food-restricted rats
and 12% in hypophysectomized animals. Some of the reduced pathology in
old age may be due to improved immune function in old hypophysectomized
rodents (Scott *et al*. 1979, Harrison *et al*. 1982).

The life duration of hypophysectomized rats is greater than that of intact
controls when maintained under good animal house conditions of low stress
and warm environment of 27°C, the thermoneutral temperature (Everitt
1988). The diminished secretion of adrenocortical hormones in hypophysectomized rats increases sensitivity to stress, and the reduced thyroid function
impairs the long-term thermogenic response to cold causing body temperature
to fall. Life-long subphysiological injections of cortisone were found to
extend the mean life duration of hypophysectomized rats to 925 days
compared with 785 days for *ad libitum* fed controls (Everitt *et al*. 1980).
Over a 25-year period the maximum life durations in the aging rat colony
at the University of Sydney were 1201 days for *ad libitum* fed male Wistar
controls, 1352 days for hypophysectomized rats and 1515 days for food-
restricted animals (Everitt and Wyndham 1982). Food restriction is better
than hypophysectomy in extending the life span of the rat, probably because
optimal hormone replacement therapy has yet to be determined for
hypophysectomized rats.

Denckla (1974) postulated that aging is due to the action of an unidentified
pituitary factor, decreasing oxygen consumption hormone (DECO). This
factor has not been isolated from the pituitary. He proposed that the
neuroendocrine system produces a death hormone which kills the organism
via actions on the cardiovascular and immune systems (Denckla 1975).

The target glands of hypophysectomized rodents also age at a slower
rate. Ovarian aging as measured by the rate of oocyte loss with age, is
halved by hypophysectomy at an early age in three strains of mice (Jones
and Krohn 1961). Adrenocortical aging is also retarded in hypophysectomized rats, whose adrenal cortex accumulates less age pigment in old age
(Walton *et al*. 1988). Adrenal, thyroid and testicular tumours are present
in reduced numbers in old hypophysectomized rats (Everitt and Wyndham
1982).

THYROID HORMONES

The thyroid gland produces the hormones thyroxine and triiodothyronine,
whose secretion is regulated by pituitary thyrotrophin (TSH). Thyroidec-

tomy, like hypophysectomy, causes large reductions in metabolic rate, food intake, growth and aging of collagen and kidney (Everitt 1976). There is a loss of thyroid hormones and also reduced secretion of pituitary hormones such as growth hormone, corticotrophin and gonadotrophins (Martin and Reichlin 1987).

The anti-aging effects of thyroidectomy on collagen and kidney aging are quantitatively the same as those of food restriction (Giles and Everitt 1967, Everitt 1976). These changes are reversed by long-term thyroxine replacement therapy. Thyroxine injections in old rats which increased food intake by 50% over a period of 5 months produced large increases in collagen (Everitt et al. 1969) and kidney aging (Everitt and Porter 1976). Thyroxine has been shown to increase bone age in hypophysectomized rats (Asling et al. 1954). Life-long hypothyroidism, like hypophysectomy, was found to extend mean life duration in the rat (Ooka et al. 1983), whereas long-term administration of non-toxic doses of thyroxine shortened life duration in the Wistar rat (Ooka and Shinkai 1986).

ADRENOCORTICAL HORMONES

The adrenal cortex secretes steroid hormones (cortisol, corticosterone, aldosterone, dehydroepiandrosterone) whose secretion is controlled by pituitary corticotrophin (ACTH). Complete adrenalectomy kills most rats within a week. Life is prolonged by 1% sodium chloride as drinking water and with the addition of a very small amount of cortisol to the water adrenalectomized rats will survive until old age (Landfield et al. 1981). Long-term adrenalectomy retards morphological age changes in the hippocampus (Landfield et al. 1981), while prolonged cortisol therapy promotes hippocampal age changes (Landfield et al. 1980, Sapolsky et al. 1986). Glucocorticoid treatment over long periods accelerates age-related changes in the cardiovascular system such as arteriosclerosis, hypertension, cardiac hypertrophy and coronary heart disease (Wexler 1976), tail tendon collagen (Everitt 1973) and promotes tumour growth (Sapolsky and Donnelly 1985).

OVARIAN HORMONES

The ovary secretes oestrogens and progesterone during the reproductive phase of life, and the secretion of these hormones is controlled by pituitary gonadotrophins (FSH and LH). Ovariectomy in young rodents delays several age-associated changes in the hypothalamus, preventing loss of oestrous cycles in rats with ovarian grafts (Aschheim 1976), loss of gonadotrophin surges (Mobbs *et al.* 1984) and increased glial activity in the arcuate nucleus of the hypothalamus (Schipper *et al.* 1981). There is good evidence showing that these hypothalamic age changes are promoted by oestrogens secreted by the ovary (Finch and Landfield 1985). Long-continued oestrogen therapy damages the neurons of the arcuate nucleus and medial basal hypothalamus (Brawer *et al.* 1978, Sarkar *et al.* 1982).

Ovariectomy inhibits while oestrogens promote a number of other age-related processes. Removal of the ovary slows the rate of collagen aging in rat tail tendon (Árvay 1976) and oestrogen therapy increases senile osteoarthrosis in mice (Silberberg and Silberberg 1970). Oestrogen promotes the development of mammary and pituitary tumours frequently seen in old rats (Sarkar *et al.* 1983). Ovariectomy reduces the incidence of mammary tumours in old mice (Bittner 1948). Oestrogen replacement therapy used in postmenopausal women to inhibit osteoporosis increases the risk of endometrial carcinoma, cardiovascular problems and gall bladder disease (Gambrell 1982, Coe and Parks 1989).

TESTICULAR HORMONE

The testis secretes testosterone, whose secretion is controlled by pituitary gonadotrophins. Despite the early rejuvenation studies of Brown-Séquard (1889) comparatively little is known of the role of testosterone in aging. The work of Hamilton (1948) suggests that testosterone accelerates aging in certain tissues and shortens life. Castration has been reported to increase the life duration of Pacific salmon (Wexler 1976), rats (Drori and Folman 1976) and human patients in a mental institute (Hamilton and Mestler 1969). Prostatic carcinoma, a major cause of death in elderly men, is not seen in eunuchs or eunuchoids (Moore 1944).

HYPOTHALAMIC FACTORS

The hypothalamus consists of 32 pairs of nuclei which regulate the vegetative functions of the body such as metabolism, temperature, feeding, cardiovascular actions, hormone secretion, sleep and fluid balance which are all necessary to sustain life. The long-term preservation of life and the development of age changes appear to be regulated by at least two different mechanisms, by the hypothalamic control of (1) pituitary hormone secretion and (2) food intake, which are interrelated.

Pituitary Hormone Secretion

The secretion of anterior pituitary hormones is controlled by specific hypophyseotrophic hormones carried in pituitary portal vessels from the hypothalamus to the pituitary. Each hypophyseotrophic hormone (also called releasing or release-inhibiting hormone) is produced in a specific area or nucleus of the hypothalamus (Ganong 1987). For example, the luteinizing hormone releasing hormone or gonadotrophin releasing hormone (LRH, GnRH) is produced by cell bodies located in the preoptic area. The production and secretion of hypophyseotrophic hormones is controlled by neurotransmitters released by nerve endings in the hypothalamus, especially catecholamines (CAs) like norepinephrine (Meites *et al.* 1987).

Reproductive decline in old rats leading to loss of oestrous cycles in females is due primarily to age changes in the hypothalamus (Aschheim 1976, Finch *et al.* 1984). A decrease in norepinephrine (noradrenaline) content of the hypothalamus (Simpkins *et al.* 1977) leads to decreased secretion of GnRH from the hypothalamus (Wise and Ratner 1980). The lack of GnRH secretion by the hypothalamus reduces pituitary LH secretion and stimulation of the ovary, with loss of oestrous cycles. Administration of drugs which increase hypothalamic CAs can reinitiate oestrous cycles in old constant oestrous rats (Clemens and Bennett 1977). The decrease in hypothalamic CAs appears to be due to loss or damage of catecholaminergic neurons caused by the chronic action of oestrogens (Brawer *et al.* 1978, Sarkar *et al.* 1982). In the old rat pituitary gonadotrophin secretion decreases due to the diminished hypothalamic GnRH stimulation of pituitary gonadotropes.

However, in aging women pituitary gonadotrophin secretion rises with age, due to the failure of the ovary rather than the hypothalamus. Thus in old age some age changes are due to a lack of hormones.

Food Intake

It is well known that long-term food restriction inhibits many physiological age changes, delays the onset of age-related pathology and prolongs life in the rodent (Masoro 1988, Snyder 1989). Food may increase the aging rate as a result of aging factors in the diet such as glucose (Cerami 1985), free radicals formed from the metabolism of food (Melhorn and Cole 1985), increased secretion of hormones which have aging actions (Everitt and Meites 1989) and other mechanisms.

Food intake is controlled by feeding centres in the lateral hypothalamus and satiety centres in the ventromedial hypothalamus, which apparently play important roles in aging and the onset of age-related disease. Destruction of the ventromedial nucleus causes overeating which leads to obesity and an

FOOD RESTRICTION

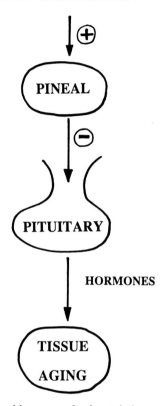

Fig. 4. The inhibitory effect of long-term food restriction on tissue aging mediated by the reduced secretion of hormones with aging effects from the pituitary and its target glands (thyroid, adrenal cortex, ovary and testis). This anti-aging effect appears to be mediated, at least in part, by the pineal gland in the brain, whose secretion of melatonin is increased by prolonged food restriction. Melatonin inhibits the secretion of most anterior pituitary hormones.

early onset of senile kidney lesions (Kennedy 1957). Since hypophysectomy is able to inhibit the development of these renal lesions in obese rats with ventromedial damage, hormonal factors are also involved (Everitt *et al.* 1983). Thus the consumption of food and the aging effects of food appear to be interrelated with neuroendocrine function. Furthermore, food restriction acting over lengthy periods is known to inhibit the secretion of many hormones from the hypothalamus, pituitary, thyroid, ovary and testis (Everitt and Porter 1976, Campbell *et al.* 1977, Merry and Holehan 1985), which have been found to promote aging in various tissues (Everitt and Meites 1989).

The secretion of melatonin from the pineal gland is increased in food restricted rats (Chick *et al.* 1987, Everitt *et al.*, submitted) (Fig. 4). Melatonin is reported to inhibit the secretion of pituitary hormones (Romijn 1978, Banerji and Kothari 1987), prevent the growth of certain tumours (Blask 1984) and prolong the life of the mouse (Maestroni *et al.* 1988). Thus the pineal hormone melatonin may mediate the anti-aging effects of food restriction acting via the pituitary endocrine axis.

CONCLUSION

Neuroendocrine factors affect aging in two ways. In young and middle-aged rodents hormones of the pituitary, thyroid, adrenal cortex, ovary and testis acting over long periods of time have been shown to promote many aging processes. These hormones increase gene expression, metabolism, the level of organ function and produce tissue damage by "wear and tear", by the actions of free radicals and other mechanisms. In old age deficiencies of some hormones produce secondary aging, which may be reversed by appropriate hormone replacement therapy.

ACKNOWLEDGEMENTS

The author is grateful to Professor G. A. Broe and Dr. J. Walton for their support of this project and to Roland Smith for photography.

REFERENCES

Árvay, A. (1976). Reproduction and aging. *In* "Hypothalamus, pituitary and aging" (A. V. Everitt and J. A. Burgess, eds) pp. 362–375. Charles C. Thomas, Springfield, IL.

Aschheim, P. (1976). Aging in the hypothalamo-hypophyseal ovarian axis in the rat. *In* "Hypothalamus, pituitary and aging" (A.V. Everitt and J.A. Burgess, eds) pp. 376–418. Charles C. Thomas, Springfield, IL.

Asling, C. W., Simpson, M. E., Li, C. H. and Evans, H. M. (1954). The effects of chronic administration of thyroxine to hypophysectomized rats on their skeletal growth, maturation and response to growth hormone. *Anatomical Record* **119**, 101–117.

Banerji, A. P. and Kothari, L. (1987). Exposure to continuous light and chronic melatonin administration affects the pituitary protein profiles of the rat. *Neuroendocrinology Letters* **9**, 315–320.

Beznák, M. (1963). Effect of growth hormone and thyroxine on cardiovascular system of hypophysectomized rats. *American Journal of Physiology* **204**, 279–283.

Bilder, G. E. and Denckla, W. D. (1977). Restoration of the ability to reject xenografts and clear carbon after hypophysectomy of adult rats. *Mechanisms of Ageing and Development* **8**, 153–163.

Bittner, J. J. (1948). The causes and control of mammary cancer in mice. *Harvey Lectures* **42**, 221–246.

Blask, D. E. (1984). The pineal: an oncostatic gland? *In* "The pineal gland" (R.J. Reiter, ed.) pp. 253–284. Raven Press, New York.

Boros-Farkas, M. and Everitt, A. V. (1967). Comparative studies of age tests on collagen fibres. *Gerontologia* **13**, 37–49.

Brawer, J. R., Naftolin, F., Martin, J. and Sonnenscheim, C. (1978). Effects of a single injection of estradiol valerate on the hypothalamic arcuate nucleus and on reproductive function in the female rat. *Endocrinology* **103**, 501–512.

Brown-Séquard, C. D. (1889). Des effects produits chez l'homme par des injections sous-cutanées d'un liquide retiré des testicules frais de cobaye et de chien. *Comptes Rendus de la Societe de Biologie* **41**, 415–422.

Campbell, G. A., Kurcz, M., Marshall, S. and Meites, J. (1977). Effects of starvation on serum levels of follicle stimulating hormone, luteinizing hormone, thyrotropin, growth hormone and prolactin; response to LH-releasing hormone and thyrotropin releasing hormone. *Endocrinology* **100**, 580–587.

Cerami, A. (1985). Hypothesis: glucose as a mediator of aging. *Journal of the American Geriatrics Society* **33**, 626–634.

Chick, C. L., Ho, A. K. and Brown, G. M. (1987). Effect of food restriction on 24-h serum and pineal melatonin content in male rats. *Acta Endocrinologica* **115**, 507–513.

Clemens, J. A. and Bennett, D. R. (1977). Do aging changes in the preoptic area contribute to loss of cyclic endocrine function? *Journal of Gerontology* **32**, 19–24.

Coe, F. L. and Parks, J. H. (1989). The risks of oral contraceptives and estrogen replacement therapy. *Perspectives in Biology and Medicine* **33**, 86–109.

Denckla, W. D. (1974). Role of the pituitary and thyroid glands on the decline of minimal O_2 consumption with age. *Journal of Clinical Investigation* **53**, 572–581.

Denckla, W. D. (1975). A time to die. *Life Sciences* **16**, 31–44.

Doren, M. and Schneider H.P.G. (1989). Overall rationale for hormonal substitution therapy after the menopause. *In* "Update on hormonal treatment in the menopause" (M. L. Hermite, ed.) pp. 1–15. S. Karger, Basel.

Drori, D. and Folman, Y. (1976). Environmental effects on longevity in the male rat: exercise, mating, castration and restricted feeding. *Experimental Gerontology* **11**, 25–32.

Everitt, A. V. (1973). The hypothalamic-pituitary control of ageing and age-related pathology. *Experimental Gerontology* **8**, 265–277.

Everitt, A. V. (1976). The thyroid gland, metabolic rate and aging. *In* "Hypothalamus, pituitary and aging" (A. V. Everitt and J. A. Burgess, eds) pp. 511–528. Charles C. Thomas, Springfield, IL.

Everitt, A. V. (1988). Hormonal basis of aging: antiaging action of hypophysectomy. *In* "Regulation of neuroendocrine aging" (A.V. Everitt and J.R. Walton, eds) pp. 51–60. S. Karger, Basel.

Everitt, A. V. and Cavanagh, L. M. (1965). The ageing process in the hypophysectomized rat. *Gerontologia* **11**, 198–207.

Everitt, A. V. and Meites, J. (1989). Aging and anti-aging effects of hormones. *Journal of Gerontology* **44**, B139–B147.

Everitt, A. V. and Porter, B. (1976). Nutrition and aging. *In* "Hypothalamus, pituitary and aging" (A. V. Everitt and J. A. Burgess, eds) pp. 570–613. Charles C. Thomas, Springfield, IL.

Everitt, A. V. and Wyndham, J. R. (1982). Hypothalamic pituitary regulation and aging. *In* "Endocrine and neuroendocrine mechanisms of aging" (R. C. Adelman and G. S. Roth, eds) pp. 123–165. CRC Press, Boca Raton, FL.

Everitt, A. V., Giles, J. S. and Gal, A. (1969). The role of thyroid and food intake in the ageing of collagen fibres II. In the old rat. *Gerontologia* **15**, 366–373.

Everitt, A. V., Seedsman, N. J. and Jones, F. (1980). The effects of hypophysectomy and continuous food restriction, begun at ages 70 and 400 days, on collagen aging, proteinuria, incidence of pathology and longevity in the male rat. *Mechanisms of Ageing and Development* **12**, 161–172.

Everitt, A. V., Wyndham, J. R. and Barnard, D. L. (1983). The anti-aging action of hypophysectomy in hypothalamic obese rats: effects on collagen aging, age-associated proteinuria development and renal histopathology. *Mechanisms of Ageing and Development* **22**, 233–251.

Everitt, A. V., Shorey, C. D. and Ficarra, M. A. (1985). Skeletal muscle aging in the hind limb of the old male Wistar rat. Inhibitory effect of hypophysectomy and food restriction. *Archives of Gerontology and Geriatrics* **4**, 401–415.

Everitt, A. V., Parks, A., Eyland, A., Cairncross, K. D., Destefanis, P. and Maxwell, K. Inhibitory effect of neonatal pinealectomy on the puberty-delaying action of food restriction on the female Wistar rat. *Journal of Pineal Research* (submitted).

Finch, C. E. and Landfield, P. W. (1985). Neuroendocrine and autonomic functions in aging mammals. *In* "Handbook of the biology of aging" 2nd edn (C.E. Finch and E. L. Schneider, eds) pp. 567–594. Van Nostrand Reinhold, New York.

Finch, C. E. Felicio, L. S., Mobbs, C. V. and Nelson, J. F. (1984). Ovarian and steroidal influences on neuroendocrine aging processes in female rodents. *Endocrinology Review* **5**, 467–497.

Gambrell, R. D. (1982). The menopause: benefits and risks of estrogen: progestogen replacement therapy. *Fertility and Sterility* **37**, 457–474.

Ganong, W. F. (1987). "Review of medical physiology" 13th edn. Lange Medical Publ., Los Altos, CA.

Giles, J. S. and Everitt, A. V. (1967). The role of the thyroid and food intake in the ageing of collagen fibres I. In the young rat. *Gerontologia* **13**, 65–69.

Hamilton, J. B. (1948). The role of testicular secretions as indicated by the effects of castration in man and by studies of pathological conditions and the short life span associated with maleness. *Recent Progress in Hormone Research* **3**, 257–322.

Hamilton, J. B. and Mestler, G. E. (1969). Mortality and survival. Comparison of eunuchs with intact men and women in a mentally retarded population. *Journal of Gerontology* **24**, 395–411.

Harrison, D. E., Archer, J. R. and Astle, C. M. (1982). The effect of hypophysectomy on thymic aging in mice. *Journal of Immunology* **129**, 2673–2677.

Jones, E. C. and Krohn, P. L. (1961). The effect of hypophysectomy on age changes in the ovaries of mice. *Journal of Endocrinology* **21**, 497–509.

Kennedy, G. C. (1957). Effects of old age and overnutrition on the kidney. *British Medical Bulletin* **13**, 67–70.

Landfield, P., Waymire, J. and Lynch, G. (1978). Hippocampal aging and adrenocorticoids: a quantitative correlation. *Science* **202**, 1098–1102.

Landfield, P. W., Sundberg, D. K., Smith, M. S., Eldridge, J. C. and Morris,

M. (1980). Mammalian aging: theoretical implications of changes in brain and endocrine systems during mid and late life. *Peptides* **1** (Suppl.), 185–196.

Landfield, P. W., Baskin, R. and Pitler, T. A. (1981). Brain aging correlates: retardation by hormonal–pharmacological treatments. *Science* **214**, 581–584.

Maestroni, G. J. M., Conti, A. and Pierpaoli, W. (1988). Pineal melatonin, its fundamental immunoregulatory role in aging and cancer. *Annals of the New York Academy of Sciences* **521**, 140–148.

Martin, J. B. and Reichlin, S. (1987). "Clinical neuroendocrinology" 2nd edn. F.A. Davis, Philadelphia.

Masoro, E. J. (1988). Minireview: Food restriction in rodents: An evaluation of its role in the study of aging. *Journal of Gerontology* **43**, B59–B64.

Meites, J. (1989). Evidence that underfeeding acts via the neuroendocrine system to influence aging processes. *In* "Dietary restriction and aging" (D. L. Snyder, ed.) pp. 169–180, Alan R. Liss, New York.

Meites, J., Goya, R. and Takahashi, S. (1987). Why the neuroendocrine system is important in aging processes. *Experimental Gerontology* **22**, 1–15.

Melhorn, R. J. and Cole, G. (1985). The free radical theory of aging: a critical review. *Advances in Free Radical Biology and Medicine* **1**, 165–223.

Merry, B. J. and Holehan, A. M. (1985). The endocrine response to dietary restriction in the rat. *In* "Molecular biology of aging" (A. D. Woodhead, A. D. Blackett and A. Hollaender, eds) pp. 117–141. Plenum Press, New York.

Mobbs, C. V., Gee, D. M. and Finch, C. E. (1984). Reproductive senescence in C57BL/6J mice: ovarian impairments and neuroendocrine impairments that are partially reversible and delayed by ovariectomy. *Endocrinology* **115**, 1653–1662.

Moore, R. A. (1944). Benign hypertrophy and carcinoma of the prostate. *Surgery* **16**, 152–167.

Mulinos, M. G. and Pomerantz, L. (1940). Pseudohypophysectomy, a condition resembling hypophysectomy, produced by malnutrition. *Journal of Nutrition* **19**, 493–504.

Oikawa, S., Maruhama, Y. and Goto, Y. (1985). Evidence for direct effect of growth hormone on capillary basement membrane thickness. *Tohoku Journal of Experimental Medicine* **146**, 167–174.

Ooka, H. and Shinkai, T. (1986). Effects of chronic hyperthyroidism on the lifespan of the rat. *Mechanisms of Ageing and Development* **33**, 275–282.

Ooka, H., Fujita, S. and Yoshimoto, E. (1983). Pituitary-thyroid activity and longevity in neonatally thyroxine-treated rats. *Mechanisms of Ageing and Development* **22**, 113–120.

Robertson, O. H. and Wexler, B. C. (1962). Histological changes in the organs and tissues of senile castrated Kokanee salmon (*Oncorhynchus nerka Kennerlyi*). *General and Comparative Endocrinology* **2**, 458–472.

Romijn, R. (1978). The pineal, a tranquilizing organ? *Life Sciences* **23**, 2257–2274.

Sapolsky, R. and Donnelly, T. (1985). Vulnerability to stress-induced tumor growth increases with age in the rat: role of glucocorticoid hypersecretion. *Endocrinology* **117**, 662–666.

Sapolsky, R. M., Krey, L. C. and McEwen, B. S. (1986). The neuroendocrinology of stress and aging: the glucocorticoid cascade hypothesis. *Endocrinology Review* **7**, 284–301.

Sarkar, D. K., Gottschall, P. E. and Meites, J. (1982). Damage to hypothalamic dopaminergic neurons is associated with the development of prolactin-secreting tumors. *Science* **218**, 684–686.

Sarkar, D. K., Gottschall, P. E. and Meites, J. (1983). Relation of the neuroendocrine system to development of prolactin-secreting pituitary tumors. *In* "Neuroendocrinology of aging" (J. Meites, ed.) pp. 353–376. Plenum Press, New York.

Schipper, H., Brawer, J. R., Melson, J. F., Felicio, L. S. and Finch, C. E. (1981). Role of the gonads in the histologic aging of the hypothalamic arcuate nucleus. *Biology of Reproduction* **25**, 413–419.

Scott, M., Bolla, R. and Denckla, W. D. (1979). Age-related changes in immune function of rats and the effect of long-term hypophysectomy. *Mechanisms of Ageing and Development* **11**, 127–136.

Silberberg, M. and Silberberg, R. (1970). Age-related modification of the effect of estrogen on joints and cortical bone of female mice. *Gerontologia* **16**, 201–211.

Simpkins, J. W., Mueller, G. P., Huang, H. H. and Meites, J. (1977). Evidence for depressed catecholamine and enhanced serotonin metabolism in aging male-rats: possible relation to gonadotrophin secretion. *Endocrinology* **100**, 1672–1678.

Snyder, D. L. (1989). "Dietary restriction and aging". Alan R. Liss, New York.

Walton, J., Pruss J. and Everitt, A. V. (1988). Adrenocortical cell turnover and aging in growth-retarded rats. *In* "Regulation of neuroendocrine aging" (A. V. Everitt and J. R. Walton, eds) pp. 74–80. S. Karger, Basel.

Wexler, B. C. (1976). Comparative aspects of hyperadrenocorticism and aging. *In* "Hypothalamus, pituitary and aging" (A. V. Everitt and J. A. Burgess, eds) pp. 333–361. Charles C. Thomas, Springfield, IL.

Wise, P. M. and Ratner, A. (1980). Effect of ovariectomy on plasma LH, FSH, estradiol and progesterone and medial basal hypothalamic LHRH concentrations in old and young rats. *Neuroendocrinology* **30**, 15–19.

Wyndham, J. R., Everitt, A. V., Eyland, A. and Major, J. (1987). Inhibitory effect of hypophysectomy and food restriction on glomerular basement membrane thickening, proteinuria and renal enlargement in aging male Wistar rats. *Archives of Gerontology and Geriatrics* **6**, 323–337.

Discussion

Hesse: Dr. Everitt, I think I have a solution for your paradox of adrenalectomized rats found 20 years ago. We examined the corticosterone production of rats which were adrenalectomized 4 weeks after the operation and found they had more corticosterone than normal rats, and we also found that they built up accessory adrenal glands. And when you give adrenalectomized rats cortisol, I think they will not develop these glands.

Everitt: Yes, this is a well-known phenomenon; actually, if the adrenalectomy is complete and there are no accessory glands developing, then the rats survive, although limited to 1 week or so. Certainly there are some strains, I understand, of rats, where this does happen more so than in others, where the accessory glands do develop.

von Hahn: As successor to Fritz Verzar, directing the Institute of Experimental Gerontology, I would very much like to thank both Prof. Frolkis and Prof. Everitt for their mentioning him here. I think he deserves every word. To us he was the father of experimental gerontology, and both Marco Ermini, who is in the chair today, and myself learned our gerontology and very many other things from him. He was a kind-hearted and terrible-tempered man at the same time, and all of us who ever worked with him—and I know that Arthur Everitt worked with him several times—have benefited tremendously.

I would like to make one point about the aging effects of hormones. It seems to me that findings like that speak quite clearly against any kind of evolutionary mechanism for the development of aging. It seems to me that hormones were made to get the animal up to the reproductive age as fit as possible to ensure reproduction, and if then the hormones later on start to damage metabolism, to kill cells, then this is, to my mind, something which nature really did not plan. As all of us know, we find old animals really only where man has interfered with the evolution— household animals, zoo animals, kept animals. In any case in wild animals, as L. Hayflick recently remarked in a very stimulating paper, you would not find a mechanism like that. Would you like to comment on that?

Everitt: In terms of the effects of the hormones on the tissues in relation to evolution, unfortunately I have not given this as much thought as I really should have. All I can say is that I thank you for drawing my attention to it.

Loss of Agonist-receptor Efficacy in Senescence: Possible Decrements in Second Messenger Function and Calcium Mobilization

J. A. Joseph and G. S. Roth

Molecular Physiology and Genetics Section, Gerontology Research Center/NIA, Baltimore, Maryland, USA

INTRODUCTION

One of the hallmarks of the aging process that has been studied for many years is a decrease in responsiveness that occurs in a variety of peripheral and central receptor-mediated systems. This loss usually takes the form of a reduced physiological response to ligand receptor activation and translates into diminished physiological adaptation to various stimuli (Shock *et al.* 1984). As of this writing there have been a host of systems that have been examined which have shown reduced responsiveness to pharmacological and hormonal stimulation in senescence. These include: decreased β-adrenergic receptor-mediated relaxation of vasculature (e.g. Deisher *et al.* 1989, Hiremath *et al.* 1989); decreased β-adrenergic receptor-mediated modulation of cardiovascular function (see Lakatta 1986); decreases in inhibitory efficacy of norepinephrine on electrophysiological responses of the cerebellar Purkinje cells (Hoffer *et al.* 1988); reduced effects of the monoamine oxidase inhibitor, nialamide on nucleus accumbens in old rats (Cousins *et al.* 1986); reduced rotational behavioural responses to the dopamine) stimulating agent, amphetamine in senescent rats (Joseph *et al.* 1978). These alterations appear to take place for a variety of reasons (e.g. reduced receptor density, altered receptor second messenger activation etc., see below). However, the interaction of this multiplicity of factors producing reductions in responsivity can translate into diminished behavioural adaptability.

Such reduced adaptation can take many forms ranging from difficulties in avoiding oncoming traffic to decreased ability to combat infectious agents, to impaired ability to withstand extremes of temperature. While we recognize that similar decrements in hormonal responsiveness can occur in various physiological and pathological states independent of senescence (e.g. Chrousos et al. 1986, Melnechuk 1978), they can also occur as part of the "normal aging process". In fact, the problem is further complicated by the fact that aging may predispose the individual to many types of disease (Johnson 1985, Shock et al. 1984). However, not all individuals manifest these types of deterioration at the same rate or with the same incidence. What, then, are the mechanisms by which the efficacy of various hormones and transmitters involved in the regulation of biological function is reduced as a function of aging? We have alluded to at least two of these possible mechanisms, i.e. decreases in receptor concentrations and impaired second messenger induction. The second of these mechanisms could be the result of decrements at several points (e.g. alterations in receptor-G-protein coupling, reduced phospholipase C activation; lowered induction of inositol trisphosphate, adenylate cyclase (see below); reduced ability to form high affinity complexes with ligands) in the signal transduction pathways which result in reduced Ca^{2+} mobilization (see Roth 1989 for review).

Given these considerations, our research has focused on trying to determine the locus or loci in the signal transduction pathways that could account for the reduced responsiveness in senescence. In order to accomplish this the work has utilized three model systems: perifused striatal slices from mature and senescent animals, parotid cell aggregates and pituitary cells. In the parotid cell aggregate system we have assessed α-adrenergic stimulated K^+ release and Ca^{2+} efflux, while in the pituitary cells determinations of luteinizing hormone releasing hormone (LHRH)-stimulated luteinizing hormone release were made. In the perifused striatal slices studies have been carried out to assess muscarinic regulation of dopamine release. This model has proven to be very sensitive for evaluating the efficacy of muscarinic agonists in senescence. A great deal of previous work has indicated only minimal success in improving performance on tasks which assess memory in senescent animals or humans through the use of agents which enhance muscarinic cholinergic function. Use of the striatal model has allowed us to observe the possible cellular basis for these minimal improvements.

CHANGES IN MUSCARINIC RESPONSIVENESS IN SENESCENCE

As indicated in the introduction central muscarinic reponsiveness declines as a function of age. Our research has attempted to determine the nature of changes that might account for this "age-induced mAChR desensitization".The loss of sensitivity manifests itself in several parameters that involve reduced: (a) basal and stimulated ACh release (Thompson *et al.* 1984) and (b) activity of muscarinic agonists to inhibit dopamine (DA)-stimulated adenylate cyclase from striatal broken-cell preparations (Coupet *et al.* 1985). The latter of these preparations showed that the muscarinic agonists oxotremorine and carbachol were effective in young (6 months old) and middle-aged (12 months old) animals in inhibiting DA-stimulated adenylate cyclase but not in old (24 months old). More recent studies have indicated an inability of muscarinic agonists to regulate striatal DA function (Joseph *et al.* 1988a, b, Joseph and Roth, in press).

It has been known for several years that striatal DA release is under the control of a group of striatal D_2 (subtype) autoreceptors (Dwoskin and Zahniser 1986). If these autoreceptors are enhanced or inhibited, K^+-evoked release of DA will be respectively enhanced or inhibited (see Joseph *et al.* 1988a, b). This control is mediated through inhibitory presynaptic cholinergic heteroreceptors presumably located on the same terminals as the autoreceptors (Raiteri *et al.* 1984). Cholinergic agonist stimulation of perifused striatal slices normally results in enhancement of K^+-evoked release of DA. However, Joseph *et al.* (1988a) demonstrated that even though no age-related differences were observed in levels of striatal DA or in K+-evoked release of DA from perifused striatal slices significant reductions in the efficacy of several muscarinic agonists (e.g. oxotremorine, carbachol) to enhance K^+-evoked release of DA were apparent. Application of some agonists (e.g. carbachol) resulted in diminished responding as early as 12 months of age.

These deficits in mAChR responsiveness to agonist stimulation appear to extend to the hippocampus as well. In this latter region, both extracellular (Lippa *et al.* 1985) and intracellular (Segal 1982) recording studies have revealed a highly selective reduction in the ability of iontophoretically applied ACh to increase the excitability of hippocampal pyramidal cells. Moreover, Lippa *et al.* (1985) also suggested that this diminished responsivity began at about 15–16 months of age, at which time reductions in the burst firing rate of these cells to applied ACh were observed. Further reductions were observed in the senescent (24 months old) group.

Thus these studies, as well as those cited above, suggest that there are profound, consistent age-related declines in the sensitivity of mAChR to agonist stimulation beginning around middle age in the rodent. Given findings such as these, it is not surprising that previous work has indicated only minimal success in improving performance on tasks which assess memory function in senescent animals or humans through use of agents which enhance cholinergic functioning (e.g. Bartus *et al*. 1985).

An important question becomes what alterations occur in the functioning of the muscarinic receptor to blunt its responsiveness to agonists? The answer to this question may have important implications for therapeutic efforts directed toward improving memory in normal aging and in dementing diseases such as Alzheimer's disease.

Previous research has assessed a variety of parameters to determine muscarinic function in senescence, including high affinity choline uptake (HACU), acetylcholinesterase (AChE) and choline acetyltransferase (ChAT) activities, muscarinic receptor binding, and cellular and neuronal densities.

ChAT, HACU and AChE

Examinations of ChAT activity have indicated decreases (McGeer *et al*. 1971, Meek *et al*. 1977 Strong *et al*. 1982) in the rodent striatum by some investigators. Others have reported no change (e.g. Morin and Wasterlain 1980). No consistent age-related findings in this parameter have been seen in cortex or hippocampus as well (e.g. see Decker 1987 for review). Generally, changes in ChAT in areas such as the hippocampus and cortex that occur as a function of normal aging are less reliable than those seen in Alzheimer's disease.

The reasons for these inconsistent findings are numerous and could include assay procedures (Waller *et al*. 1983) or sex/strain/species differences (Luine *et al*. 1986, Strong *et al*. 1980). One other important consideration is the precise localization of the neural area utilized for the assay. This appears to be especially true when HACU is assessed. While several studies have reported no age-related differences in this parameter in cortex (e.g. Consolo *et al*. 1986) or hippocampus (Sherman *et al*. 1981), an additional study (Strong *et al*. 1986) indicated significant intrastriatal differences in HACU.

The results with respect to AChE have been even more contradictory than those for ChAT. Various studies have indicated that declines in this parameter range from 0 to 26% in the rodent (e.g. Morin and Wasterlain 1980) and are less than 20% in the aged human. Thus, the variability of these results makes it difficult to explain loss of responsiveness using these parameters.

Muscarinic Receptor Binding

If this parameter is considered, there is better general agreement that there are decreases in the number of binding sites in several brain areas, including the striatum as a function of age. Using the ligand ^{3}H $(-)$ [^{3}H]-quinuclidinyl benzilate (^{3}H-QNB), these studies have generally shown changes in the concentration of muscarinic receptors (mAChR) of about 11–36% in the hippocampus (Kubanis et al. 1982, Waller and London 1983, Lippa et al. 1985) and cortex (Strong et al. 1980, Kubanis et al. 1982, Pedigo and Polk 1985, Norman et al. 1986). More recent studies have generally supported these findings (e.g. cortex and hippocampus, Bigeon et al. 1988, Gurwitz et al. 1987) and extended them to the striatum where reductions similar to those observed in cortex and hippocampus were observed (10–20%, Bigeon et al. 1988, 19%, Gurwitz et al. 1987).

Distribution of these receptors within the striatum was similar to that seen for the DA (D_2 subtype) receptors, being highest in the rostral region and lowest in the caudal portion of the striatum. Muscarinic (m) AChR were lost as a function of age primarily from the medial and caudal portions of the striatum (Strong et al. 1982). However, in a later study using Fischer rather than Sprague Dawley rats by this group (Strong et al. 1986) significant mAChR loss of about 20% throughout the striatum was observed. Strain differences appear again to be important in this regard.

There have been no attempts to determine the pattern of loss of mAChR subtypes (see below) (M_1 and M_2) as a function of normal aging. Bigeon et al. (1988) utilized 100 μM carbachol in the incubation medium (see Mash and Potter 1986) for preliminary autoradiographic analysis of M_1 receptor distribution, but no significant differences as a function of age were seen. These findings support a previous experiment using the putative M_1 antagonist, pirenzepine (Norman et al. 1986). Detailed analyses of alterations in muscarinic receptor subtypes in senescence are likely to be facilitated by the use of AF-DX 116, a selective M_2 antagonist and the development of specific cDNA probes which, when used with in situ hybridization, can determine age differences in regional expression of four muscarinic receptor subtypes (m_1–m_4). At present pharmacologic agents which distinguish only between the M_1 may consist of three gene products (m_1, m_3, m_4: Bonner et al. 1987; Brann et al. 1988) and M_2 mAChR subtypes.

Autoradiographic analysis by Bigeon et al. (1988) and Blake et al. (in press) also revealed that the pattern of mAChR loss throughout the brain was highest in areas such as the striatum which contain high concentrations of cholinergic perikaryon. Thus, a selective loss of cholinergic neurons could be a contributing factor to the decline in mAChR concentration. Studies by Albanese et al. (1985) and Gozzo et al. (1986) have indicated, using AChE staining techniques, a loss of forebrain cholinergic neurons as a function of age. Armstrong *et al.* (1988), using immunocytochemical staining for ChAT, observed swollen cholinergic profiles and "grapelike clusters of immunoreactivity" in the neocortex and cingulate of the aged Fischer rat. Similar findings have been reported in aged humans and non-human primates (Struble *et al.* 1982, Kitt *et al.* 1984, Armstrong *et al.* 1986, Tago *et al.* 1987). In support of these latter findings, Adams (1987) reported decreases in the number of synapses and increases in the length of the postsynaptic contact zone in human precentral motor cortex. Additional experiments by Altavista *et al.* (1988) using AChE staining extended these findings to the striatum to show that the size of the neostriatum as well as the number of putative, cholinergic, AChE-positive perikaryon are significantly reduced as of 24 months in the rat. Cell density deceased by approximately 16%. The loss is most pronounced in the dorsal, lateral, and ventromedial areas of the striatum. Unfortunately, this study employed only four animals from two age groups (3 and 24 months) to make these determinations so the results are inconclusive. Nevertheless, when taken together with previous studies cited above, they suggest that nearly all of the mAChR loss in the aged striatum can be accounted for by neuronal loss. In this respect, these findings differ from the striatal D_1 and D_2 results wherein only 50% of the age-related decline could be accounted for by neuronal loss (Han *et al.* 1989). It is interesting to note in this regard that a recent assessment in our laboratory of mRNA activity for m_1, m_2, m_3, and m_4 mAChR subtypes using *in situ* hybridization has indicated no age-related declines in any brain region examined (Blake *et al.* in press). These findings suggest that although there is a small decline in mAChR concentration this decrement is not the result of a transcription deficit and may also argue against neuronal loss unless a compensatory mechanism is involved.

In summary the studies cited thus far in this section indicate that, generally, there are variable changes in these rather static indices. Such small changes (which are species and strain dependent) provide little insight as to the nature of the rather profound decline in muscarinic responsivity described above.

Cross-talk among Second Messenger Systems

It would be tempting to speculate that the rather small decline in central mAChR is at least partially responsible for the reductions in agonist/receptor efficacy. However, previous research in at least one other receptor system has indicated that significant age-related reductions occur in the concentrations of both dopamine D_1 and D_2 receptor subtypes (see Joseph and Roth 1988) but few indications are found in the literature to suggest loss of responsiveness to pharmacological stimulation even in the face of this significant result ($> 30\%$ loss, see Joseph and Roth 1988 for review). Joseph *et al.* (1988a, b) observed no reductions in K^+-evoked release of DA in striatal tissue from senescent animals. These findings support those of earlier work (Thompson *et al.* 1981) in the striatal slice, and at least partially support a study by Rose *et al.* (1986) in which DA release was assessed in the striatal slice using *in vivo* voltometry. Very preliminary findings from our laboratory, using microdialysis, indicate no decrements in striatal DA release following direct cocaine application to this area. Moreover, Joseph *et al.* (1988a) have shown that if DA autoreceptors are directly inhibited by haloperidol, or inhibited via activation of nicotinic heteroreceptors, no age-related decrements are observed in the enhancement of K^+-evoked release of DA. Therefore, simple explanations implying that receptor loss in a striatal cholinergic system are sufficient to explain functional loss in agonist responsiveness are not adequate. Rather, it may be necessary to examine possible age-related reductions in signal transduction parameters to explain decrements in responsiveness in this system.

An enormous amount of data has accumulated in recent years showing that ligand activation of mAChRs results in Ca^{2+} mobilization brought about through a signal transduction process involving ligand-induced increases in the turnover of phosphatidylinositol (PI) (through the activation of G proteins), a product which may be further phosphorylated to break down phosphatidylinositol 4,5-bisphosphate (PIP_2). Phospholipase C, activated by the ligand–receptor complex, cleaves PIP_2. One product resulting from this cleavage is 1,4,5-inositol trisphosphate (IP_3) which diffuses into the cytoplasm, releases Ca^{2+} from storage and ultimately induces a physiological response (see Fisher and Agranoff 1987). As of this writing, few experiments have attempted to make these determinations in central mAChR systems. However, findings from at least one suggest that if the mAChR is bypassed and Ca^{2+} mobilized directly with the Ca^{2+} ionophore A23187 or IP_3 no age-related deficits in enhancement of K^+-evoked release are observed (Joseph *et al.* 1988b). These observations suggest that the deficits may occur at the receptor/ligand interface or very early in the signal transduction process. Indeed, a greater number of receptors probably exist in desensitized states in both hippocampus (Lippa *et al.* 1985) and possibly striatum (Joseph *et al.*, in preparation). These receptors may be permanently coupled to G proteins and are unable to uncouple upon stimulation. Thus, the α subunits of the G proteins could not be uncoupled from the respective β–γ subunits and the first step of the transduction sequence cannot be initiated. Numerous studies have indicated that depending upon the particular mAChR subtype, these receptors may be coupled to G_p(2) or G_i (Weiss *et al.* 1988). At present, pharmacological agents which would distinguish among these mAChR

J. A. Joseph and G. S. Roth

Table 1

Effects of various combinations of carbachol, oxotremorine and arachidonic acid on dopamine and IP_3 release (pmol mg^{-1} protein, $\pm$ SEM) from striatal tissue

	DA release			IP_3 release	
	6 months	24 months	ns	6 months	24 months
KCl	104 $\pm$ 7	104 $\pm$ 7	9,11	0	0
Carbachol	155 $\pm$ 12	100 $\pm$ 8	12,11	80 $\pm$ 2	40 $\pm$ 3
Oxotremorine	161 $\pm$ 9	103 $\pm$ 10	10,9	32 $\pm$ 3	10 $\pm$ 2
Oxotremorine + carbachol	163 $\pm$ 12	175 $\pm$ 15	4,4	30 $\pm$ 1	50 $\pm$ 5
Arachidonic acid	158 $\pm$ 13	85 $\pm$ 10	14,13		
Arachidonic acid + oxotremorine	159 $\pm$ 11	160 $\pm$ 5	4,4		
Arachidonic acid + carbachol	178 $\pm$ 4	157 $\pm$ 13	4,4		

KCl 30 mM, oxotremorine 500 μM, carbachol 500 μM, arachidonic acid 10 μM.

subtypes do not exist. The specifications of these agents and the determinations of which mAChR subtypes couple to respective G_p or G_i proteins await further specification.

However, even given these considerations, recent evidence from our laboratory has indicated that it is possible to "resensitize" the mAChR in striatal tissue from senescent animals by taking advantage of "cross talk" (Hill and Kendall 1989) that exists between second messenger systems. To elaborate, following mAChR agonist stimulation second messengers such as IP_3 must reach a certain threshold for a response to take place. Since this does not appear to occur in old animals, we attempted to lower the second messenger threshold necessary for a response to take place by simultaneously activating and inhibiting more than one second messenger system. It is known that carbachol stimulates PI hydrolysis (Fisher and Agranoff 1987). In addition, this mAChR agonist also inhibits cyclic AMP activity (Harden et al. 1986, Anderson and Mckinney 1988, Schoffelmeer et al. 1988, McKinney et al. 1989), while oxotremorine primarily inhibits cyclic AMP activity (Anderson and Mckinney 1988, Cockcroft and Stutchfield 1988, Schoffelmeer et al. 1988) and has little effect on PI hydrolysis. Thus, we determined the effects of combined application of carbachol and oxotremorine to perifused striatal slices from old anaimals on K^+-evoked DA release. The results indicated that, as reported previously (Joseph et al. in press), enhancement of K^+-evoked DA release was lower in striatal tissue from 24-month-old animals to either of these agents applied alone and this was accompanied to reduced IP_3 activation (Table 1).

However simultaneous application of these agonists enhanced K^+-evoked DA release to the same extent in the striatal tissue from young and old animals even though age differences in IP_3 activation remained (Table 1). Moreover coapplication of arachidonic acid which has a variety of direct and indirect second messenger effects (e.g. see Axelrod et al. 1988 for review) with either carbachol or oxotremorine also produced enhancement of K^+-evoked DA release to the same extent in striatal tissue from young and old animals (Table 1).

Thus, these findings suggest that until research efforts determine the locus (i) of the age-related deficits in muscarinic function (i.e. G protein coupling, alterations in receptor structure etc.) methods to improve mAChR functioning might utilize procedures which can affect more than one second messenger system simultaneously. Synergistic activity among these systems may greatly facilitate nervous transmission and subsequent physiological responses. At present, these explorations have not been done with respect to aging.

Alpha₁-adrenergic and Muscarinic Stimulation of Parotid Secretion

In order to gain a more generalized understanding of the effects of aging on IP_3/Ca^{2+}-dependent signal transduction, we have paralleled our studies in the brain with a well-characterized model of stimulus–secretion coupling, the parotid cell aggregate system (for a review see Baum et al. 1983). Both α-adrenergic and muscarinic receptors are coupled to phospholipase C via G proteins in a manner somewhat analogous to that in the striatal system (Aub and Putney 1985, Putney 1986, Merritt and Rink 1987). Likewise, IP_3 stimulates mobilization of Ca^{2+} from intracellular stores and the resultant increase in cytosolic Ca^{2+} elicits secretion of water and electrolytes (Putney 1986, Merritt and Rink 1987). Both α-adrenergic and muscarinic responses are reduced as rats age from 3 to 26 months, but the former exhibits the greatest decrement; 40–50% as opposed to approximately 20% (Bodner et al. 1983, Ishikawa et al. 1988).

As with the striatal dopamine release system, age deficits can be completely reversed by elevation of extracellular Ca^{2+} levels in the presence of the ionophore A23187 (Ito et al. 1982). Figure 1 compares α-adrenergic-stimulated K^+ release from parotid cell aggregates of 3- and 24-month-old Wistar rats. It is also obvious that cells of both age groups have a greater but essentially equal capability to respond to increased levels of Ca^{2+} than to epinephrine. Thus, as in the brain, aged cells retain the capacity for Ca^{2+}-dependent responses, but exhibit selective impairments in the signal transduction events leading to calcium mobilization.

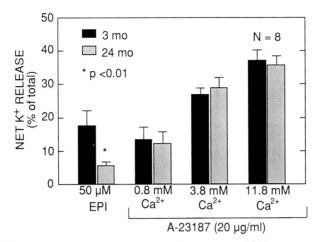

Fig. 1. Effects of calcium concentration and ionophore A23187 on potassium release from rat parotid cell aggregates. Parotid cell aggregates were prepared from 3- and 24-month-old Wistar rats and potassium release assessed under the indicated conditions as described in Ito *et al.* (1982). Values represent the means ± standard errors from eight separate experiments. EPI: epinephrine.

Figure 2 confirms this age-related decline in ability to mobilize Ca^{2+} and stimulation by epinephrine. A similar decrement can be detected using the fluorescent dye Quin 2 to assess free intracellular Ca^{2+} concentrations (Table 2). Again, the age change in response to epinephrine is much greater than that to carbachol, the muscarinic agonist.

This differential effect presented an interesting paradox since both α_1-adrenergic and muscarinic signal transduction pathways were believed to utilize the same G proteins and phospholipase C enzymes (Downes 1989). Differences could not be attributed to preferential loss of α_1-adrenergic receptors or high affinity agonist displacement since no age differences in these parameters were detected (Ito *et al.* 1982, Ishikawa *et al.* 1989). Instead, it now appears that epinephrine- and carbachol-stimulated responses may utilize different G proteins and/or phospholipase Cs (Kowatch and Roth 1989). This concept is based in the fact that neomycin, which acts at least partially at the phospholipase C level, has minimal effect on α_1-adrenergic-stimulated IP_3 generation and Ca^{2+} mobilization, while the corresponding muscarinic responses are almost completely abolished (Kowatch and Roth 1989). Preliminary data suggest that carbachol- and epinephrine-stimulated IP_3 production may indeed be additive. However, both responses appear equally sensitive to pertussis toxin inhibition, offering no evidence for, but not eliminating the possibility of multiple G protein involvement (Kowatch and Roth 1989). Whether or not different phospholipase C enzymes are involved will be dependent upon separation

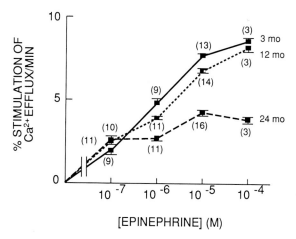

Fig. 2. Effect of age on α-adrenergic-stimulated calcium mobilization in rat parotid cells. Parotid cell aggregates were prepared from 3-, 12- and 24-month-old Wistar rats and epinephrine–stimulated $^{45}Ca^{2+}$ release determined as described in Ishikawa et al. (1988). Values represent the means ± standard errors from the numbers of experiments indicated in parentheses.

Table 2

Effects of age on epinephrine- and carbachol-stimulated free calcium concentration assessed by Quin 2 fluorescence

	Free Ca²⁺ (nM)			
	3 months	n	24 months	n
Epinephrine	518 ± 83	12	284 ± 40	11
Carbachol	611 ± 113	11	489 ± 103	11

Parotid cell aggregates were prepared and epinephrine- and carbachol-stimulated Ca^{2+} mobilization assessed by Quin 2 fluorescence as described in Ishikawa et al. (1988). Values represent the means ± standard errors for the numbers of experiments (n).

and quantitation of the isozyme forms which are present (for a review see Rhee et al. 1989).

With respect to the primary cause of age-associated reductions in α_1-adrenergic stimulation of Ca^{2+} mobilization, evidence for both impaired phosphoinositide metabolism and IP_3-stimulated Ca^{2+} release has been presented (Ito et al. 1982, Ishakawa et al. 1988). However, no age changes in either the concentration or binding affinity of microsomal IP_3 receptors have been detected (Maki et al. 1989). Thus at present the former possibility

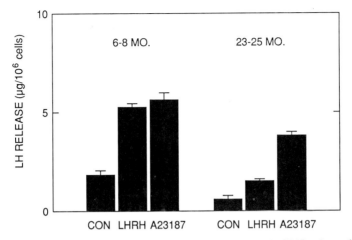

Fig. 3. Effect of age on LHRH- and A23187-stimulated LHRH release from rat pituitary cells. Anterior pituitary cell cultures were prepared and LH release stimulated by LHRH and A23187 as described in Chuknyiska *et al.* (1987). Values represent the means ± standard errors from 2–3 individual experiments employing 10–12 pituitaries from each age group.

seems to be the more convincing and in general agreement with the muscarinic-stimulated striatal dopamine release system.

GONADOTOTROPIN RELEASING HORMONE STIMULATION OF PITUITARY GONADOTROPIN SECRETION

Like the muscarinic- and α_1-adrenergic-stimulated striatum and parotid, gonadotropin or luteinizing hormone releasing hormone (LHRH) stimulates rapid release of luteinizing hormone (LH) through an IP_3/Ca^{2+}-dependent mechanism (Hanson *et al.* 1987, Kiesel *et al.* 1987, Shangold *et al.* 1988, Tasaka *et al.* 1988). However, after approximately 15 min, sustained LH release requires entrance of extracellular Ca^{2+} into the cytoplasm via voltage-dependent membrane Ca^{2+} channels (Hanson *et al.* 1987, Kiesel *et al.* 1987, Shangold *et al.* 1988, Tasaka *et al.* 1988). This longer term response exhibits a marked reduction with increasing age (Fig. 3). As with the brain and parotid systems, the age-related secretory impairment can be largely abolished in the presence of the ionophore A23187 (Fig. 3).

The exact mechanism responsible for the age change in Ca^{2+} mobilization is not yet clear. Conflicting results concerning possible age-associated loss of LHRH receptors have appeared (Marian *et al.* 1981, Sonntag *et al.*

1984, Limonta *et al.* 1988). Thus, further examination of these receptors as well as the stoichiometric relationships between receptor occupancy and LH release needs to be performed. If receptor alterations cannot be causally linked to secretory deficits it will be necessary to examine those signal transduction events which elicit Ca^{2+} entry through plasma membrane channels as a function of age.

SUMMARY AND CONCLUSIONS

Various adaptive systems exhibit reductions in responsiveness during aging. Such decrements may be the result of diminished effectiveness of agonists at both the receptor and post-receptor levels of signal transduction. Our laboratory has focused on three model systems which require calcium mobilization at the post-receptor level. These are the striatal slices, the pituitary cells, and parotid cell aggregates. Release of dopamine, LH, and water and electrolytes are impaired respectively with increasing age in these three systems. In all cases, such reductions in response can be fully or partially abolished if Ca^{2+} is mobilized directly (rather than by the respective agonists), or if the Ca^{2+} signal is amplified by other second messenger signals. The loci of the age-associated deficits may be at the G protein interface with either receptors, phospholipase C or both in the striatum and parotid, while pituitary dysfunction may occur at the voltage-dependent Ca^{2+} channels in the cell membrane. Further work will be necessary to precisely identify these loci; however, the amelioration of age-related functional deterioration by manipulations of Ca^{2+} signals through simultaneous second messenger activation/inhibition described in this review may offer an extremely useful therapeutic strategy in the future.

REFERENCES

Adams, I. (1987). *Brain Research* **424**, 343–351.

Albanese, A., Gozzo, S., Iacopino, C. and Altavista, M. C. (1985). *Brain Research* **334**, 380–384.

Altavista, M. C., Bentivoglio, A. R., Crociani, P., Rossi, P. and Albanese, A. (1988). *Brain Research* **455**, 177–181.

Anderson, D. J. and Mckinney, M. (1988). *Brain Research* **475**, 28–34.

Armstrong, D. M., Bruce, G., Gersh, L. B. and Terry, R. D. (1986). *Neuroscience Letters* **71**, 229–234.

Armstrong, D. M., Hersh, L. B. and Gage, F. H. (1988). *Neurobiology and Aging* **9**, 199–205.

Aub, D. L. and Putney, J. W. (1985). *Biochemical Journal* **225**, 263–266.

Axelrod, J., Burch, R. M. and Jelsema, C. L. (1988). *Trends in Neurological Science* **11**, 117–123.

Bartus, R. T., Dean, R. L., Pontecorvo, M. J. and Flicker, C. (1985). *Annals of the New York Academy of Science*, **444**, 332–358.

Baum, B. J., Ito, H. and Roth, G. S. (1983). *In* "Adrenoreceptors and catecholamine action—Part B" (G. Kunos, ed.), pp. 265–294. John Wiley, New York.

Bigeon, A., Duvdevani, R., Greenberger, V. and Segal, M. (1988). *Journal of Neurochemistry* **51**, 1381–1385.

Blake, M. J., Appel, N. M., Joseph, J. A., Stagg, C., Anson, M., De Souza, E. B. and Roth, G. S. (in press). *Neurobiology and Aging*.

Bodner, L., Hoopes, M. T., Gee, M., Ito, H., Roth, G. S. and Baum, B. J. (1983). *Journal of Biological Chemistry* **258**, 2774–2777.

Bonner, T. I., Buckley, N. J., Young, A. C. and Brann, M. R. (1987). *Science* **237**, 527–532.

Brann, M. R., Buckley, N. J. and Bonner, T. I. (1988). *FEBS Letters* **230**, 90–94.

Chuknyiska, R. S., Blackman, M. R. and Roth, G. S. (1987). *American Journal of Physiology* **253**, E233–E237.

Cockcroft, S. and Stutchfield, J. (1988). *Biochemical Journal* **256**, 343–350.

Consolo, S., Wang, J-W., Fiorentini, F., Vezzani, A. and Ladinsky, H. (1986). *Brain Research* **374**, 212–218.

Coupet, J., Rauh, C. E. and Joseph, J. A. (1985). *Society of Neuroscience Abstracts* **11**, 573.

Cousin, K. M., Gerald, M. C. and Uretsky, N. J. J. (1986). *Journal of Pharmacology and Experimental Therapeutics* **237**, 25–30.

Decker, M. J. (1987). *Brain Research Reviews* **12**, 423–438.

Deisher, T. A., Mankani, S. and Hoffman, B. B. (1989). *Journal of Pharmacology and Experimental Therapeutics* **249**, 812–819.

Downes, C. P. (1989). *Trends in Pharmacological Science*, Dec. Suppl. 39–42.

Dwoskin, L. P. and Zahniser, N. R. (1986). *Journal of Pharmacology and Experimental Therapeutics* **239**, 442–454.

Fisher S. K. and Agranoff, B. W. (1987). *Journal of Neurochemistry* **258**, 7358–7363.

Gozzo, S., Iacopino, C., Altavista, M. C. and Albanese, A. (1986). "Symposia in neuroscience", vol 3, pp. 299–303. Liviana, Padua.

Gurwitz, D., Egozi, Y., Henis, Y. I., Kloog, Y. and Sokolovsky, M. (1987). *Neurobiology and Aging* **8**, 115–122.

Han, Z., Kuyatt, B. L., Kochman, K.A., De Souza, E.B. and Roth, G. S. (1989). *Brain Research* **498**, 299–307.

Hansen, J. R., McArdle, C. A. and Conn, P. M. (1987). *Molecular Endocrinology* **1**, 808–815.

Harden, T. K., Heng, M. M. and Brown, J. H. (1986). *Molecular Pharmacology* **30**, 200–206.

Hiremath, A. N., Pershe, R. A., Hoffman, B. B. and Blaschke, T. F. (1989). *Journal of Gerontology* **44**, M13–17.

Hill, S. J. and Kendall, D. A. (1989). *Cell Signal* **1**, 135–141.

Hoffer, B. J., Rose, G., Parfitt, K., Freedman, R. and Bickford-Wimer, P. C. (1988). *In* "Central determinants of age-related declines in motor function" (J. A. Joseph, ed.), pp. 269–287.

Ishikawa, Y., Gee, M. V., Ambudkar, I. S., Bodner, L., Baum, B. J. and Roth, G. S. (1988). *Biochimica et Biophysica Acta* **968**, 203–210.

Ishikawa, Y., Gee, M. V., Baum, B. J. and Roth, G. S. (1989). *Experimental Gerontology* **24**, 25–36.

Ito, H., Baum, B. J., Uchida, T., Hoopes, M. T., Bodner, L. and Roth, G. S. (1982). *Journal of Biological Chemistry* **257**, 9532–9538.

Johnson, H. A. (ed.) (1985). "Relations between normal aging and disease". Raven Press, New York.

Joseph, J. A. and Roth, G. S. (1988). *In* "Proceedings of the First International Conference on Neuroimmunomodulation" (W. Pierpaoli, ed.), vol. 521, pp. 110–122. Annals of the New York Academy of Sciences, New York.

Joseph, J. A., Roth, G. S., Kowatch, M. A. and Maki, T. (In press). *Brain Research*.

Joseph, J. A., Berger, R. E., Engel, B. T. and Roth, G. S. (1978). *Journal of Gerontology* **33**, 643–649.

Joseph, J. A., Dalton, T. K. and Hunt, W. A. (1988a). *Brain Research* **454**, 140–148.

Joseph, J. A., Dalton, T. K., Roth, G. S. and Hunt, W. A. (1988b). *Brain Research* **454**, 149–155.

Kiesel, L., Lukacs, G. L., Eberhardt, I., Runnebaum, B. and Spat, A. (1987). *FEBS Letters* **217**, 85–88.

Kowatch, M. A. and Roth, G. S. (1989). *Biochemical and Biophysical Research Communications* **162**, 347–351.

Kubanis, P., Zornetzer, S. F. and Freund, G. (1982). *Pharmacology, Biochemistry and Behavior* **17**, 313–322.

Kitt, C. A., Price, D. L., Struble, R. G., Cork, L. C., Wainer, B, H., Becher, M. W. and Mobley, W. C. (1984). *Science* **226**. 1443–1444.

Lakatta, E. G. (1986). *Cardiology Clin.* **4**, 185–200.

Limonta, P., Donatella, D., Maggi, R., Martin, L. and Piva, F. (1988). *Life Sciences* **42**, 335–342.

Lippa, A. S., Loullis, C. C., Rotrosen, J., Cordasco, D. M., Critchett, D. J. and Joseph, J. A. (1985). *Neurobiology and Aging* **6**, 317–325.

Luine, V. N., Renner, K. J., Heady, S. and Jones, K. L. (1986). *Neurobiology and Aging* **7**, 193–198.

Maki, T., Kowatch, M. A., Baum, B. J., Amudkar, I. S. and Roth, G. S. (1989). *Biochimica et Biophysica Acta* **1014**, 73–77.

Marian, J., Cooper, R. L. and Conn, P. M. (1981). *Molecular Pharmacology* **19**, 399–405.

Mash, D. C. and Potter, L. T. (1986). *Neuroscience* **19**, 551–564.

McGeer, E. G., Fibiger, H. C., McGeer, P. L. and Wickson, V. (1971). *Experimental Gerontology* **6**, 391–396.

McKinney, M., Anderson, D. and Vella-Rountree, L. (1989). *Molecular Pharmacology* **35**, 39–47.

Meek, J. L., Bertilsson, L., Cheney, D. L., Zsilla, G. and Costa, E. (1977). *Journal of Gerontology* **32**, 129–131.

Merritt, J. E. and Rink, T. J. (1987). *Journal of Biological Chemistry* **262**, 4958–4960.

Morin, A. M. and Wasterlain, C. G. (1980). *Neurochemistry Research* **5**, 301–308.

Norman, A. B., Blaker, S. N., Thal, L. and Creese, I. (1986). *Neuroscience Letters* **70**, 289–294.

O'Mally, K., Docherty, J. R. and Kelly, J. G. (1988). *Journal of Hypertension Supplement* **6**, S59–62.

Pedigo, N. W. Jr and Polk, D. M. (1985). *Life Sciences* **37**, 1443–1449.

Putney, J. W. (1986). *Annual Review of Physiology* **48**, 75–88.

Raiteri, M., Riccardo, L. and Marchi, M. (1984). *Journal of Pharmacology and Experimental Therapeutics* **228**, 209–215.

Rhee, S. G., Suh, P-G, Ryu, S-H and Lee, S. Y. (1989). *Science* **244**, 546–550.

Rose, G. M., Gerhardt, G. L., and Hoffer, B. J. (1986). *Neurobiology and Aging* **7**, 77–82.

Roth, G. S. (1989). *In* "Endocrine function and aging" (H. J. Armbrect, R. H. Coe and N. Wangsurawat, eds), pp. 26–34. Springer, New York.

Schoffelmeer, A. N. M., Hogenboom, F. and Mulder, A. H. (1988). *Journal of Pharmacology and Experimental Therapeutics* **245**, 658–663.

Segal, M. (1982). *Neurobiology and Aging* **5**, 323–333.

Shangold, G. A., Murphy, S. N. and Miller, R. J. (1988). *Proceedings of the National Academy of Sciences of the USA* **85**, 6566–6570.

Sherman, K. A., Kuster, J. E., Dean, R. L., Bartus, R. T. and Friedman, E. (1981). *Neurobiology and Aging* **2**, 99–104.

Shock, N. W., Greulich, R. C., Andres, R. A., Arenberg, D., Costa, P. T., Lakatta, E. G. and Tobin, J. D. (1984). The Baltimore Longitudinal Study of Aging, NIH, Bethesda, MD 57–58.

Sonntag, W. E., Forman, L. J., Fiori, J. M., Hylka, W. W. and Meites, J. (1984). *Endocrinology* **114**, 1657–1663.

Strong, R., Hicks, P., Hsu, L., Bartus, R. T. and Enna, S. J. (1980). *Neurobiology and Aging* **1**, 59–63.

Strong, R., Samorjski, T. and Gottesfeld, Z. (1982). *Journal of Neurochemistry* **39**, 831–836.

Strong, R., Rehwaldt, C. and Wood, G. W. (1986). *Experimental Gerontology* **21**, 177–186.

Struble, R. G., Cork, L. C., Whitehouse, P. J. and Price, D. L. (1982). *Science* **216**, 413–415.

Tago, H., McGeer, P.L. and McGeer, E.G. (1987). *Brain Research* **406**, 363–369.

Tasaka, K., Stojikovic, S. S., Izumi, S-I. and Catt, K. J. (1988). *Biochemical and Biophysical Research Communications* **154**, 398–403.

Thompson, J. M., Whitaker, J. and Joseph, J. A. (1981). *Brain Research* **224**, 436–440.

Thompson, J. M., Makino, C., Whitaker, J. and Joseph, J. A. (1984). *Brain Research* **299**, 169–173.

Waller, S. and London, E. D. (1983). *Experimental Gerontology* **18**, 419–425.

Waller, S. B., Ingram, D. K., Reynolds, M. A. and London, E. D. (1983). *Journal of Neurochemistry* **41**, 1421–1428.

Weiss, E. R., Kelleher, D. J., Woon, C. W., Soparkar, S., Osawa, S., Heasly, L. E. and Johnson, G. L. (1988). *FASEB Journal* **2**, 2841–2848.

Discussion

Robert: I enjoyed both presentations, but I was a little bit surprised that you did not speak at all about the phosphokinase. I wonder whether the phosphokinase steps are impaired or not, at least in your experiment, because one of the early indications, e.g. from Vince Cristofalo and others, concerns just this uncoupling of receptor function and phosphorylation. Is there any evidence in your experiments for or against this step being impaired somehow?

Roth: I am not sure that all types of receptors are phosphorylated as a polyreaction.

Certainly, in Vince Cristofalo's experiments looking at the growth factor with the fibroblast growth factor receptor, a necessary polyreaction is autophosphorylation in the receptor. In the case of the muscarinic and the α-adrenergic receptors I am not sure that these are actually phosphorylated as a polyreactivation process. Do you have some data on that?

Robert: No, I don't have any data. We study a completely different receptor, the elastine receptor. I had the chance to speak about it in your Institute a few weeks ago with George Martin and we do not have any evidence yet that there is an age-dependent decrease of the phosphorylation. Perhaps there is not, because we really believed that this receptor, the elastine receptor, is responsible for the age-dependent increase in calcium influx in the aorta for instance. But just because of these data of Vince Cristofalo I wondered if you happened to go one step further and study the responses in the parotid gland where protein excretion is a very important function. Is that impaired at all?

Roth: We do not have any data, sorry.

Birren: I am embarrassed to ask that question, but I have to ask it as a general orientation to aging. What was the state of the animals at the time the tissues were drawn so that the results are not a reflection of activity and disuse rather than senescence example. The work at Berkeley by Bennett, Rosenzweig, indicate that the activity levels in the older animals are important in that the active older animals show greater brain weight, larger neurons and greater level of cholinesterase, suggesting that some of the phenomena that were observed previously were due to caging effect, isolation and low activity. Is this senescence we are observing, or are these animal-related circumstances?

Roth: Since we did not talk about motor behaviour I was hoping we would not get this question. Ask me this question in one year because we are starting these experiments in animals that have been exercised. Now I don't know about the study by Rosenzweig. But you know, Marilyn Diamond talks about this too, and she gets some 4% increase in the cortex, but I am not sure that would make a difference here. We also would like to study this, at least the muscarinic part of it in the animals that have been dietarily restricted and possibly would be more active that way. But we are just getting started with what we call exercise experiments. We are going to look at a lot of these parameters in exercised animals.

Scuderi: Prof. Roth, as you showed, we have many control mechanisms of intracellular calcium. Among these we have pumps. Do you know if, under basal condition, we have an alteration of intracellular sodium concentration that could be responsible for the alteration of calcium extrusion?

Roth: I am not sure. I don't know of many cases like that. We have measured pump activity in the parotid, and I know that Richard Miller in Boston has done this in lymphocytes also. We get different results. The calcium pump pumps the calcium out of the cell. In the case of the parotid it's not sodium sensitive. We did some experiments with monoenzymes and this one was not sodium-sensitive, but I really cannot answer your question as to whether there are any changes in intracellular sodium levels in either of the systems.

Yesavage: From the clinical implications of what you are saying I understand that there are some of us who would spend a lot of time giving little old ladies who have been beating their heads against a stone wall various drugs which are receptor agonists. But what you are saying is that the receptors may be there but the next step behind the receptors is defected.

Roth: I keep going on with the literature searches, hoping to find something where somebody has given one of these muscarinic agonists, or physostigmine, or something that works, and I have not seen anything. There was a review by Sherman recently and the drugs she talks about may be given at certain times. On the other hand, there are some old data by Flood and Cherkin in rats, looking at performance in the maze, in which they gave combinations of different things, tacrin, arecolin etc. They have done this in old animals and this is the only data I know of. Anybody has done anything which has actually affected an increase and it was by similar combinations that we looked at *in vitro* here. If anybody knows of data where anybody has got an increase in cognitive functions "in people", by stimulating the cholinergic system in the elderly or the elderly demented, I'd like to hear about it because I have never seen it.

Morphofunctional Changes of Synaptic Terminals in Physiological Aging and Alzheimer's Disease

Carlo Bertoni-Freddari, Patrizia Fattoretti,
Tiziana Casoli, William Meier-Ruge* and Jürg
Ulrich*

*Centre for Surgical Research, INRCA Research Department,
Ancona, Italy and *Division of Neuropathology, Institute of
Pathology, University of Basel, Switzerland*

INTRODUCTION

In industrially developed countries, the steep growth of the population aged 65 and over has raised the awareness of the increasing incidence of age-related diseases. Among these, senile dementia of the Alzheimer type (SDAT) has been reported to affect 5–10% of this part of the population in the United States and this percentage is predicted to increase in the future due to the increasing number of elderly people. Senile plaques, neurofibrillary tangles, congophilic angiopathy, Hirano bodies, vacuolation and loss of neurons in specific areas of the CNS are the most investigated histopathological hallmarks of SDAT (Tomlinson 1980, Ulrich *et al.* 1986). Despite the efforts and the results of many investigators from different laboratories, the aetiology of this devastating disease of the senile brain is still unknown, but pieces of the puzzle are being continuously identified and hopefully, will lead to the final solution. For the time being, in order to tackle the problems of senile dementia, it is of primary importance to characterize in detail which are the changes occurring in the SDAT brain as compared with the physiologically aged one. In demented patients, loss

Challenges in Aging
ISBN 0-12-090163-3

of memory and impairment of cognitive functions are the early, subtle and often undiagnosed symptoms, which may also occur in normal aging (e.g. benign forgetfulness). Despite the identification of these precocious alterations in behaviour, the pattern of subcellular changes occurring in SDAT is still far from complete.

Synaptic contact zones have been shown to be deeply involved in brain performances such as learning and memory (Carlin and Siekevitz 1983, Lynch and Baudry 1984). While being well-differentiated areas of the neuronal membrane, synaptic junctions undergo relevant adaptive changes even in the fully developed adult nervous system, in order to enable the neuronal circuitries to give the best response to environmental stimuli (Cotman *et al.* 1981). Synaptic plasticity is the widely used term to denote such a plastic condition of the synaptic terminals and also includes changes which take place at the ultrastructural level. In the present paper we report the results of a computer-assisted morphometric investigation on the synaptic junctions of autoptic hippocampi from adult, old and SDAT patients. This study was undertaken to seek whether synaptic alterations may contribute to the pathogenesis of SDAT.

THE ANATOMICAL MODEL AND MORPHOLOGICAL CATEGORIZATION OF SYNAPTIC JUNCTIONAL DENSITIES

Although senile plaques have also been found recently in the cerebellum of SDAT patients (Braak *et al.* 1989) and amyloid β-protein deposition has been demonstrated in tissues other than brain (Joachim *et al.* 1989), this disease has been long reported to selectively affect discrete areas of the CNS such as frontal cortex, amygdala, nucleus basalis of Meynert and hippocampus. The reasons why such zones are more sensitive to SDAT pathology are still debated, however the characteristic hallmarks of the demented brains are consistently found in higher density in these areas. With regard to the involvement of neurotransmitter systems in SDAT pathology, cholinergic innervation from the nucleus basalis of Meynert and associated areas, noradrenergic fibres from the locus coeruleus, serotoninergic input from the raphe and dopaminergic innervation from the ventral tegmentum are seriously deteriorated in the demented brain (Hardy *et al.* 1985, Mann and Yates 1986). It is still controversial as to which of these transmitter systems suffers the most dramatic changes, however the cholinergic one appears to be much more vulnerable than any other system both during aging and to a higher extent, in SDAT (Perry and Perry 1980, Bartus *et al.* 1982, Coyle *et al.* 1985). In looking for a reliable anatomical model to perform our morphometric investigation on synaptic junctions, we considered the above points and chose the dentate gyrus molecular layer. This zone of the hippocampal formation is particularly suitable to perform quantitative morphological studies since fibre inputs coming to this area are organized in a laminar distribution and do not overlap (Mosko *et al.* 1973, Hyman *et al.* 1987). Thus, very discrete and homogeneous areas (with regard to the transmitter used at the synapses) can be sampled. It has been clearly shown that the narrow band immediately above the granular cells receives cholinergic fibres from the septum and that this zone is intensely and finely stained when histochemical procedures are applied to detect the activity of choline acetyltransferase (CAT), a key enzyme in the synthesis of the neurotransmitter acetylcholine. Our study was performed in this area, known as the dentate gyrus supragranular layer, in order to sample a SDAT-sensitive zone both from the anatomical and the neurotransmitter point of view.

Qualitative synaptic ultrastructural changes, if not extreme, are not detectable and do not allow statistical group comparisons. Conversely, recently developed computer-assisted morphometric procedures applied by means of sophisticated image analysers have enabled the researchers to perform reliable measurements of several synaptic ultrastructural parameters (Bertoni-Freddari *et al.* 1988). The commonly recognized limits of these procedures are that fully or semi-automatized analysers should be equipped to identify the anatomical or cytological structures the investigator is interested in evaluating quantitatively and that specific programmes for the aim of the study should be prepared. Morphological studies of the synaptic contact zones are currently carried out either by staining the tissue by means of the conventional osmium/lead procedure which visualizes synaptic contacts, vesicles and background tissue or by the ethanol-phosphotungstic acid (E-PTA) preferential technique (Bloom and Aghajanian 1968) which only stains the synapses leaving the background electron lucent. It is well known that histochemical methods do not permit the staining of isolated compounds, but can show reactive groups and molecules arranged in a biological structure. In this context, although it remains to be completely clarified, the E-PTA specificity for synaptic paramembranous material is well proven (Bertoni-Freddari *et al.* 1986, 1988, 1989). In agreement with these findings the E-PTA procedure proved to be very suitable for our purposes. As shown in Fig. 1, E-PTA-stained synapses appear as pre- and postsynaptic dark densities separated by a cleft. According to morphological categorization of the E-PTA-stained contacts proposed by Dyson and Jones (1976), three main types of synapses can be recognized (Fig. 2). Type A represents only the postsynaptic density and is commonly referred to as a maturing or degenerating contact. Against this, types B and C show both pre- and postsynaptic densities, the only difference being that in B the

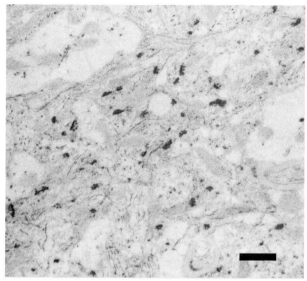

Fig. 1. Electron microscopic picture of E-PTA-stained synapses in the human dentate gyrus. The junctional areas are visualized as black densities against an electron lucent background. Bar = 1 μm,

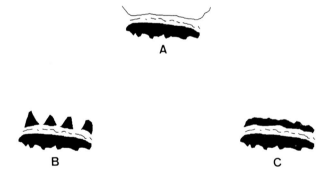

Fig. 2. Schematic drawing of the ultrastructural features of E-PTA-stained synapses. Further details in the text.

presynaptic element looks like a mountain range with peaks commonly known as dense projections, whereas in type C each pre- and postsynaptic apposition is a continuous band of lengthwise uniform thickness. As the onset of electrical activity has been related to the presence of a definable presynaptic density (Woodward *et al.* 1971), we considered types B and C as functional contacts, at least from a morphological standpoint, and set up

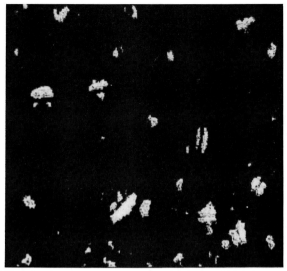

Fig. 3. E-PTA-stained synapses as reproduced by the ASBA image analyser. The pre- and postsynaptic appositions are clearly identified by the computer program. Unspecific material was deleted during analysis.

a computer program able to identify these junction types (Fig. 3). As schematically drawn in Fig. 4, we measured: (1) the number of synapses in a unit volume of tissue (Nv), i.e. their numerical density; (2) the average area of the single contact (S) considering the synaptic appositions as circular disks; (3) the total area of the synaptic contact zones in a unit volume of tissue (Sv), or in morphometric terms, the synaptic surface density.

SYNAPTIC CHANGES DURING AGING AND SDAT

Table 1 summarizes the results from our study. During physiological aging, Nv and Sv significantly decrease, whereas S increases. In a comparison between demented and age-matched controls Nv and Sv undergo a further decrease, but S is unchanged. If we consider the adult values as 100%, SDAT patients demonstrate 61% and 44% decreases of Nv and Sv, respectively, but also a 40% increase in S.

Recently proposed structural theories regarding the anatomical basis of learning and memory support the fact that major modifications occur in the brain's basic wiring diagram and that these changes take place at synaptic junctional areas (Carlin and Siekevitz 1983, Lynch and Baudry 1984, Petit 1988). In the light of these assumptions, the three synaptic parameters measured in the present study have raised great interest among

Numeric Density of Synapses per μm³

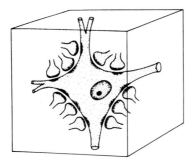

Average Area
of a Single
Synaptic Contact
Zone in μm²

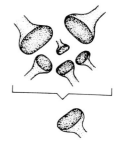

Nv: No. Syn./μm³

$\overline{S}$: μm²

Surface Density of Synaptic
Contact Zones
per μm³

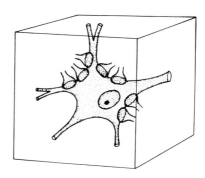

Sv: μm²/μm³

Fig. 4. Schematic drawing of the synaptic ultrastructural parameters studied.
Further details in the text.

neurobiologists. Overproduction and subsequent elimination of synapses
take place in the cerebral cortex during the developmental period and are
aimed at the functional stabilization of the currently used junctions (Purves
and Lichtman 1980). Even in the adult CNS, the number of contacts
appears to be modifiable following electrical stimulation, leading to long-
term potentiation (LTP) or after recurrent presynaptic activation (kindling)
(de Toledo-Morrell *et al.* 1988). Thus, it is commonly accepted that the

Table 1

Synaptic parameters from hippocampal dentate gyri. Mean (± SEM)

	Nv (No. synapses μm^{-3})	S (μm^2)	Sv ($\mu m^2\ \mu m^{-3}$)
Adult	1.5991 (0.1331)	0.1149 (0.0041)	0.1798 (0.0097)
Old	0.8308 (0.0424)	0.1756 (0.0096)	0.1399 (0.0025)
Demented	0.6270* (0.0270)	0.1780 (0.0098)	0.1083* (0.0081)

Statistical comparisons: demented and old parameters are all significantly different when compared with adult values, respectively.
*Statistically significant vs the old group.

growth of novel connections represents a real possibility for the nervous system to adapt to the changing environmental and experiential framework. Although largely expected on the basis of well-documented cognitive and electrophysiological impairments, the decrease in the number of contacts in aging and SDAT is still controversial, probably due to several factors (tissue processing, age of the patients, sampling procedures, individual bias etc.) involved in the correct measurement of this important synaptic parameter (Bertoni-Freddari *et al.* 1988, 1990a). In our opinion, a marked improvement in the estimation of the actual situation in the tissue has been achieved by relating the synaptic Nv to the numerical density of neurons in the sampled area. The number of contacts per neuron is independent of factors such as tissue shrinkage due to experimental processing, age and/or pathology, therefore it helps to define synaptic efficacy from a morphological point of view (Bertoni-Freddari *et al.* 1990a, b). Figure 5 shows that the numerical density of dentate gyrus granular cells does not change when comparing aging with SDAT patients, but it is significantly decreased vs the adult group. Figure 6 reports the synapse to neuron ratios in the three groups analysed: by considering the adult value as 100%, the decrease in old and demented patients is 15.6% and 48%, respectively. From these results it is evident that the reduction in synaptic numbers represents *per se* a prominent feature of the old and demented CNS.

Changes in synaptic size have been as intensely investigated as the alterations in the number of contacts and it is accepted that any manipulation purported to alter neural activity is able to modify synaptic size (Petit 1988). Modifications in the length of postsynaptic density have been documented in experimental models of learning, memory, visual training,

Neuronal density: No. cells x10³/mm³

Human dentate gyrus

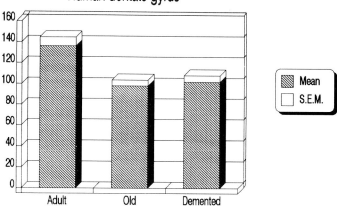

Fig. 5. Number of dentate gyrus granular cells during aging and SDAT Statistical comparisons (Student's *t*-test): adult/old, $P < 0.001$; adult/demented, $P < 0.001$; old/demented, not significant.

Synapse/Neuron x10³/mm³

Human dentate gyrus

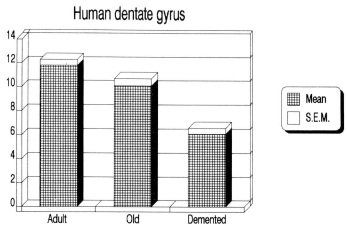

Fig. 6. Number of synapses per dentate gyrus granular cell during aging and SDAT. Statistical comparisons (Student's *t*-test): adult/old, $P < 0.05$; adult/demented, $P < 0.001$; old/demented, $P < 0.01$.

alcohol withdrawal, environmental enrichment or deprivation etc. (Vrensen and Nunes-Cardozo 1981, Siekevitz 1985, Phillips 1985, Sirevaag and Greenough 1985). The biological significance of the changes in synaptic size has been based on the hypothesis that larger junctional areas can release more transmitter and activate more postsynaptic receptors, thus strengthening the transmission of information (Petit 1988). According to electrophysiological experiments in animal models this appears to be the case (Barnes and McNaughton 1980), but conversely to these tenets, it has been clearly demonstrated that when the synaptic contact area exceeds a still undefined limit, some discontinuities or perforations appear in the synaptic contact zones. These perforations are hypothesized to be involved in the plastic changes occurring at synapses and are thought to represent a CNS mechanism to modify the connectivity by increasing the number of contacts (Nieto-Sampedro et al. 1982, Carlin and Siekevitz 1983, Dyson and Jones 1984). The functional meaning of the splitting of large junctional areas into smaller contacts is still unclear, but loss of perforated synapses has been shown in memory disorders (Geinisman et al. 1986) whereas an increase of this type of junction is reported with CNS maturation and experience (Greenough et al. 1978).

Any possible explanation of synaptic size enlargements reported in Table 1 must take into account the above reported literature data regarding this synaptic parameter. In order to verify whether the increase in synaptic size during aging and SDAT represents the first step in the mechanism leading to subsynaptic plate perforations (Carlin and Siekevitz 1983, Petit 1988), we performed a percentage distribution of S as shown in Fig. 7. It is evident that in the adult group the number of small contacts (< 0.12 μm^2) accounts for about 50% of the whole synaptic population, whereas in the old and SDAT patients the percentage of junctions measuring less than 0.12 μm^2 is below 10%. Since the number of small contacts in aging and SDAT is very low, there is scarce possibility that the enlarged junctional areas measured by us are part of a splitting programme. Conversely, we believe that the growth in the average synaptic area may be interpreted in terms of synaptic structural remodelling, also considering Nv and Sv.

The three parameters we investigated, besides reporting on discrete ultrastructural features of the synapses, are closely related to each other. Namely, in morphological studies including human brain aging and SDAT it has been found that decrease in Nv is associated with a parallel increase in S (Davies et al. 1987, Bertoni-Freddari 1989, 1990a). This reciprocal relationship between synaptic number and size has also been documented in animal models and has led Hillman and Chen (1984) to propose that Sv is the final result of this inverse balance. According to these authors, maintaining Sv constant is a necessary prerequisite in stabilizing the functional circuitries in CNS and it is accomplished by compensations vs

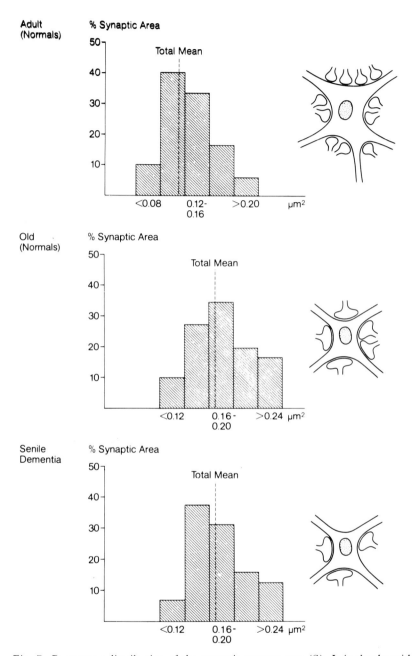

Fig. 7. Percentage distribution of the synaptic average area (S). It is clearly evident that in aging and SDAT the majority of synaptic junctions have an enlarged size as compared with adult values. The schematic drawings on the right visualize the situation in the tissue according to the present data: many small contacts in adults, a decreased number of larger junctional areas in physiological aging, a further reduction in the number of large synapses in SDAT.

reductions between Nv and S. Conceivably, when considered all together per group of samples, Nv, S, and Sv are a reliable index of the ultrastructural synaptic plasticity (Bertoni-Freddari et al. 1988, 1990a, Bertoni-Freddari 1989). When comparing adult vs old and SDAT patients, reduced Sv appears to be due to the marked decrease in Nv since S is increased. On the basis of the reciprocal relationship among these parameters and of the results shown in Fig. 7 reporting a high percentage of larger contacts in aging and SDAT, we interpret the enlargement of S as a compensative phenomenon counteracting the reduction in Sv. Although speculative, our interpretation finds support in recent data documenting increased staining of synapsin I and synaptophysin (two proteins found in active synaptic terminals) in the inner molecular layer of the hippocampus from SDAT patients (Hamos et al. 1989). In addition, the reactive capabilities of SDAT brain seem to involve the whole synaptic regions as demonstrated by the consistent sprouting of septal afferents in the hippocampus (Geddes et al. 1985, Hyman et al. 1987), by some neurites retaining functional activity even in the neuritic plaques (Probst et al. 1983) and by the increase in the number of dendritic segments in the dentate gyrus granular cells (Flood et al. 1987). To conclude, it seems clear that despite the fact that structural dynamics of synaptic membranes are seriously compromised both in physiological and pathological aging, our present findings on S enlargement should be regarded as a recovery intervention brought about even in the SDAT brain.

In looking for causative events leading to these morpho-functional changes, it must be stressed that several factors are reported to play a role in synaptic plasticity and among these, an age-dependent deficit in energy production could contribute to a high extent. The nervous system has a high metabolic rate, thus a proper and actual supply of oxygen and glucose are needed to cope with its energy requirements. Because no tissue stores of oxygen and only small amounts of glucose are available in the brain, short supply of either or both leads to neuronal dysfunction and may cause serious and irreversible damage to nerve cell structures according to the severity and time course of the alteration. With regard to the data shown in Table 1, a fine distribution of many small contacts, while providing a fine tuning of neuronal circuitries, would need a higher metabolic rate than a reduced number of large junctional zones. Thus, in the old and demented CNS a reduced energy supply could contribute to the impairment in synaptic morphology documented by our results. No data are available to directly support this latter assumption, nevertheless it is well demonstrated that a reduced capacity to step up glycolitic and oxidation chain processes takes place in the old and demented brain (Siesjo and Rehncrona 1980, Smith 1984, Meier-Ruge 1985).

Finally, not forgetting that synaptic junctions are very sensitive areas of neuronal membrane, the present findings are of relevance in the light of recent findings on membrane alterations, aging and SDAT. Namely, growing evidence is now being documented that β-amyloid precursor is a degeneration product of a protein spanning the cell membrane. This protein is supposed to play a role in establishing the contacts among nerve cells at synaptic terminals where it seems to be abundant (Masters *et al.* 1985, Kang *et al.* 1987, Marx 1989; Majocha *et al.* 1989). It is still to be ascertained whether the release of β-amyloid peptide from neuronal and synaptic membranes is a key step in nerve terminal degeneration or is an event subsequent to cell death, however these biochemical data and our present findings support a very important role of neuronal membrane deterioration in the pathogenesis of SDAT (Bertoni-Freddari 1988).

ACKNOWLEDGEMENT

The authors wish to thank Mr Marcel Bruhlmann for his skilful technical help and Mrs Lesley Vowden for reading this manuscript.

REFERENCES

Barnes, C. A. and McNaughton, B. L. (1980). Physiological compensation for loss of afferent synapses in rat hippocampal granule cells during senescence. *Journal of Physiology* **309**, 473–485.

Bartus, R. T., Dean, R. L. III, Beer, B. and Lippa, A. S. (1982). The cholinergic hypothesis of geriatric memory disfunction. *Science* **217**, 408–417.

Bertoni-Freddari, C. (1988). Age-dependent deterioration of neuronal membranes and the pathogenesis of Alzheimer's disease: a hypothesis. *Medical Hypotheses* **25**, 147–149.

Bertoni-Freddari, C. (1989). Synaptic plasticity in the cerebellar glomeruli of rats: effects of aging and vitamin E deficiency. *In* "Handbook of free radicals and antioxidants in biomedicine" (J. Miquel, A. T. Quintanilha and H. Weber), pp. 255–267. CRC Press Inc., Boca Raton FL.

Bertoni-Freddari, C., Giuli, C., Pieri, C. and Paci, D. (1986). Quantitative investigation of the morphological plasticity of synaptic junctions in rat dentate gyrus during aging. *Brain Research* **366**, 187–192.

Bertoni-Freddari, C., Meier-Ruge, W. and Ulrich, J. (1988). Quantitative morphology of synaptic plasticity in the aging brain. *Scanning Microscopy* **2**, 1027–1034.

Bertoni-Freddari, C., Fattoretti, P., Meier-Ruge, W. and Ulrich, J. (1989). Computer-assisted morphometry of synaptic plasticity during aging and dementia. *Pathology Research and Practice* **185**, 799–802.

Bertoni-Freddari, C., Fattoretti, P., Casoli, T., Meier-Ruge, W. and Ulrich, W. (1990a). Morphological adaptive response of the synaptic junctional zones in the human dentate gyrus during aging and Alzheimer's disease. *Brain Research*, **517**, 69–75.

Bertoni-Freddari, C., Fattoretti, P., Casoli, T., Meier-Ruge, W. and Ulrich, J.

(1990b). The role of neuronal membranes deterioration in the pathogenesis of Alzheimer's disease: an ultrastructural perspective. *In* "Alzheimer's and Parkinson's disease II: basic and therapeutic strategies" (T. Nagatsu, A. Fisher and M. Yoshida, eds), in press.

Bloom, F. E. and Aghajanian, G. K. (1968). Fine structural and cytochemical analysis of the staining of synaptic junctions with phosphotungstic acid. *Journal of Ultrastructure Research* **22**, 361–375.

Braak, H., Braak, E., Bohl, J. and Lang, W. (1989). Alzheimer's disease: mismatch between amyloid plaques and neuritic plaques. *Journal of Neurological Science* **93**, 277–287.

Carlin, R. K. and Siekevitz, P. (1983). Plasticity in the central nervous system: do synapses divide? *Proceedings of the National Academy of Sciences of the USA* **80**, 3517–3521.

Cotman, C. W., Nieto-Sampedro, N. and Harris, E. W. (1981). Synapse replacement in the nervous system of adult vertebrates. *Physiological Reviews* **61**, 684–784.

Coyle, J. T., Price, D. L. and DeLong, M. R. (1985). Alzheimer's disease: a disorder of cortical cholinergic innervation. *In* "Neuroscience" (P. H. Abelson, E. Butz and S. H. Snyder, eds), pp. 418–431.

Davies, C. A., Mann, D. M. A., Sumpter, P. Q. and Yates, P. O. (1987). A quantitative morphometric analysis of the neuronal and synaptic content of frontal and temporal cortex in patients with Alzheimer's disease. *Journal of Neurological Science* **78**, 151–164.

de Toledo-Morrell, L., Geinisman, Y. and Morrell, F. (1988). Age-dependent alterations in hippocampal synaptic plasticity: relation to memory disorders. *Neurobiology of Aging* **9**, 581–590.

Dyson, S. E. and Jones, D. G. (1976). The morphological categorization of developing synaptic junctions. *Cell and Tissue Research* **167**, 363–371.

Dyson, S. E. and Jones, D. G. (1984). Synaptic remodelling during development and maturation: junction differentiation and splitting as a mechanism for modifying connectivity. *Developmental Brain Research* **13**, 125–137.

Flood, D. G., Buell, S. J., Horwitz, G. J. and Coleman, P. D. (1987). Dendritic extent in human dentate gyrus granule cells in normal aging and senile dementia. *Brain Research* **402**, 205–216.

Geddes, J. W., Monaghan, D. T., Cotman, C. W., Lott, I. T., Kim, R. C. and Chang Chui, H. (1985). Plasticity of hippocampal circuitry in Alzheimer's disease. *Science* **230**, 1179–1181.

Geinisman, Y., de Toledo-Morrell, L. and Morrell, F. (1986). Loss of perforated synapses in the dentate gyrus: morphological substrate of memory deficit in aged rats. *Proceedings of the National Academy of Sciences of the USA* **83**, 3027–3031.

Greenough, W. T., West, R. W. and Devoogd, T. J. (1978). Subsynaptic plate perforations: changes with age and experience in the rat. *Science* **202**, 1096–1098.

Hamos, J. E., DeGennaro, L. J. and Drachman, D. A. (1989). Synaptic loss in Alzheimer's disease and other dementias. *Neurology* **39**, 355–361.

Hardy, J. A., Adolfsson, R., Alafuzoff, I., Bucht, G., Marcusson, J., Nyberg, P., Pendall, E., Wester, P. and Winblad, B. (1985). Transmitter deficits in Alzheimer's disease. *Neurochemistry International* **7**, 545–563.

Hillman, D. E. and Chen, S. (1984). Reciprocal relationship between size of postsynaptic densities and their number: constancy in contact area. *Brain Research* **295**, 325–343.

Hyman, B. T., Kromer, L. J. and Van Hoesen, G. W. (1987). Reinnervation of the hippocampal perforant pathway zone in Alzheimer's disease. *Annals of Neurology* **21**, 259–267.

Joachim, C. L., Mori, H. and Selkoe, D. J. (1989). Amyloid β-protein deposition in tissues other than brain in Alzheimer's disease. *Nature* **341**, 226–230.

Kang, J., Lemaire, H. G., Unterback, A., Salbaum, J. M., Masters, C. L., Grzeschik, K. H., Multhaup, G., Beyreuther, K. and Muller-Hill, B. (1987). The precursor of Alzheimer's disease amyloid A4 protein resembles a cell-surface receptor. *Nature* **325**, 733–736.

Lynch, G. and Baudry, M. (1984). The biochemistry of memory: a new and specific hypothesis. *Science* **224**, 1057–1063.

Majocha, R. E., Jungalwala, F. B., Rodenrys, A. and Marotta, C. A. (1989). Monoclonal antibody to embryonic CNS antigen A2B5 provides evidence for the involvement of membrane components at sites of Alzheimer degeneration and detects sulfatides as well as gangliosides. *Journal of Neurochemistry* **53**, 953–961.

Mann, D. M. A. and Yates, P. O. (1986). Neurotransmitter deficits in Alzheimer's disease and in other dementing disorders. *Human Neurobiology* **5**, 147–158.

Marx, J. L. (1989). Brain protein yields clues to Alzheimer's disease. *Science* **243**, 1664–1666.

Masters, C. L., Multhaup, G., Simms, G., Pottgiesser, J., Martins, R. N. and Beyreuther, K. (1985). Neuronal origin of cerebral amyloid: neurofibrillary tangles of Alzheimer's disease contain the same protein as the amyloid of plaque cores and blood vessels. *EMBO Journal* **4**, 2757–2763.

Meier-Ruge, W. (1985). Neurochemistry of the aging brain and senile dementia. *In* "Aging 2000: our health care destiny" (C. M. Gaitz and T. Samorajski, eds), pp. 101–112. Springer, New York.

Mosko, S., Lynch, G. and Cotman, C. W. (1973). The distribution of septal projections to the hippocampus of the rat. *Journal of Comparative Neurology* **152**, 163–174.

Nieto-Sampedro, M., Hoff, S. F. and Cotman, C. W. (1982). Perforated postsynaptic densities: probable intermediates in synapse turnover. *Proceedings of the National Academy of Sciences of the USA* **79**, 5718–5722.

Perry, E. K. and Perry, R. H. (1980). The cholinergic system in Alzheimer's disease. *In* "Biochemistry of dementia" (P. J. Roberts, ed.), pp. 135–183. John Wiley, New York.

Petit, T. L. (1988). Synaptic plasticity and the structural basis of learning and memory. *In* "Neural plasticity: a lifespan approach" (T. L. Petit and G. O. Ivy, eds), pp. 201–234. Alan R. Liss, New York.

Phillips, S. C. (1985). Qualitative and quantitative changes of mouse cerebellar synapses after chronic alcohol consumption and withdrawal. *Experimental Neurology* **88**, 748–756.

Probst, A., Basler, V., Bron, B. and Ulrich, J. (1983). Neuritic plaques in senile dementia of Alzheimer type: a Golgi analysis in the hippocampal region. *Brain Research* **268**, 249–254.

Purves, D. and Lichtman, J. V. (1980). Elimination of synapses in the developing nervous system. *Science* **210**, 153–157.

Siekevitz, P. (1985). The postsynaptic density: a possible role in long-lasting effects in the central nervous system. *Proceedings of the National Academy of Sciences of the USA* **82**, 3494–3498.

Siesjo, B. K. and Rehncrona, S. (1980). Adverse factors affecting neuronal metabolism: relevance to the dementias. *In* "Biochemistry of dementia" (P. J. Roberts, ed.), pp. 91–120. John Wiley, New York.

Sirevaag, A. M. and Greenough, W. T. (1985). Differential rearing effects on rat visual cortex synapses. *Developmental Brain Research* **19**, 215–226.

Smith, C. B. (1984). Aging and changes in cerebral energy metabolism. *Trends in Neurosciences*, **6**, 203–208.

Tomlinson, B. E. (1980). The structural and quantitative aspects of the dementias. *In* "Biochemistry of dementia" (P. J. Roberts, ed.), pp. 15–52. John Wiley, London.

Ulrich, J., Probst, A., Anderton, B. H. and Kahn, J. (1986). Dementia of Alzheimer type (DAT)—a review of its morbid anatomy. *Klinische Wochenschrift* **64**, 103–114.

Vrensen, G. and Nunes-Cardozo, J. (1981). Changes in size and shape of synaptic connections after visual training: an ultrastructural approach of synaptic plasticity. *Brain Research* **218**, 79–97.

Woodward, D. J., Hoffer, B. J., Siggins, G. R. and Bloom, F. E. (1971). The ontogenetic development of synaptic junctions. Synaptic activation and responsiveness to neurotransmitter substances in rat cerebellar Purkinje cells. *Brain Research* **34**, 73–98.

Discussion

Williams: Thinking back to Dr Birren's comment earlier about the state of activity of rats, I wonder whether in these human situations some of the decline you might have seen in the normal brains might have been due to lessened mental activity as compared to the younger, whether there be any way to control the state of youth of the brain. The other question is whether, given your findings, it would not be likely that a nerve growth factor might have a really beneficial effect on the synapses.

Bertoni: I cannot comment on the first question, so I would like to reply to the second question. I have read just a few days ago a paper in *Science* by Hefti and co-workers which stresses that the nerve growth factor can be detrimental if not given at the proper moment. So it seems that it can improve just the deteriorative events rather than ameliorate the reactive capacities of the brain. It is still a matter of debate, but I personally believe that the position of Hefti is much more tenable than giving nerve growth factor without any rule.

Robert: How far do you think that vascular changes which you studied can also be responsible for these modifications you described?

Bertoni: I am sure that they are involved in such changes. For instance, with regard to the hippocampus, Hatchinsky reported 1977 in *Mechanisms of Ageing and Development* that the vascular bed of the hippocampus is supplied by a rake-like capillary network. And this is very sensitive to changes in blood supply. So I would support this pretention that changes in vascular bed may probably induce the changes I observed.

M. Ermini

I would like to conclude this afternoon's session with a few words, not to summarize the individual talks but rather to try to draw an overall conclusion from what we have heard.

First, I think it was fascinating to see the focus of research on the rather holistic aspect of aging at the integrated system level narrowing in on the very specific cellular and molecular structures of the CNS. This reflects the classical reductionistic approach and shows both its merits and problems: the more we approach the single components of a system the closer we may come to the basic principle of its functioning. However, at the same time it becomes increasingly difficult to bridge back to the complex systems of higher order. How to tie the observations by Roth and Joseph on the calcium-dependent mechanisms of receptor function of striatal neurons with the synaptic changes in the hippocampus described by Bertoni, or, even more problematic, with the apparently overall deleterious effects of hormones as evidenced by Everitt and the neuroendocrine regulatory disturbances as pictured by Frolkis? Only by experimental manipulation of the systems will it be possible to bridge the gaps of understanding between the various levels of structural organization. One approach has been shown by Everitt using hypophysectomy or removal of other hormonal glands to prove the effects of hormones; another one, closer to therapeutic applicability, was exemplified by Joseph and Roth who used specifically acting substances, e.g. the ionophores alleviating intracellular calcium mobilization, to prove the correctness of their hypothesis of an impairment of calcium mobilization in aging nerve cells.

This leads to my second point. In contrast to earlier years of basic research, when scientists tended to defend their position as independent "pure scientists", nowadays practical considerations seem to be not any more "taboo" to them. This may be in part due to the fact that our body of knowledge has greatly increased, allowing such practical, i.e. therapeutical aspects to be considered more readily, but also due to the increasing involvement of pharmacological techniques in gerontological research, particularly in neurobiology. As pharmacologically active substances play an important role in the elucidation of neurobiological processes, their consideration as therapeutics is a logical consequence. This can be deduced from the presentations given by Joseph and Roth as well as by the other speakers.

Finally, the Sandoz Lectures are explicitly designed to bridge the gaps between the various disciplines in gerontology. I think that this much needed bridging, which seems particularly difficult between biological research and psychological or even social research, became nicely evident today. For example, if we think about the talks by Birren on speed of behaviour, or by Yesavage on memory we can say that these psychological phenomena clearly have a biological basis which at least in part could be linked to some of the observations discussed this afternoon. More direct, of course, are such relationships with research on dementia, or, generally, with the medical aspects of aging, as will be seen in the next session.

Part III

Chronic Illness in the Elderly: Clinical Strategies

Aging and the Bladder

J. C. Brocklehurst

Department of Geriatric Medicine, University of Manchester

In discussing micturition problems that are faced by people growing older we really have to look at the bladder and the brain, their interrelationship and the effects of aging and age-associated diseases. A rather beautiful definition of the bladder is that given by the Scottish anatomist Bell, in his monograph "Anatomy of the human body" published in 1826. He writes:

Of the bladder of urine
The bladder of urine must be classed with the membraneous or hollow viscera. It is a bag or receptacle into which the urine slowly distils through the ureters that it may be expelled at convenient seasons.

The bladder consists of two muscles, the detrusor and the trigone (and Bell in his book accurately described the function of the trigone in closing the ureteric orifices when the bladder contracts). The principal nerve receptors in the detrusor are cholinergic and those in the trigone α-adrenergic.

While there is no real difference between the sexes in the urinary bladder there are obvious differences in the form and structure of the urethra. In the female, the urethra has an average length of 3.4 cm. It consists of two muscle layers—a smooth muscle innermost layer which is a continuation of the detrusor muscle and runs mainly in a longitudinal direction and a striated muscle, the external sphincter which surrounds the urethra. The external sphincter appears to be a somewhat unusual striated muscle in that it contains no spindles. The fibres are almost all of the slow twitch variety and it would appear to share its innervation between the somatic and autonomic nervous systems—that is the pudendal nerve and the pelvic (parasympathetic) nerves (Gosling *et al.* 1981). It is not clear to what extent this muscle is under voluntary control since voluntary cessation of micturition in the female seems to be predominantly an action of the

Challenges in Aging
ISBN 0-12-090163-3

pubococcygeus muscle (part of the pelvic diaphragm) which may both elevate the bladder neck and squeeze the urethra. In the male, the smooth muscle forms a circular sphincter at the bladder neck and the receptors are α-adrenergic. Its main function appears to be in the prevention of retrograde ejaculation and it is the external sphincter lying below the prostate which maintains the main closing pressure on the urethra. As in the female, this is an unusual striated muscle which appears to derive its innervation from the pelvic nerve predominantly but possibly in part from the pudendal nerve. The pubococcygeus muscle impinges its closure pressure on the urethra below the prostate and appears to be the main muscle concerned in voluntary cessation of micturition. The unusual qualities of the striated muscle sphincters have only recently been described (Gosling et al. 1981) and their role is still not clearly understood.

Closure of the urethra in both sexes is also maintained by the rich network of elastic tissue around the length of the urethra in the female and the upper urethra in the male and possibly also by the rich periurethral vascular networks.

It is known that the closing pressure of the female urethra becomes lower in old age and we have shown (Carlile et al. 1988) that this is due to a relative loss of striated muscle fibres.

In the male the urethra is lined by cuboidal or transitional epithelium but in the female during the reproductive period, this becomes stratified squamous epithelium (which is oestrogen sensitive) (Walter et al., 1979). We have also shown (Carlile et al. 1987) that the proportion of stratified squamous epithelium in the female urethra diminishes with age.

While functional disorders of the lower urinary tract and particularly urinary incontinence may result from pathological changes in the bladder and urethra (for instance, cystitis, prostatism and pelvic floor weakness), the most important causes of these problems in old age lie in the central nervous system. The nervous control of micturition has been a hugely researched subject for 150 years or more and controversy still remains. By 1939 there was a fairly clear and simple concept that two main centres governed micturition—one in the sacral spinal cord and one in the forebrain. It has long been known, of course, that many other areas are involved and electrical stimulation experiments in animals in the diencephalon and mesencephalon have shown variable effects of inhibition and facilitation on micturition. However, the relatively simple state of affairs illustrated in Fig. 1 allowed micturition to be thought of in terms of upper and lower motor neurons, very much as in control of skeletal muscle. Lesions affecting the autonomic nerves and their connections in the sacral spinal cord may lead to loss of sensation or loss of contractility causing the "atonic bladder". Destruction of the sacral segments of the cord (e.g. in spinal artery occlusion or metastatic carcinoma) removed both sensation and contractility. Lesions

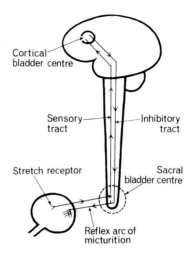

Fig. 1. Simple representation of neurological control of micturation.

above the sacral cord whether rising in the spinal cord or in the brain, on the other hand, allowed the sacral reflex and micturition to emerge uncontrolled and so uninhibited bladder contractions developed as the bladder filled up. The individual may or may not have been aware of these depending on whether or not the afferent nervous connections were affected. In paraplegia associated with total spinal cord transection, the bladder would be entirely reflex. However, in most diseases affecting the hindbrain, midbrain and forebrain, sensation is retained but the ability to inhibit the sacral reflex of micturition is lost, a condition described as the uninhibited neurogenic bladder producing the symptoms of urgency and urge incontinence.

More recently it has been realized that the main controlling centre for micturition lies not in the sacral part of the spinal cord but rather in the reticular formation in the pons. This is the effective switch through which consciousness may impinge its action on micturition through the connections between the frontal cerebral cortex and the pontine centre. Lesions between this pontine centre and the sacral centre produce the condition of detrusor sphincter dyssynergia in a majority of cases. In the normal process of micturition, contraction of the detrusor muscle is due to withdrawal of central inhibition through a conscious act of will relayed to the pontine centre. In the condition of detrusor sphincter dyssynergia, the contraction of the detrusor muscle is not co-ordinated with relaxation of the striated muscle of the external sphincter and so micturition is imperfect, high intravesical pressures are generated and a high residual urine remains. The bladder muscle becomes hypertrophied leading to trabeculation and diverticula.

It is not clear what the temporal associations are in normal micturition as far as this synergy is concerned. In the past, it has been thought that relaxation of the striated sphincter and contraction of the trigone closing the ureteric orifices precedes detrusor contraction by at least 1 s (Blaivas *et al.* 1981). The alternative theory is based on a gate mechanism, namely that elevation of intravesical pressure operates a gate through the afferent impulses in the sympathetic nerves to the posterior horn cells. This allows descending impulses to fire off parasympathetic efferents to the detrusor muscle only when a certain intravesical pressure has been reached (McMahon and Spillane 1982).

A normal and complete process of micturition occurs with lesions above the pontine centre but in this case the bladder may empty at inappropriate times over which the individual has no control.

The effect of aging on these neural processes of micturition is again uncertain. Work which I carried out in 1965 in a series of 24 elderly females who were not incontinent nor had neurological disease indicated the presence of uninhibited contractions in 50% (Brocklehurst and Dillane, 1966). This suggested that loss of neurons particularly in the cingulate gyrus and prefrontal areas with aging impaired cortical inhibition and so allowed the reflex (acting through the sacral or the pontine centres) to be activated producing uninhibited bladder contractions. Thus it seemed that normal elderly individuals were predisposed to urinary incontinence by possessing bladders already functioning imperfectly. However, work published in 1988 by Diokno and colleagues has indicated the presence of uninhibited bladder contractions in only 3.6% of normal women under 75 and 7.7% over 75. The figures for males, however, are strikingly different since they found 31% of males aged 60–74 and 37.5% over 75 had uninhibited contractions. This remarkable sex difference can only be due to the effect of changes in the prostate gland causing detrusor instability in males. The effects of aging elsewhere in the central nervous system are still unexplored in relation to the process of micturition.

Diseases in the central nervous system, particularly cerebrovascular disease and Alzheimer's disease but less spectacularly normal pressure hydrocephalus, may all impair cortical control of micturition producing uninhibited neurogenic bladders (detrusor instability) and urge incontinence. Other diseases which are age associated and may cause micturition disturbances are Parkinsonism (which may lead to detrusor instability or pseudodyssynergia due to a slow relaxation of the pelvic musculature) and spondylosis producing detrusor sphincter dyssynergia or an acontractile bladder.

The predominant cause of incontinence in old people in institutions is hyperreflexia leading to urge incontinence. However, Resnick and his colleagues (1989) indicated that this is not straightforward. They reported that hyperreflexia was associated with impaired contractility in 50% of women and 66% of men in this situation, a condition which they described as hyperreflexia with impaired contractility.

I will turn now to the practical management of incontinence in old people. By the process which has come to be known as urodynamics (or urodynamic assessment) a number of sophisticated investigations are now available to record changes in intravesical pressure and the development of bladder contractions in relation to filling and to provocative stimuli such as coughing and moving. These can be related to urethral closing pressure (for in the simplest terms incontinence equals a stage when intravesical pressure exceeds urethral closing pressure). These findings can also be linked to electromyogram recordings. Urodynamic assessment provides valuable information but is certainly not a first or second line form of investigation for most elderly people. Instead an algorithmic (or simple clinical) method of diagnosis and management has come to be accepted generally and this in turn will indicate the relatively small number of times when a full urodynamic assessment is necessary. The clinical approach is that of history together with examination of the central nervous system, the abdomen (for retention), the vulva (for cough leak and atrophic vaginitis), the rectum (for constipation and prostatic disease) and culture of a midstream specimen of urine. On the basis of this procedure, a number of immediately treatable conditions will have emerged which may be causing incontinence (cystitis, constipation, senile vaginitis, retention due to drugs or prostatic disease and obvious stress incontinence). There may be added to these some simple tests such as ultrasound measurement of residual urine, measurement of flow rate and a pad weighing test to determine that incontinence is actually present and its extent over a number of hours. If this simple approach has not indicated the cause then the second stage is to instigate empirical treatment for a period of a few weeks on the basis of the presenting symptom whether it is urgency (urge incontinence), stress incontinence (pelvic floor weakness) or incontinence of which the patient is unaware. In the first case, a programme of bladder re-education possibly with the use of anticholinergic drugs, should be undertaken; in the second case a programme of pelvic floor exercises, possibly with the use of electrical (interferential) stimulation and a form of biofeedback and in the third case, a further examination to determine whether chronic brain failure is present (the most likely cause) and if so to instigate a programme of timed voiding (these programmes are dealt with in the supplement to *Geriatric Medicine*).

If these are unsuccessful then further investigation and surgery may be indicated or the incontinence may be regarded as intractable and a containment programme using pads or catheters instigated.

Table 1
Histological findings in mid-urethra of six sheep after 7 days of indwelling catheters
(three comformable, three control)

	Control			Conformable		
	1	2	3	4	5	6
Epithelium						
Surface damage	+ +	+ +	±	−	−	−
Inflammatory cells	+	+	+	−	−	−
Lymphocytes, plasma cells, etc	±	±	±	−	±	±
Red blood cells	−	−	−	−	−	±
Lamina propria						
Inflammatory cells	±	±	±	±	±	±
Lymphocytes, plasma cells, etc	±	±	±	−	±	−
Red blood cells	±	±	−	−	−	−

In general, catheters are seen as a last resort in the management of urinary incontinence in old people and this is particularly because of the inevitability of associated bladder infection and the presence in many cases of bypassing due to encrustation and bypassing or extrusion due to urethral or bladder irritation leading to spasm. With these matters in mind we have produced a new catheter—the Conformacath—which attempts to overcome some of these limitations. In studying changes in the aging female urethra we began with a mouse model and found, in addition to loss of smooth muscle and an increase in connective tissue, that the urethra of the female mouse underwent a whole series of cross-sectional shape changes at different levels within the urethra. In our subsequent human studies it was shown that the upper half of the female urethra is a transverse slit which then becomes cruciate and finally a vertical slit at the external meatus. In order to obviate the traumatizing effect of a relatively rigid round tube of which the normal urethral catheter consists, we produced a catheter with a flexible or compliant intraurethral part which adapts to the changing shape of the urethra. Experiments in sheep have shown this to be less traumatizing to the urethra than control catheters (Table 1) and a comparative cross-over trial in a large number of geriatric long-stay female patients indicated that the Conformacath was more comfortable, remained *in situ* longer and encrusted less than the control. It also caused less bypassing but this was not statistically significant (Brocklehurst *et al.* 1988).

From this short survey it will be apparent that there are still no final answers as to the neurological control of micturition and the effect of aging upon it and the optimal method of managing incontinence in old people.

REFERENCES

Blaivas, J. G., Sinaha, H. P., Zied, A. A. H. and Labib, K. B. (1981). Detrusor external sphincter dyssynergia. *Journal of Urology* **125**, 542–544.
Brocklehurst, J. C. and Dillane, J. (1966). Cystometrograms in non incontinent women. *Geront. Clin.* **8**, 285–305.
Brocklehurst, J. C., Hickey, D. S., Davies, I., Kennedy, A. P. and Morris, J. A. (1988). A new urethral catheter. *British Medical Journal* **296**, 1691–1693.
Carlile, A., Davies, I., Faragher, E. and Brocklehurst, J. C. (1987). The epithelium in the female urethra: a quantitative study. *Journal of Urology* **138**, 775–777.
Carlile, A., Davies, I., Rigby, A. and Brocklehurst, J. C. (1988). Age changes in the human female urethra: a morphometric study. *Journal of Urology* **139**, 532–535.
Diokno, A. C., Brown, M. B., Brock, B. M., Herzog, A. R. and Normolle, D. P. (1988). Clinical and cystometric characteristics of continent and incontinent non-institutionalised elderly. *Journal of Urology* **140**, 567–571.
Gosling, J.A., Dixon, J. S., Critchley, H. O. D. and Thompson, S. A. (1981). A comparative study of the human external sphincter and periurethral levator ani muscles. *British Journal of Urology* **53**, 35–41.
McMahon, S. B. and Spillane, K. (1982). Brainstem influences on the parasympathetic supply to the urinary bladder of the cat. *Brain Research* **234**, 237–249.
Measuring and Managing Incontinence. Proceedings of a workshop held in Manchester on 14 July 1988 sponsored by Kabi Vitrum Ltd. Supplement to *Geriatric Medicine*.
Resnick, N. M., Yalla, S. V. and Laurino, E. (1989). The pathophysiology of urinary incontinence among institutionalised elderly persons. *New England Journal of Medicine* **320**, 1–7.
Walter, S., Olesen, K. P., Nordling, J. and Hald, T. (1979). Bladder function in urologically normal middle-aged females. *Scandinavian Journal of Urology and Nephrology* **13**, 249–258.

Discussion

Nordin: I want you to expand on the atrophic vaginitis side of the story. I have been surprised at the number of women with non-specific bladder symptoms, which you would of course be able to classify much better than I can. I think urgency and frequency would be the main features, and then those who have responded to oestrogen pessaries. When you say that one must exclude atrophic vaginitis perhaps you are being too rigorous in your definition. Perhaps there may be more elderly people with varying degrees of oestrogen insufficiency, who might benefit from a trial of an oestrogen pessary.

Brocklehurst: That was really one of the reasons why we are interested to examine the epithelium of the urethra in old and young women. Certainly nearly all women of all ages from the puberty on have some oestrogen-sensitive epithelium. In the reproductive period of most women, the whole urethra is lined with the stratified squamous epithelium which is similar to the external genital tract and which contains the oestrogen receptors. And therefore with atrophic vaginitis there will be an atrophic urethritis and treatment with oestrogens is appropriate. Jean Robinson from our department did some studies on the use of oestrogens in a whole series, and the results were not as good as we would have hoped. It may be that a tendency to revert to cuboidal epithelium as women get older was the reason in part for that.

Nordin: Did you apply these oestrogens in the form of tablets or was it local oestrogen?

Brocklehurst: It was mainly stilboestrol cream that they were using, which has its problems of course in elderly ladies.

Nordin: I have no idea what stilboestrol is—there is now an oestrol cream. I think it might be worthwhile to look at some of those. Stilboestrols are very peculiar compounds indeed.

Brocklehurst: Of course, oestrogens present problems in old ladies, they are quite often not welcome because of the breast swelling and so on.

Birren: Is there a nucleus, such as at the thalamic level, that involves the gating of sensory information from the bladder? In this manner, the normal person may be unaware of a full bladder until the phase of distracting excitement is over.

Brocklehurst: Yes, I think there are many connections, e.g. with the cerebellum, with the basal ganglia, with the hypothalamus, and there are certainly connections at many levels, and their function is by no means clear. I think the charting of the three centres simply provides the basis of our understanding of simply basic micturition. For instance, as the bladder fills the blood pressure rises and as the bladder empties the blood pressure drops; there is probably some hypothalamic link-up causing that for instance.

Hypertension in the Elderly—How Innocent a Bystander?

Franz H. Messerli

Department of Internal Medicine, Section on Hypertensive Diseases, Ochsner Clinic and Alton Ochsner Medical Foundation, New Orleans, Louisiana, USA

INTRODUCTION

Blood pressure progressively increases with aging in Westernized populations, and after the age of 65, up to 50% of otherwise healthy people will ultimately reach arbitrarily set criteria for being hypertensive (National Health Survey 1964, 1975). Since life expectancy in these populations also continues to increase (Fries 1980), we can expect that by the turn of the century more than 10% of the total population will fulfil the criteria of being hypertensive and elderly. Despite these impressive epidemiologic numbers, there is still a great deal of confusion about the significance of blood pressure elevation in the geriatric population. Several preconceived notions have contributed to this confusion: (1) it was thought that hypertension in the elderly was "essential" to compensate for diminished organ perfusion and to force blood through sclerotic vessels; (2) elderly patients often have predominantly systolic hypertension, and it was thought and taught that only diastolic blood pressure elevation was a harbinger of cardiovascular morbidity and mortality; (3) data attesting to the benefits of antihypertensive therapy in the elderly are contradictory and do not allow a firm conclusion and recommendation.

These preconceived notions notwithstanding, a variety of studies have shown that there is nothing benign in hypertension in the elderly. In fact, hypertension seems to be a more powerful risk factor in the elderly than

Challenges in Aging
ISBN 0-12-090163-3

in the middle-aged or younger patient (Veterans Administration Cooperative Study Group on Antihypertensive Agents 1972, Shekelle *et al.* 1974, Svardsudd and Tibblin 1979). Thus, we are facing a formidable health problem affecting millions of otherwise healthy senior citizens and leading all too often to premature strokes, heart attacks, and sudden death.

THE CHICKEN OR THE EGG?

Our research in geriatric hypertension was stimulated by the fact that the elderly hypertensive patient represents a puzzle of at lesat two different pathogenetic processes. On one side, progressive aging *per se* affects the cardiovascular system and can result in age-specific changes. On the other side, the cardiovascular system of the elderly hypertensive patient has been exposed to long-standing hypertension that by itself damages various target organs. The main target organs that are affected by long-standing hypertension are the brain, the heart and the kidneys—the very organs that are predominantly affected by the aging process. A dissociation of the two pathogenetic processes, i.e. aging and arterial hypertension, therefore becomes increasingly difficult. In an attempt to untangle this puzzle, we matched 30 patients over the age of 65 with essential hypertension with an equal number of patients under 42 years of age with regard to mean arterial pressure, body habitus, race and sex (Messerli *et al.* 1983b). In contrast to younger patients with borderline hypertension in whom cardiac output is often elevated, the elderly patients were characterized by a low cardiac output caused by a low stroke volume and relative bradycardia. At the same time, the elderly patients had higher systolic and lower diastolic pressures, elevated left ventricular stroke work, and a distinctly increased total peripheral resistance when compared to younger patients. Similarly, renal blood flow, intravascular volume, and plasma renin activity were low and renal vascular resistance was elevated in the old when compared to the younger hypertensive subjects, indicating volume contraction and nephrosclerosis.

HYPERTENSIVE HEART DISEASE AND SUDDEN DEATH

The heart adapts to a persistent increase in afterload such as occurs in essential hypertension by adding contractile elements to its muscle mass.

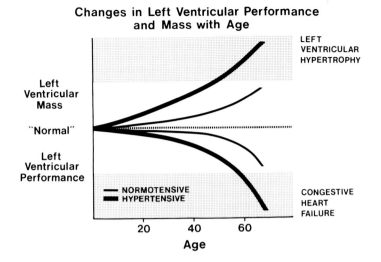

Changes in Left Ventricular Performance and Mass with Age

Fig. 1. Left ventricular mass increases with age, a process that is greatly accelerated by the occurrence of arterial hypertension. Reproduced with permission from Messerli, F. H. (1983). *American Journal of Medicine* **75** (3A), 53.

Not surprising, left ventricular hypertrophy (LVH) is, therefore, a common finding in geriatric hypertension (Fig. 1), and as many as 50% of elderly patients with mild essential hypertension have been documented to fulfil echocardiographic criteria of left ventricular hypertrophy. These context data from the Framingham Cohort must be quoted, indicating that the occurrence of left ventricular hypertrophy greatly and independently of pressure increases the risk of sudden death, acute myocardial infarction, and other cardiovascular morbidity and mortality (Kannel *et al.* 1969, Kannel 1983). Thus, left ventricular hypertrophy cannot be considered as a benign compensatory process serving to normalize wall stress or as an innocent bystander. We documented that hypertensive patients with left ventricular hypertrophy had a greatly increased prevalence of premature ventricular beats and more serious ventricular arrhythmias than patients without LVH or normotensive subjects (Messerli *et al.* 1984). Our findings were recently corroborated and expanded by an epidemiologic study of more than 4000 patients from Framingham (Levy *et al.* 1987) and a clinical report from Glasgow (McLenachan *et al.* 1987). This arrhythmogenicity of the hypertrophied myocardium may well be the predominant risk factor for the occurrence of sudden death.

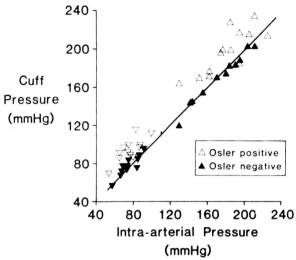

Fig. 2. Comparison of intra-arterial pressure with cuff blood pressure in Osler-positive patients (with pseudohypertension) and Osler-negative patients. Reprinted by permission of *The New England Journal of Medicine* **312**,1550 (1985).

ARTERIAL STIFFNESS, PSEUDOHYPERTENSION AND OSLER'S MANOEUVRE

Not only are the heart and kidneys damaged by long-standing hypertension, but an increase in arterial stiffness throughout the vascular tree further compromises blood flow and adds to the haemodynamic burden on the left ventricle. Arterial stiffness (diminished compliance) can become pronounced enough to give rise to pseudohypertension (Spence *et al.* 1978)—an entity that was hinted at by Sir William Osler in 1892 in his famous textbook *The Principles and Practice of Medicine* (Osler 1892):

> It may be difficult to estimate how much of the hardness and firmness is due to the tension of the blood within the vessel and how much to the thickening of the wall. If, for example, when the radial is compressed with the index finger, the artery can be felt beyond the point of compression, its walls are sclerosed.

From the eloquent description of Osler, we derived a manoeuvre (baptized the "Osler manoeuvre") that was used to classify 35 patients older than 65 years of age as being either Osler-positive or Osler-negative (Messerli *et al.* 1985, Messerli 1986b). We found that Osler-positive patients had cuff pressures that averaged 16 mmHg above intra-arterial pressure, with the greatest discrepancy amounting to 54 mmHg in one patient (Fig. 2). Arterial stiffness as measured inversely by pulse wave velocity and by the diastolic decay of the pulse tracing was consistently higher in Osler-positive than in Osler-negative subjects and correlated directly with the degree of pseudohypertension (difference between cuff pressure and arterial pressure); thus, pseudohypertension became progressively more pronounced as the arteries became stiffer. Our findings have been confirmed and extended by other publications, and Osler's manoeuvre was found to be an elegant bedside technique to differentiate patients with pseudohypertension due to excessive atheromatosis of the large arteries from those with true blood pressure elevation.

Clinical consequences arising from such spurious elevation of arterial pressure are most important. Subjects misdiagnosed as having essential hypertension may be subjected needlessly to the inconvenience, cost, risk, and adverse effects of antihypertensive therapy. Elderly hypertensive patients have been reported to be particularly susceptible to the adverse effects of antihypertensive therapy. Could part of this susceptibility be due to the fact that arterial pressure is often overestimated and therefore overtreated in this age group because of the concomitant or sole presence of pseudohypertension?

OBESITY HYPERTENSION: THE DOUBLE BURDEN

Overweight is a common complicating factor of long-standing hypertension in the elderly. We have documented that obesity, independent of arterial pressure, leads to a dilated form of cardiopathy, i.e. eccentric LVH, by predominantly increasing the preload to the left ventricle (Messerli et al. 1983a, Messerli 1986a). Thus, obesity provides an additional haemodynamic burden to the left ventricle that is already working hard because of the elevated afterload from arterial hypertension (Messerli, 1984). The combination of the two burdens (preload from obesity, afterload from hypertension) takes a heavy toll on the heart and often leads to premature congestive heart failure. Indeed, the Framingham study has identified obesity as a powerful determinant of congestive heart failure (Gordon and Kannel 1976). Not only is congestive heart failure common in obese patients with an enlarged heart, but these patients also are prone to ventricular arrhythmias. We have documented that the prevalence of ventricular ectopy and more serious arrhythmias was significantly more common in obese patients with LVH than in those without LVH or lean subjects (Messerli et al. 1987) (Fig. 3). These data in context with the observations from Framingham of a higher rate of sudden death lend credence to the notion of Hippocrates that "sudden death is more common in those who are naturally fat than in the lean".

Franz H. Messerli

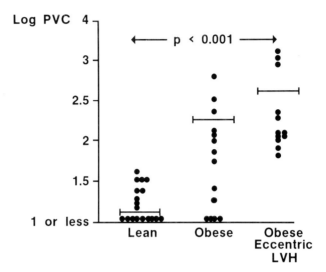

Fig. 3. Ventricular ectopy in obese patients with and without eccentric left ventricular hypertrophy as compared with lean subjects. Reproduced with permission from Messerli, F. H. *et al.* (1987). *Archives of Internal Medicine* **147**, 1725.

CLINICAL IMPLICATIONS

Although it is clear that the occurrence of hypertension in the elderly greatly increases the risk of heart attack, stroke, sudden death, and congestive heart failure, it is not so clear whether lowering of arterial pressure into the normotensive range will prevent cardiovascular morbidity and mortality. In fact, treatment of hypertension in the elderly has proved to be difficult and often frustrating. We submit that a part of this lack of success is due to the fact that cardiovascular findings in elderly patients are distinct from the ones in young patients and therefore necessitate a different age-specific approach. Unfortunately, in most of the studies that examined the effects of antihypertensive therapy in the elderly, no concessions were made in this regard. Moreover, the presence of pseudohypertension in a small percentage of our senior citizens will lead to miscalculation of cardiovascular risk factors and may become responsible for adverse effects caused by inappropriately lowered blood pressure. Clearly, before we label as many as half of our oldsters as hypertensive and subject them for the remainder of their days to the risk, inconvenience, and cost of hypertensive therapy, the presence of pseudohypertension should be ruled out. Regardless of pseudohypertension, however, any increase in arterial pressure serves to accelerate the aging process of the cardiovascular system. Conversely, a close match between cardiovascular pathophysiology in the geriatric patient

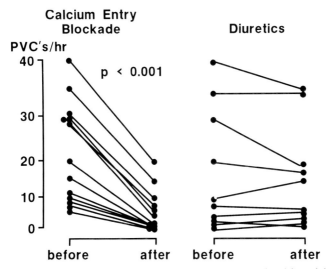

Fig. 4. Decrease in ventricular ectopy in patients treated with calcium entry blockade. No decrease in ventricular ectopy (nor in left ventricular hypertrophy) in patients treated with a diuretic despite a similar fall in arterial pressure. Reproduced with permission from Messerli, F. H. *et al.* (1989). *Archives of Internal Medicine* **149**, 1263–1267.

and the pharmacologic effects of an antihypertensive drug will increase flow to and function of target organs and thereby will hopefully decelerate the aging process and reset the biological clock at a slower pace. Figure 4 illustrates an example of such a specific approach: antihypertensive therapy with calcium entry blockade reduces arterial pressure and left ventricular hypertrophy and diminishes ventricular ectopy (Messerli *et al.* 1989). In contrast, antihypertensive therapy with a diuretic had no effect on left ventricular hypertrophy or on ventricular ectopy despite a similar fall in arterial pressure.

OUTLOOK

Research over the past few years has allowed us to better define mechanisms of pressure elevation in the elderly hypertensive patient and to identify early development of target organ disease such as left ventricular hypertrophy with its ominous prognosis and nephrosclerosis. Hopefully, specific anti-hypertensive therapy closely targeted to mechanisms of pressure elevation will prevent or reverse such target organ disease. This targeted approach should not only lower millimetres of mercury but should improve the patient's well-being and quality of life and thereby add meaningful years to the life spans of our senior citizens.

REFERENCES

Fries, J. F. (1980). Aging, natural death, and the compression of morbidity. *New England Journal of Medicine* **303**, 130–135.

Gordon, T. and Kannel, W. B. (1976). Obesity and cardiovascular diseases: the Framingham study. *Clinics in Endocrinology and Metabolism* **5** (2), 367–375.

Kannel, W.B. (1983). Prevalence and natural history of electrocardiographic left ventricular hypertrophy. *In* "Proceedings of a symposium: left ventricular hypertrophy in essential hypertension" (F. H. Messerli and R. C. Schlant, eds), *American Journal of Medicine* **76**, 4–11.

Kannel, W.B., Gordon, T. and Offutt, D. (1969). Left ventricular hypertrophy by electrocardiogram: prevalence, incidence, and mortality in the Framingham study. *Annals of Internal Medicine* **71**, 89–105.

Levy, D., Anderson, K. M., Savage, D. D., Balkus, S. A., Kannel, W. B. and Castelli, W. P. (1987). Risk of ventricular arrhythmias in left ventricular hypertrophy: The Framingham heart study. *American Journal of Cardiology* **60**, 560–565.

McLenachan, J. M., Henderson, E., Morris, K. I. and Dargie, H. J. (1987). Ventricular arrhythmias in patients with hypertensive left ventricular hypertrophy. *New England Journal of Medicine* **317**, 787–792.

Messerli, F. H. (1983). Clinical determinants and consequences of left ventricular hypertrophy. Proceedings of a symposium: left ventricular hypertrophy in essential hypertension—mechanisms and therapy. *American Journal of Medicine* **75** (3A), 51–56.

Messerli, F. H. (1984). Obesity in hypertension: how innocent a bystander? *American Journal of Medicine* **77**, 1077–1082.

Messerli, F. H. (1986a). Cardiopathy of obesity—a not-so-Victorian disease. *New England Journal of Medicine* **314** (6), 378–380.

Messerli, F. H. (1986b). Osler's maneuver, pseudohypertension, and true hypertension in the elderly. *American Journal of Medicine* **80**, 906–910.

Messerli, F. H., Sundgaard-Riise, K., Reisin, E. D., Dreslinski, R. D., Ventura, H. O., Oigman, W., Frohlich, E. D. and Dunn, F. G. (1983a). Dimorphic cardiac adaptation to obesity and arterial hypertension. *Annals of Internal Medicine* **99**, 757–761.

Messerli, F. H., Ventura, H. O., Glade, L. B., Sundgaard-Riise, K., Dunn, F. G. and Frohlich, E. D. (1983b). Essential hypertension in the elderly: haemodynamics, intravascular volume, plasma renin activity, and circulating catecholamine levels. *Lancet* **2**, 983–986.

Messerli, F.H., Ventura, H. O., Elizardi, D. J., Dunn, F. G. and Frohlich, E. D. (1984). Hypertension and sudden death: increased ventricular ectopic activity in left ventricular hypertrophy. *American Journal of Medicine* **77**, 18–22.

Messerli, F. H., Ventura, H. O. and Amodeo, C. (1985). Osler's maneuver and pseudohypertension. *New England Journal of Medicine* **312**, 1548–1551.

Messerli, F. H., Nunez, B. D., Ventura, H. O. and Snyder, D. W. (1987). Overweight and sudden death: increased ventricular ectopy in cardiopathy of obesity. *Archives of Internal Medicine* **147**, 1725–1728.

Messerli, F. H., Nunez, B. D., Nunez, M. M., Garavaglia, G. E., Schmieder,

R. E. and Ventura, H. O. (1989). Hypertension and sudden death: disparate effects of calcium entry blocker and diuretic therapy on cardiac dysrhythmias. *Archives of Internal Medicine* **149**, 1263–1267.

National Health Survey. (1964). Vital and Health Statistics USA. Blood pressure of adults by age and sex. US Government Printing Office, p. 9. Washington, DC.

National Health Survey. (1975). Vital and Health Statistics Series 11, No. 150. Blood pressure of persons 18 to 74 years. US Department of Health, Education and Welfare, Bethesda, MD.

Osler, W. (1892). "Principles and Practice of Medicine". Appleton-Century & Croft, New York.

Shekelle, R. B., Ostfeld, A. M. and Klawans, H. F. Jr (1974). Hypertension and risk of stroke in an elderly population. *Stroke* **5**, 71–75.

Spence, J. D. Sibblad, W. J. and Cape, R. D. (1978). Pseudohypertension in the elderly. *Clinical Science and Molecular Medicine* **5** (4), 399s–402s.

Svardsudd, K. and Tibblin, G. (1979). Mortality and morbidity during 13.5 years' follow up in relation to blood pressure. *Acta Medica Scandinavica* **205**, 483–484.

Veterans Administration Cooperative Study Group on Antihypertensive Agents. (1972). Effect of treatment on morbidity in hypertension: III. Influence of age, diastolic pressure, and prior cardiovascular disease. *Circulation* **45**, 991–1004.

Discussion

Dall: I would like to congratulate you on your overview and I would like to ask a little more about left ventricular hypertrophy in relation to blood pressure and particularly to the measurement of left ventricular hypertrophy before and after treatment. There is some evidence to suggest that the function of the left ventricle changes as you bring the blood pressure down and that what we may be seeing is an alteration in the form of contraction rather than a change in real wall thickness and I wonder if you have any comment on that.

Messerli: I know what you are referring to. It is quite clear that when you lower arterial pressure you unload the left ventricle, therefore there is a change in structure as well as a change in function. Now this, however, depends a good deal on what kind of antihypertensive therapy you use. When you give a beta-blocker for instance, you have a relative ventricular dilatation; when you give a diuretic, then, on the contrary, you have a relative ventricular contraction. Overall, it is probably true that the change in millimetres of wall thickness that we measure is due to this ventricular dilatation or ventricular contraction. That's correct.

The Measurement Paradox of Disability and its Implications for Gerontology

Matthew H. Liang

*Robert B. Brigham Multipurpose Arthritis Center, Brigham
and Women's Hospital, and Departments of Medicine and
Rheumatology/Immunology, Harvard Medical School,
Harvard School of Public Health, Boston, Massachusetts,
USA*

INTRODUCTION

Modern medicine has focused quite appropriately on impairment or
anatomical, biological and physiological abnormalities, and increasingly, at
genetic aberrations. But having described human disease in these terms
much seems missing in describing human ailments. A biosocial view of
human disease illuminates the illness experience, the consequences of
impairment on individuals and permits an understanding of functionality,
or its converse, disability and handicap. The disability model which
distinguishes impairment, disability and handicap provides a useful framework for identifying the important features of any organized system of care
for the elderly (Wood 1980).

Functional disability is the common result of all diseases and surgical
conditions and, inevitably, also of aging. Over 27 years since Katz and
colleagues standardized the assessment of biological and psychological
functioning in the elderly (Katz *et al.* 1963), the measurement of
function, health status and quality of life has evolved to the point where
psychometrically reliable, valid, sensitive measures can be applied to a

Challenges in Aging
ISBN 0-12-090163-3

variety of problems. These include community morbidity surveys, case-finding (Liang *et al.* 1981), evaluation of health services (Liang *et al.* 1984), cost-benefit/cost-effectiveness analysis (Liang *et al.* 1986), needs assessment (Fortinsky *et al.* 1981) and clinical trials (Liang *et al.* 1990).

Surveys of disability provide a simple and economic way to document community morbidity or identify potential subjects in need of services. In 1981 we used this approach in a population-based study of 11 000 subjects to establish the prevalence of musculoskeletal disability and to do case identification and needs assessment, and showed that a community ombudsman could be effective in reducing barriers and in improving function (Liang *et al.* 1981). Since then, the use of function as a survey focus has been used by the World Health Organization in the Third World, in the People's Republic of China, and in Taiwan.

The study taught us that reported function in the elderly could very often be at variance with observed ability and that functional problems were not recognized nor dealt with by the subject's physician in a quarter of the individuals.

Quantitative measures of function have been used to evaluate the impact and cost effectiveness of services and treatments in the elderly. For example, total joint arthroplasty is a major advance in the management of end-stage joint disease, and yet in some countries, has been restricted or debated in the elderly. We showed it to be cost effective, that cost effectiveness was related to function at baseline, and challenged the appropriateness of using *only* cost-benefit analysis in formulating policy for the elderly (Liang *et al.* 1986).

The debate over home care, its effectiveness, its cost effectiveness, and what components should be supported has engendered heated debate with scant objective data. We evaluated the effectiveness of intensive rehabilitation services in homebound elderly (Liang *et al.* 1984). This controlled clinical trial showed that in frail homebound elderly patients, intensive social and rehabilitation services did not change utilization, function or mental health for the group as a whole, but that such services, done for a minimal marginal cost, enabled most clients to achieve functional goals, and in some patients, to achieve dramatic functional improvement.

The patients also taught us that simple things, particularly aids and devices, could improve independence, that function is relative, and that functional problems once established cannot easily be dissected into component causes. The experience also showed that the measurement of function and health status in groups of subjects is very different from the problems presented to clinicians who are involved with the care of the elderly. There are abundant assessment schemes for the elderly but these are largely for elderly in institutional settings (Kane and Kane 1981) and not for the aged population in the community. We have developed a rapid functional evaluation scheme based on observed tasks for evaluating the elderly in the community (Liang *et al.* 1983). This instrument is now an integral part of the routine assessment by community nurses in Boston and by some family practitioners in Europe.

In each case, the paradox of disability, its imperfect relationship to "objective" impairment, is evident and these exceptions tell us something as we respond to the challenge of caring for the elderly.

FUNCTION AS A MULTIFACTORIAL PHENOMENON

Functional ability is determined by the mental and physical capabilities to perform complex integrated tasks of self-care, work and recreation; by the motivation and will to do so; and by the necessity to do so as dictated by the social support system and the physical environment. The conceptual model which assumes that function can be captured validly by a closed-ended questionnaire ignores this basic problem.

Correcting impairments is a necessary but not sufficient strategy for improving function. Fixing things may not be acceptable ("I'm too old to have surgery") or done safely. A preoccupation with impairment overlooks the opportunities to manipulate the environment to allow a subject with diminished physical capacity to adapt or to be maximally independent.

The community environment is, after all, under man's control to a large degree and means that we can rationally improve it to minimize the effects of normal aging or aging in the rheumatic disease patient. These include improved access to public transportation, public buildings, housing options which permit autonomy with surveillance and meaningful social interactions, and reimbursement of rehabilitation services.

DISABILITY AS A NON-LINEAR PHENOMENON

Disability is a non-linear phenomenon like an argument whose antecedent events, misunderstandings, and differences cannot be pieced together. Once established it cannot be easily dissected or treated. In the elderly, the reason for a fall, for example, may be impossible to sort out. A detailed examination shows no gross deficits or small problems that do not add up or cannot be reversed. We attribute it to aging. Similarly, multiple factors *might* be causative. A report by Wolf-Klein detailing a comprehensive evaluation of 36 patients who had fallen showed multiple diagnosis and associated problems, with the majority having more than one aetiological factor (Wolf-Klein *et al.* 1988).

The discontinuous development of disability suggests that regular assessment of function might allow one to intercede at an earlier point in which it might be prevented. If this were true this assessment is unlikely to be done effectively by physicians since they usually see patients for problems and when functional loss is advanced. Even when patients are closely followed by physicians functional problems are often not recognized or treated (Liang *et al.* 1981, Hart *et al.* 1988). Rather, a more effective public health strategy might be educational, directed at the elderly, or their caretakers to enable them to identify these problems themselves. More research on the course of functional decline (Weg, 1973, Bergstrom *et al.* 1985) and attention to identifying areas in which early intervention might make a difference are desperately needed.

THE INEVITABILITY OF FUNCTIONAL DECLINE

Decline in functional ability in normal aging is insidious and inevitable and the only issue for an individual is the slope of that trajectory. For the individual the decline imperceptibly unfolds while expectations and activities constrict, and their social network adapts and the individual gets used to diminished ability. What trajectory functional decline takes is a matter of genes and chance but social and health policy should not miss treatable functional decline. Critical incidents put an individual on a steeper slope of declining function and could be amenable to focused interventions.

More research needs to be done, but we already know something about this area, and I would like to illustrate two important milestones.

The first example is PM, an 80-year-old Irish surveyor, who was homebound because of "arthritis" which, on evaluation, proved to be severe flexion contractures of the knees and hips with normal joints and neuromotor function. PM's wife died 6 years before our visit. Shortly after her death, PM had a urinary tract infection which prompted hospitalization. PM was treated successfully and discharged home. Once home, he fell several times and was convinced that he would never walk again. When we saw him, his apartment was bare except for a cockpit around his couch on which he stayed 24 hours a day. He slept, drank, and toileted there, and his knees took the shape of his couch. He could not walk unaided.

Full recovery after a major illness or hospitalization is a critical event. A discharged patient is often assumed to be recovered and is not followed up. With the pressure to reduce hospital stay to reduce costs many patients will experience what this patient did. Recovery occurs more slowly in the elderly but in our experience is an important opportunity to ensure that the patient has an active programme to regain his or her baseline. Intercurrent illness or hospitalization can also reduce the ability of the elderly patient to respond to an increase in activity or programmed exercises to improve endurance (Naso *et al.* 1990).

> The second milestone may be illustrated by a woman we visited. The subject was a 75-year-old woman of Swedish ancestry whom we visited in a retirement home. Her health was good but she complained of decreased stamina. A medical evaluation showed no abnormalities. A social history revealed that she had thrived for many years in the home. She started to deteriorate 3 years before our visit after the home had been bought by a for-profit company. At this point her neighbours changed dramatically and instead of people she could socialize with, demented and emotionally troubled residents were accepted—to take advantage of government reimbursement—and our patient became withdrawn and stopped going to group activities and on walks.

It's difficult to know for sure whether her diminished stamina was related to diminished social reinforcement of physical activity which could have led to deconditioning. Studies indicate that elderly subjects can respond to endurance training. We surmise that the change in her social environment may have been the critical incident in her decline.

BARRIERS TO IMPROVING FUNCTION

One practical problem is that a functional evaluation, especially in multi-need, elderly patients with sensory deficits, can be time consuming. We find no one technique completely satisfactory. Self-administered questionnaires, whether they be short screening or comprehensive ones, may give false negative replies in elderly patients who perceive no discrepancy between what they do and what they are expected to do, or who have become used to their disability. Stated problems with functional risks may have nothing to do with actual ability but may be related to lack of confidence or fear that performing the task, for example, might put them at risk of falling or fracturing osteoporotic bones. Self-reported function and performance tests may be difficult to interpret in the cognitively impaired. Self-reported function is probably insensitive to early or mild deficits. We have developed a performance-based physical capacity evaluation for morbidity surveys but it would not be convenient in the office setting. We believe that any functional evaluation of the elderly must include both questions and performance tests to be a sensitive, reliable measure (Table 1).

Having a practical and sensitive functional assessment technique is only

Table 1
Screening for functional problems*

Test	Areas tested	Suspected functional problem
1. Touch first knuckle to top of head	Shoulder abduction, flexion and external rotation, elbow flexion	Oral hygiene, grooming, eating
2. Touch back of waist	Shoulder internal rotation, wrist flexion	Dressing
3. Place palm to opposite trochanter	Wrist flexion, shoulder internal rotation, elbow flexion	Perineal care
4. Touch index finger to palmar crease	Finger flexion	Grip
5. Touch index finger to thumb	Thumb opposition, finger abduction	Grip
6. Sitting, touch toes	Back, hip, knee flexion, elbow extension	Lower body dressing
7. Stand up from chair without use of hands	Hip girdle and quadriceps strength	Transfer ability
8. Stand unassisted, clear 6″ block	Quadriceps strength. Hip, knee, ankle subtalar flexion	Walking, stairclimbing
9. Tandem stand†	Balance	Mobility
10. Copy sentence‡	Fine hand co-ordination, cognition	Cognitive

*Examiner asks subject to imitate tasks and observes ability, rhythm or pain.
†Subject is asked to stand toe to heel for 10 seconds.
‡Subject is asked to copy the following sentence as quickly as possible: "John saw the red truck coming". (Observe for slow response, difficulty in seeing, or copying one word at a time.) The letters are 1/8″ high and in bold print.

part of the solution. Although much can be done by educating health care providers in doing better functional assessment, there is little formal training in medicine on how to improve function or what to do after discovering a problem. A recent study of a geriatric assessment team illustrates this (McVey et al. 1989). Among elderly patients admitted to an acute-care facility 60% had some and a third had serious functional difficulties. The multidisciplinary team did not alter the functional outcomes; it was thought to be due to inability to deliver or follow-up recommendations.

Rubenstein also showed that physician education and regular reports of health status on their patients did not result in improved function for the patients although the information was found to be of use (Rubenstein *et al.* 1989).

RECOMMENDATIONS

The model of disability provides a framework on which to plan for effective elder care. Home care is largely provided by significant others and an organized approach should do everything possible to support the caregivers (Andolsek *et al.* 1988, Zola 1990). These include providing "travel agent" functions to help the uninitiated take advantage of community resources; back-up home rehabilitation, no-fault admissions to minimal care units. Assistive devices are inappropriately prescribed, maintained and followed. Many devices and assistive aids are never used. Finally, we should not miss treating reversible functional decline and improving the social and physical environment to optimize function.

ACKNOWLEDGEMENT

I am indebted to my colleagues Martha Logigian, Holley Eaton, Alison Partridge and Charlotte Phillips, for their insights and to Jacqueline Mazzie for assistance in the preparation of this manuscript.

Supported by NIH grants No. AR36308, Biomedical Research Support Grant RR–05950 and NIH grant No. AG07459–01.

REFERENCES

Andolsek, K. M., Clapp-Channing, N. E., Gehlbach, S. H., Moore, I., Proffitt, V. S., Simon, A. and Warshaw, G. A. (1988). Caregivers and elderly relatives: The prevalence of caregiving in a family practice. *Archives of Internal Medicine* **1481**, 2177–2180.

Bergstrom, G., Aniansson, A., Bjelle, A. *et al.* (1985). Functional consequences of joint impairment at age 79. *Scandinavian Journal of Rehabilitation Medicine* **17**, 183–190.

Fortinsky, R. H., Granger, C. V. and Seltzer, G. B. (1981). The use of functional assessment in understanding homecare needs. *Medical Care* **19**, 489–493.

Hart, D., Bowling, A., Ellis, M. and Silman, A. (1988). Potentially reversible joint-related handicap in an elderly population. *British Journal of Rheumatism* **27** (suppl. 2), 68.

Kane, R. A. and Kane, R. L. (1981). "Assessing the elderly: a practical guide to measurement". Lexington Books, Lexington, Massachusetts.

Katz, S., Amasa, B. F., Moskowitz, R. W., Jackson, B. A. and Jaffe, M. W. (1963). Studies of illness in the aged. The index of ADL: a standardized measure of biological and psychological function. *Journal of the American Medical Association* **185**, 914–919.

Liang, M. H., Phillips, E. E., Scamman, M. D., Lurye, C. S., Keith, A., Cohen, L. and Taylor, G. (1981). Evaluation of a pilot program for rheumatic disability in an urban community. *Arthritis and Rheumatism* **24**, 937–943.

Liang, M. H., Gall, V., Partridge, A. and Eaton, H. (1983). Management of functional disability in homebound patients. *Journal of Family Practice* **17**, 429–435.

Liang, M. H., Cullen, K. E., Larson, M. G., Thompson, M. S. and Schwartz, J. A. (1986). Cost-effectiveness of total joint arthroplasty in osteoarthritis. *Arthritis and Rheumatism* **29**, 937–943.

Liang, M. H., Partridge, A. J., Larson, M. G., Gall, V., Taylor, J. E. and Master, R. (1984). Evaluation of comprehensive rehabilitation services for elderly homebound patients with arthritis and orthopedic disability. *Arthritis and Rheumatism* **27**, 258–266.

Liang, M. H., Katz, J. N. and Ginsburg, K. S. (1990). *In* "Chronic rheumatic disease in quality of life assessments in clinical trials" (B. Spilker, ed.), pp. 441–458. Raven Press, New York.

McVey, L. J., Becker, P. M., Saltz, C. C., Feusnner, J. R. and Cohen, H. J. (1989). Effect of a geriatric consultation team on functional status of elderly hospitalized patients: a randomized, controlled clinical trial. *Annals of Internal Medicine* **110**, 79–84.

Naso, F., Carner, E., Blankfort-Doyle, M. A. and Coughey, K. (1990). Endurance training in the elderly nursing home patient. *Archives of Physical Medicine and Rehabilitation* **71**, 241–243.

Rubenstein, L. V., Calkins, D. R., Young, R. T., Cleary, P. D., Fink, A., Kosecoff, J., Jette, A. M., Davies, A. R., Delbanco, T. L. and Brook, R. H. (1989). Improving patient function: a randomized trial of functional disability screening. *Annals of Internal Medicine* **111**, 836–842.

Weg, R. B. (1973). The changing physiology of aging. *American Journal of Occupational Therapy* **27**, 213–217.

Wolf-Klein, G. P., Silverstone, F. A., Basavaraju, N., Foley, C. J., Pascaru, A. and Ma, P. H. (1988). Prevention of falls in the elderly population. *Archives of Physical Medicine and Rehabilitation* **69**, 689–691.

Wood, P. H. N. (1980). Appreciating the consequences of disease: the international classification of impairments, disabilities, and handicaps. *WHO Chronicle* **34**, 376–380.

Zola, I. K. (1990). Aging, disability and the home-care revolution. *Archives of Physical Medicine and Rehabilitation* **71**, 93–96.

Discussion

E. Steinhagen-Thiessen: Have you data about the patients who were evaluated for the 2-month treatment programme [Liang *et al.* 1984] about their objective health status in comparison with their subjective health status, i.e. do you have a scale or ranking about their objective health status?

Liang: Their subjective health status measured by a modified Functional Status Instrument did not improve *as a group* although some patients improved tremendously on objective measures.

The Role of Calcium in the Pathogenesis of Atherosclerosis

Hajime Orimo and Yasuyoshi Ouchi

Department of Geriatrics, Faculty of Medicine, University of Tokyo, Tokyo 113, Japan

INTRODUCTION

Pathological examinations have revealed that various changes such as intimal thickening, fatty deposits, and proliferation of smooth muscle cells are observed in atherosclerotic lesions. As atherosclerosis advances, necrotic lesions are formed, and free cholesterol and calcium accumulate in the atherosclerotic lesion. The biological process involved in the development of atherosclerosis is, thus, quite complex. Moreover, because of the slow development, to elucidate the pathogenesis has been difficult. However, recent advances in cell biology and molecular biology have facilitated the research of atherosclerosis from new standpoints.

Previously, the role of calcium in atherogenesis has been overlooked, because calcium deposits were believed to occur in the final stage of atherogenesis, precluding its possible involvement. However, Blumenthal *et al.* (1950) reported that calcium deposits are present in the media of the aorta in the early stage of atherosclerosis. Strickberger *et al.* (1988) also reported the increase, by 4.8-fold, of Ca transport across the aortic plasma membrane and the increase of both intracellular and extracellular Ca in cholesterol-fed rabbits. Evidence has accumulated that calcium is crucial in the various cellular functions such as cell proliferation, secretion and contraction (Campbell 1983). Moreover, calcium antagonists, including lanthanum (Kramsch *et al.* 1980), nifedipine (Henry and Bentley 1981), nicardipine (Willis *et al.* 1985), verapamil (Blumlein *et al.* 1984), diltiazem

Challenges in Aging
ISBN 0-12-090163-3

(Ginsburg *et al.* 1983), and nilvadipine (Koibuchi *et al.* 1989) have been reported to prevent the development of atherosclerosis in cholesterol-fed rabbits. These findings strongly suggest that calcium plays an important role in atherogenesis.

The pathogenesis of atherosclerosis is nowadays explained based on the "response-to-injury" hypothesis (Ross and Glomset 1976, Ross 1986). According to this hypothesis, the following major phenomena occur in the process of atherogenesis:

1. Endothelial cells lining the arterial intima are injured.
2. Permeability of endothelial cells increases.
3. Platelets aggregate at the injured site.
4. Smooth muscle cells migrate from the media to the intima and subsequently proliferate in response to growth factors released from platelets such as platelet derived growth factor (Ross *et al.* 1974) and epidermal growth factor (Oka and Orth 1983, Ouchi *et al.* 1988).

However, the role of calcium in the procss of atherogenesis has not been fully elucidated. Therefore, we investigated the function of arterial cells with special reference to intracellular Ca metabolism. We also investigated the effect of long-term use of nifedipine on the progression of coronary artery stenosis in humans.

ENDOTHELIAL CELLS

Endothelial cells (ECs) have some important functions in maintaining blood vessel homeostasis. One of the major functions of ECs is an antithrombotic action, which can be largely attributed to the prostaglandin I_2 (PGI_2)producing activity. PGI_2 is known to be a potent vasodilator and, also, a potent platelet aggregation inhibitor, thus preventing thrombus formation on arterial walls. The PGI_2-producing activity of ECs depends on calcium; PGI_2 synthesis increases when intracellular calcium concentration is increased by calcium ionophore (Brotherton *et al.* 1982). PGI_2 is synthesized from arachidonic acid which is a breakdown product of cell membrane phospholipid. The reaction is known to be catalysed by phospholipase A_2. PGI_2 is finally synthesized via PGG_2 and PGH_2 by the action of PGI_2 synthetase. The rate-limiting step of this sequential reaction is the arachidonic acid synthesis from phospholipid, and calcium ions are reported to accelerate this reaction (Pickett *et al.* 1977). On the other hand, calcium antagonists, acting as a voltage-dependent calcium channel blocker, increase PGI_2 release from cultured ECs (Toyoda *et al.* 1984) and aortic smooth muscle cells (SMCs) (Terashita and Orimo 1986). We assessed the mechanism of action of diltiazem, a calcium antagonist that increases PGI_2 release from cultured aortic SMCs (Terashita and Orimo 1986). Our first study was designed to assess the effect of diltiazem on the activity of phospholipase A_2, a rate-limiting enzyme in PGI_2 synthesis. Cultured rat aortic SMCs were incubated along with ^{14}C-arachidonic acid (0.05 μCi ml^{-1}) for 24 h. After washing out unincorporated ^{14}C-arachidonic acid, diltiazem (100 μM) was then added to the culture media, and phospholipase activity was measured by the amount of released ^{14}C-arachidonic acid. We found that diltiazem produced no significant change in the enzyme activity. Next, we investigated the effect of diltiazem on the PGI_2 synthetic pathway after arachidonic acid synthesis. We measured the amount of PGI_2 (assayed as the amount of 6-keto-$PGF_{1\alpha}$ released into the culture media) when arachidonic acid was added after inhibiting endogenous arachidonic acid production with quinacrine (50 mM). Diltiazem (100 μM) again had no effect on PGI_2 production. Based on these results, we concluded diltiazem does not affect the PGI_2 synthetic process, but may accelerate the release of synthesized PGI_2 from SMCs. Toyoda et al. (1984) also reported the similar result that diltiazem and verapamil increase PGI_2 release in cultured ECs derived from human umbilical vein. They suggested that the increased release of PGI_2 might be mediated by a decrease in cyclic GMP production in ECs provoked by nifedipine.

Another important biological function of ECs is to regulate the vascular permeability. We found that lipid peroxide and superoxide, both members of active oxygen species, increase low-density lipoprotein (LDL) transport across ECs. LDL transport across ECs was assessed according to the method described by Territo et al. (1984). ECs from pig aorta were cultured on gelatin-coated polycarbonate filter (pore size 5 μm) placed in a modified Boyden chamber. At confluency, ^{125}I–LDL was added to the medium in the upper chamber with and without linoleate hydroperoxide (3.2 μM) and was incubated at 37°C for 60 min. Radioactivity in the lower chamber was then measured and was considered to be the amount of transported LDL. We also found that lipid peroxide and superoxide increase intracellular calcium levels, measured by using quin 2, in ECs in a dose-dependent manner (Hirosumi et al. 1988). Nifedipine (3 μM) inhibited both the increase in intracellular calcium levels and the increase in LDL transport. Such members of active oxygen species as lipid peroxide and superoxide are known to damage ECs both morphologically (Weiss et al. 1981, Sasaguri et al. 1984) and functionally, which in turn promotes atherosclerosis. Our results indicate that the atherogenic activity of active oxygen species might be, at least in part, mediated by calcium influx into ECs, and calcium antagonist may prevent the endothelial cell damage provoked by active oxygen.

Other important functions of ECs include the synthesis of proteoglycan, which possesses anticoagulation activity (Shimada and Ozawa 1987), plasminogen activators, and thrombomodulin (Maruyama and Majerus

1985). Moreover, ECs are known to produce various biologically active substances, such as endothelium derived relaxing factor (Furchgott and Zawadzki 1980), endothelin (Yanagisawa *et al.* 1988), and platelet-activating factor (Benveniste *et al.* 1972). The role of calcium in the production and the action of these substances remains to be elucidated.

SMOOTH MUSCLE CELLS

The fundamental function of vascular smooth muscle cells (SMCs) in the media of arteries is contracting and relaxing arteries, and this type of SMC is thus called the "contractile type". In contrast, SMCs migrated from the media to the intima in the process of atherogenesis are somehow changed to the "synthetic type", which produces various substances such as collagen and elastin and proliferates. Migration of SMCs and the subsequent proliferation in the intima are important phenomena in atherogenesis (Ross 1986). Nakao *et al.* (1983a) revealed that calcium plays an important role in the migration of SMCs. They investigated the effect of 12-hydroxy-5,8, 10,14-eicosatetraenoic acid (12-HETE) on migration of rat aortic SMCs cultured on a Millipore filter (pore size 8 μm) which was placed in the upper compartment of a Boyden chamber. The number of SMCs reaching a depth of 30 μm were used as the index of migrating activity. 12-HETE significantly increased the migration of SMCs; this migration was inhibited by reducing extracellular calcium concentration and by pretreating SMCs with nicardipine and trifluoroperazone. These results indicate that 12-HETE-induced migration of SMCs is calcium dependent. They also showed that platelet-derived growth factor (PDGF) increases the migration of SMCs and that the effect disappears in the presence of lipoxygenase inhibitor (Nakao *et al.* 1983b). These results clearly indicate that lipoxygenase products, such as 12-HETE, are actually involved in the mechanism of migration-accelerating activity of PDGF. Calcium antagonists are reported to inhibit smooth muscle cell migration provoked also by interleukin-1, leukotriene B_4, PDGF and inflammatory cell products (Nomoto *et al.* 1988).

   The proliferation of SMCs is also closely related to calcium. We investigated the effect of growth factors on DNA synthesis and intracellular calcium concentration of cultured SMCs derived from rat aortic media (Hirosumi *et al.* 1989). DNA synthesis of SMCs was measured as the incorporation of [3H]-thymidine into SMCs and intracellular calcium concentration in SMCs was measured by using a fluorescent calcium

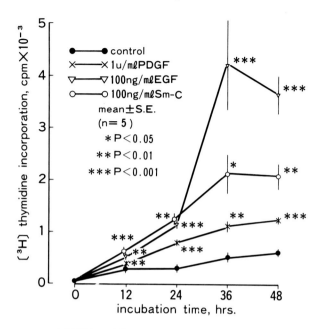

Fig. 1. Time course of [³H]thymidine incorporation into cultured rat aortic smooth muscle cells stimulated by platelet-derived growth factor (1 unit ml⁻¹; $\triangle$———$\triangle$), epidermal growth factor (100 ng ml⁻¹; $\blacktriangle$———$\blacktriangle$) and somatomedin-C (100 ng ml⁻¹; $\bullet$———$\bullet$). *$P < 0.05$, **$P < 0.01$ vs control ($\circ$———$\circ$). The amount of [³H] thymidine incorporation is expressed as the radioactivity (cpm) per well of culture dish. Mean ± SE from five experiments. (Reproduced from Hirosumi et al. 1989, with permission.)

indicator, quin 2 (Tien et al. 1982). Epidermal growth factor (EGF) and PDGF rapidly increased intracellular calcium concentration (Fig. 1), which was followed by increased DNA synthesis in SMCs (Fig. 2). The mechanism which links increased intracellular calcium concentration with increased DNA synthesis is not yet known. Be that as it may, calcium might be a second messenger of the biological action of EGF and PDGF. We also found that the effect of nifedipine on intracellular calcium concentration and DNA synthesis increased by EGF and PDGF. As shown in Figs 3 and 4, nifedipine significantly inhibited the EGF-induced increase in intracellular calcium concentration and DNA synthesis, but did not inhibit the PDGF-induced increase in DNA synthesis. Intracellular calcium is known to be mobilized via two routes: (1) influx of extracellular calcium and (2) release of calcium from intracellular storage sites such as endoplasmic reticulum and mitochondria. EGF was considered to increase intracellular calcium concentration by stimulating influx of extracellular calcium, because the EGF-induced increase in intracellular calcium concentration disappeared

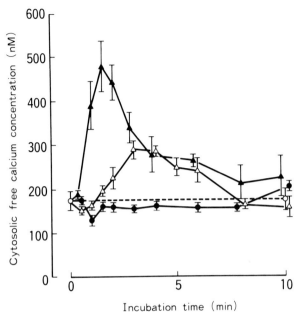

Fig. 2. Time course changes in cytosolic free calcium concentration in cultured rat aortic smooth muscle cells stimulated by platelet-derived growth factor (1 unit ml^{-1}; △——△), epidermal growth factor (100 ng ml^{-1}; ▲——▲) and somatomedin-C (100 ng ml^{-1}; ●——●). Results from control experiments are designated as ○-----○. Mean ± SE from four experiments. (Reproduced from Hirosumi *et al.* 1989, with permission.)

after eliminating extra-cellular calcium by EGTA. Similar findings were obtained on Swiss 3T3 cells (Hesketh *et al.* 1985). In contrast, PDGF is known to produce inositol trisphosphate, which mobilizes calcium from intracellular calcium store (Berridge and Irvine 1984). The different calcium sources may explain the reason why nifedipine was ineffective in inhibiting the increased DNA synthesis by PDGF. On the other hand, somatomedin-C stimulated DNA synthesis without affecting intracellular calcium concentration (Figs 1 and 2). Moreover, nifedipine did not inhibit somatomedin-C-stimulated DNA synthesis (Fig. 4). This result indicates that somatomedin-C stimulates proliferation of SMCs by a calcium-independent mechanism.

We also investigated the effect of a calcium agonist (BAY K 8644) on DNA synthesis of cultured rat aortic SMCs, and found that BAY K 8644 increased DNA synthesis in a dose-dependent manner. This result indicates the direct relationship between intracellular calcium and proliferation of SMCs.

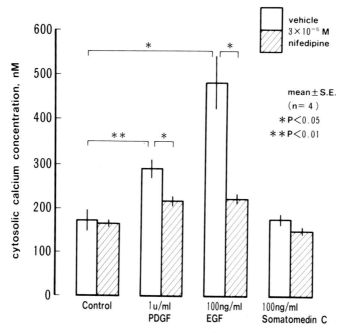

Fig. 3. Effects of nifedipine on cytosolic free calcium concentration in cultured rat aortic smooth muscle cells. Open columns represent the peak values of cytosolic free calcium concentration after the addition of platelet-derived growth factor (1 unit ml^{-1}), epidermal growth factor (100 ng ml^{-1}) and somatomedin-C (100 ng ml^{-1}). Hatched columns represent the peak values when nifedipine (3 × 10^{-6} M) was simultaneously added. Mean ± SE from four experiments. *$P < 0.05$; **$P < 0.01$ vs control without nifedipine. (Reproduced from Hirosumi *et al.* 1989, with permission.)

PLATELETS

According to the "response-to-injury" hypothesis (Ross and Glomset 1976, Ross 1986), platelets play an important role in atherogenesis. Actually, many pathological studies have revealed that platelets adhere to the injured endothelial site and aggregate at the site. Platelet aggregation has been shown to be calcium dependent. Stimulators for platelet aggregation such as collagen, ADP, thrombin, and epinephrine are reported to increase intracellular calcium concentration in human platelets in a dose-dependent manner (Ware *et al.* 1986a). Furthermore, calcium antagonists have been reported to inhibit platelet aggregation (Ware *et al.* 1986b). Rink *et al.* (1983) suggested the presence of a calcium-independent pathway for platelet activation, but this observation might have arisen from the calcium chelating action and low K_d value of quin 2. Recent study showed that the intracellular calcium concentration, measured by using aequorin, was increased in

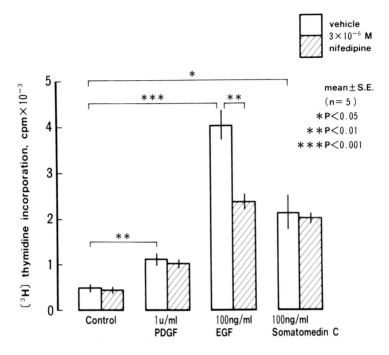

Fig. 4. Effects of nifedipine on [³H]thymidine incorporation into cultured rat aortic smooth muscle cells. Open columns represent the peak values of cytosolic free calcium concentration after the addition of platelet-derived growth factor (1 unit ml⁻¹), epidermal growth factor (100 ng ml⁻¹) and somatomedin-C (100 ng ml⁻¹). Hatched columns represent the peak values when nifedipine (3 × 10⁻⁶ M) was simultaneously added. The amount of [³H] thymidine incorporation is expressed as the radioactivity (cpm) per well of culture dish. Mean ± SE from five experiments. *P < 0.05; **P < 0.01; ***P < 0.001 vs control without nifedipine. (Reproduced from Hirosumi et al. 1989, with permission.)

response to ADP and epinephrine at a concentration which provoked platelet aggregation (Ware et al. 1986a). Moreover, the calcium ionophore, A23187-induced platelet aggregation provides strong evidence that platelet aggregation is calcium dependent (Ware et al. 1986a).

A molecular mechanism of platelet aggregation has recently been clarified (Phillips et al. 1988). Briefly, when platelet activators, such as collagen, bind to the receptors on a platelet surface, a fibrinogen (Fbg)-binding site on glycoprotein (GP) IIIa in the GP IIb/IIIa complex becomes active. Fbg released from α granules in platelets then binds to GP IIIa. Fbg possesses two binding sites for GP IIIa, and constructs a bridge formation between platelets. A protein called thrombospondin (TSP), also released from α granules of platelets, binds to GP IV in the vicinity of the GP IIb/IIIa complex. The tip of TSP has a binding site for Fbg, and the TSP–Fbg complex makes the bridge formation stronger. Calcium is reported to be required for the formation of GP IIb/IIIa complex, and release of Fbg and TSP from α granules in platelets. Thus, calcium is essential for platelet aggregation.

Aggregated platelets release PDGF, EGF, 12-HETE, β-thromboglobulin, and platelet factor 4. These biologically active substances are released by the activation of contractile proteins (actin and myosin) in platelets, which is provoked by an increase in intracellular calcium concentration. Another important substance released from aggregated platelets is thromboxane A_2 (TXA_2). TXA_2 is synthesized from arachidonic acid catalysed by thromboxane synthetase. In contrast to PGI_2, TXA_2 is a potent substance which is known to cause platelet aggregation and to constrict blood vessels. Calcium antagonists are reported to inhibit TXA_2 synthesis in platelets (Kariya et al. 1987).

CLINICAL EFFECT OF CALCIUM ANTAGONIST ON THE PROGRESSION OF CORONARY ARTERY STENOSIS

Many experimental studies have suggested the suppressive effect of calcium antagonist on atherogenesis. However, few studies have been done to elucidate the clinical effect of calcium antagonist on the course of human atherosclerosis. Therefore, we performed a retrospective and preliminary study to determine the effect of calcium antagonist on the progression of coronary atherosclerosis. Patients with ischaemic heart disease, on whom coronary angiography (CAG) was repeatedly performed, were randomly selected. Sixteen subjects were on nifedipine therapy (40 mg/day; nifedipine group; 14 males and 2 females, age 53 ± 2 years) and 13 subjects were not on nifedipine therapy (control group; 11 males and 2 females, age 58 ± 3 years). No significant differences were observed between the two groups in clinical backgrounds including age, sex, cardiac diagnosis, presence of coronary risk factors and medication other than nifedipine. The severity of coronary artery stenosis was also similar. The interval between two CAG examinations was 733 ± 237 days for the control group and 561 ± 103 days for the nifedipine group. The first CAG was carefully observed, and all lesions with 25–75% stenosis were defined as region of interest (ROI). The regions which were judged to have more than 75% stenosis were excluded from this study to avoid the possible influence of vasospasm and thrombus formation. The magnitude of coronary artery stenosis was quantitatively measured with videodensitometry (Nichols et al. 1984) by using an XR-70 coronary analyser (Vanguard, Mellville, USA). The magnitude of coronary artery stenosis was measured from a single plane angiogram which provided the details of the stenotic site. The magnitude of stenosis for each ROI on the first CAG was again measured on the same view of the second CAG, and the change in the magnitude was compared between the control group and the nifedipine group.

The magnitude of stenosis showed a small and statistically insignificant increase for the 37 ROIs in the control group (54.1 ± 2.6 to 58.6 ± 3.3%). In contrast, it showed a significant decrease for 33 ROIs in the nifedipine group (52.5 ± 3.8 to 46.2 ± 4.3%, $P < 0.05$). These results suggest the possibility that the long-term use of the calcium antagonist nifedipine might be effective against the progression of coronary atherosclerosis in humans. The effect of nifedipine was more apparent on the lesions of the left coronary artery than on those of the right coronary artery. The reason for this is not clear. It is unlikely that nifedipine is more effective on the lesions of the left coronary artery. Moreover, the location of coronary artery stenosis was not found to affect the progression and regression rate (Bruschke *et al.* 1981). The possible cause might be the difference in the magnitude of stenosis between the right and left coronary arteries on the first CAG (45.4 ± 3.6% for the right coronary artery, 57.8 ± 3.2% for the left coronary artery). Although this study was retrospectively done, the results obtained were encouraging. A large-scale clinical trial named International Nifedipine Trial on Antiatherosclerotic Therapy (INTACT) has been done (Lichtlen *et al.* 1987). The results from another large-scale clinical trial, performed in Canada and the United States, showed that nicardipine given for 2 years did not influence the course of established coronary artery stenosis, however nicardipine significantly inhibited the progression of minimal coronary artery lesions with less than 20% stenosis (Waters *et al.* 1989). A prospective and multi-centric double-blind study like these studies should be performed further to obtain a final conclusion regarding the anti-atherogenic action of calcium antagonist in humans.

CONCLUSION—CALCIUM AS A MEDIATOR OF ATHEROSCLEROSIS

We described the possible role of calcium in atherogenesis, focusing on calcium's role in regulating cellular functions in the vascular wall. Based on the findings presented in this study, we propose the hypothesis that abnormal handling of calcium in the arterial wall could be associated with development of atherosclerosis. Figure 5 shows a schematic illustration of the hypothesis. The presence of risk factors such as hypertension, hyperlipidemia, and smoking may increase the influx of calcium into vascular ECs. We have shown that active oxygen species, which are considered to be a risk factor for the development of atherosclerosis, actually increase intracellular free calcium concentration in vascular ECs. Increased intracellu-

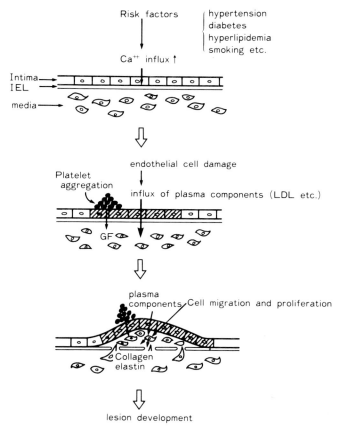

Fig. 5. Schematic illustration showing the hypothetical role of calcium in the process of atherogenesis. For legend, see text. IEL = internal elastic lamella, GF = growth factors, LDL = low-density lipoprotein.

lar calcium may damage the function of ECs, resulting in platelet aggregation at the damaged site. Increased intracellular calcium may also increase uptake of macromolecules in plasma such as LDL, eventually forming atherosclerotic plaques. We have also shown that the influx of calcium into vascular ECs is associated with LDL transport across vascular ECs. The pretreatment by nifedipine inhibited both the increase in cytosolic free calcium concentration and the increase in LDL transport, suggesting that intracellular calcium modulates LDL transport across ECs. Growth factors released from platelets may provoke migration and proliferation of medial SMCs in the arterial intima. It has been reported that migration of SMCs from arterial media to intima is enhanced by the presence of calcium, and can be inhibited by the pretreatment of calcium antagonist. As demonstrated in this study, calcium also plays an important role in the proliferation of SMCs provoked by some kinds of growth factors such as EGF.

The evidence presented in this study, however, would not be sufficient to fully explain the aetiological role of calcium in atherogenesis. Further studies are required to elucidate the mechanism of the contribution of calcium to atherogenesis. The efficacy of calcium antagonist for the prevention of atherosclerosis in humans should also be investigated further.

REFERENCES

Benveniste, J., Henson, P. M. and Cochrane, C. G. (1972). Leukocyte-dependent histamine release from rabbit platelets. *Journal of Experimental Medicine* **138**, 1356–1377.

Berridge, M. J. and Irvine, R. F. (1984). Inositol trisphosphate, a novel second messenger in cellular signal transduction. *Nature* **312**, 315–321.

Blumenthal, H. T., Lansing, A. I. and Wheeler, P.A. (1950). The interrelation of elastic tissue and calcium in the genesis of atherosclerosis. *American Journal of Pathology* **26**, 989–1009.

Blumlein, S. L., Sievers, R., Kidd, P. and Parmley, W.W. (1984). Mechanism of protection from atherosclerosis by verapamil in the cholesterol-fed rabbits. *American Journal of Cardiology* **54**, 884–889.

Brotherton, A. F. A. and Hoak, J. C. (1982). Role of Ca^{2+} and cyclic AMP in the regulation of the production of prostacyclin by the vascular endothelium. *Proceedings of the National Academy of Sciences of the USA* **79**, 495–499.

Bruschke, A. V. G., Wijers, T. S., Kolsters, W. and Landmann, J. (1981). The anatomic evolution of coronary artery disease demonstrated by coronary arteriography in 256 nonoperated patients. *Circulation* **63**, 527–536.

Campbell, A. K. (1983). The natural history of calcium. *In* "Intracellular calcium: its universal role as regulator" (Gutfreund, H. ed.), John Wiley, Chichester.

Furchgott, R. F. and Zawadzki, J. V. (1980). The obligatory role of endothelial cells in the relaxation of arterial smooth muscle by acetylcholine. *Nature* **288**, 373–376.

Ginsburg, R., Davis, K., Bristow, M. R., McKennet, K., Kodsi, S. R., Billingham, M. E. and Schroeder, J. S. (1983). Calcium antagonists suppress atherogenesis in aorta but not in the intramural coronary artery. *Laboratory Investigation* **49**, 154–158.

Henry, P. D. and Bentley, K. I. (1981). Suppression of atherogenesis in cholesterol-fed rabbit treated with nifedipine. *Journal of Clinical Investigation* **6**, 1366–1369.

Hesketh, T. R., Moore, J. P., Morris, J. D. H., Taylor, M. V., Rongers, J., Smith, G. A. and Metcalfe, J. C. (1985). A common sequence of calcium and pH signals in the mitogenic stimulation of eukaryotic cells. *Nature* **313**, 481–484.

Hirosumi, J., Ouchi, Y., Watanabe, M., Kusunoki, J., Nakamura, T. and Orimo, H. (1988). Effect of superoxide and lipid peroxide on cytosolic free calcium concentration in cultured pig aortic endothelial cells. *Biochemical and Biophysical Research Communications* **152**, 301–307.

Hirosumi, J., Ouchi, Y., Watanabe, M., Kusunoki, J., Nakamura, T. and Orimo, H. (1989). Effects of growth factors on cytosolic free calcium concentration and DNA synthesis in cultured rat aortic smooth muscle cells. *Tohoku Journal of Experimental Medicine* **157**, 289–300.

Kariya, T., Sakai, T., Yatomi, H. and Kume, S. (1987). Inhibitory effect of calcium-antagonist on thromboxan A_2 production in human platelets. *Japanese Pharmacology and Therapeutics* **15** (suppl. 3), 819–824 (in Japanese).

Koibuchi, Y., Sakai, S., Miura, S., Ono, T., Shibayama, F. and Ohtsuka, M. (1989). Suppression of atherogenesis in cholesterol-fed rabbits treated with nilvadipine, a new vasoselective calcium entry blocker. *Atherosclerosis* **79**, 147–155.

Kramsch, D. M., Aspen, A. J. and Apstein, C. S. (1980). Suppression of experimental atherosclerosis by the Ca^{2+}-antagonist lanthanum. *Journal of Clinical Investigation* **65**, 967–981.

Lichtlen, P. R., Nellessen, U., Rafflenbeul, W., Jost, S. and Hecker, H. (1987). International nifedipine trial on antiatherosclerotic therapy (INTACT). *Cardiovascular Drugs Therapy* **1**, 71–80.

Maruyama, I. and Majerus, P. W. (1985). The turnover of thrombin-thrombomodulin complex in cultured human umbilical vein endothelial cells and A549 lung cancer cells. *Journal of Biological Chemistry* **260**, 15432–15438.

Nakao, J., Itoh, H., Ohyama, T., Chang, W.-C. and Murota, S. (1983a). Calcium dependency of aortic smooth muscle cell migration induced by 12-L-hydroxy-5,8,10,14-eicosatetraenoic acid. *Atherosclerosis* **46**, 309–319.

Nakao, J., Ito, H., Chang, W.-C, Koshihara, Y. and Murota, S. (1983b). Aortic smooth muscle cell migration caused by platelet-derived growth factor is mediated by lipoxygenase product(s) of arachidonic acid. *Atherosclerosis* **112**, 866–871.

Nichols, A. B., Christopher, F. O., Gabrieli, B. A., Fenoglio, J. J. and Esser, P. D. (1984). Quantification of relative coronary arterial stenosis by cinevideo-densitometric analysis of coronary arteriograms. *Circulation* **69**, 512–522.

Nomoto, A., Mutoh, H., Hagihara, H. and Yamaguchi, I. (1988). Smooth muscle cell migration induced by inflammatory cell products and its inhibition by a potent calcium antagonist, nilvadipine. *Atherosclerosis* **72**, 213–219.

Oka, Y. and Orth, D. N. (1983). Human plasma epidermal growth factor-β/urogastrone is associated with blood platelets. *Journal of Clinical Investigation* **72**, 249–259.

Ouchi, Y., Hirosumi, J., Watanabe, M., Hattori, A., Nakamura, T., and Orimo, H. (1988). Inhibitory effect of transforming growth factor-β on epidermal growth factor-induced proliferation of cultured rat aortic smooth muscle cells. *Biochemical and Biophysical Research Communications* **157**, 301–307.

Phillips, D. R., Charo, I.F., Parise, L. V. and Fitzgerald, L. A. (1988). The platelet membrane glycoprotein IIb/IIIa complex. *Blood* **71**, 831–843.

Pickett, W. C., Jesse, R. L. and Cohen, P. (1977). Initiation of phospholipase A_2 activity in human platelets by the calcium ion ionophore A23187. *Biochimica et Biophysica Acta* **486**, 209–213.

Rink, T. J., Sanchez, A. and Hallam, T. J. (1983). Diacylglycerol and phorbol ester stimulate secretion without raising cytoplasmic-free calcium in human platelets. *Nature* **305**, 317–319.

Ross, R. (1986). The pathogensis of atherosclerosis—an update. *New England Journal of Medicine* **314**, 488–500.

Ross, R. and Glomset, J. A. (1976). The pathogensis of atherosclerosis. *New England Journal of Medicine* **295**, 420–425.

Ross, R., Glomset, J. A., Kariya, B. and Harker, L. A. (1974). A platelet-dependent serum factor that stimulates the proliferation of arterial smooth muscle cells in vitro. *Proceedings of the National Academy Sciences of the USA* **71**, 1207–1210.

Sasaguri, Y., Nakashima, T., Morimatsu, M. and Yagi, K. (1984). Injury to cultured endothelial cells from human umbilical vein by linoleic acid hydro peroxide. *Journal of Applied Biochemistry* **6**, 144–150.

Shimada, K. and Ozawa, T. (1987). Modulation of glycosaminoglycan production and antithrombin III binding by cultured aortic endothelial cells treated with 4-methylumbelliferyl-β-D-xyloside. *Arteriosclerosis* **7**, 627–636.

Strickberger, S. A., Russek, L. N. and Phair, R. D. (1988). Evidence for increased aortic plasma membrane calcium transport caused by experimental atherosclerosis in rabbits. *Circulation Research* **62**, 75–80.

Terashita, K. and Orimo, H. (1986). The effect of calcium antagonists on the release of epoprostenol from cultured rat aortic smooth muscle cells. *In* "Proceedings of 6th International Adalat Symposium" (Lichtlen, P.R. ed.), pp. 472–477. Excerpta Medica.

Territo, M., Berliner, J. A. and Fogelman, A. M. (1984). Effect of monocyte migration on low density lipoprotein transport across aortic endothelial cell monolayers. *Journal of Clinical Investigation* **74**, 2279–2284.

Tsien, R. Y., Pozzan, T. and Rink, T. J. (1982). Calcium homeostasis in intact lymphocyte: cytoplasmic free calcium monitored with a new, intracellularly trapped fluorescent indicator. *Journal of Cell Biology* **94**, 325–335.

Toyoda, T., Sawada, S., Niwa, I., Maebo, N., Tsuji, H., Hayashi, K., Kaimasu, I., Nakagawa, M. and Ijichi, H. (1984). *Japanese Pharmacology and Therapeutics* **12** (suppl. 7), 1325–1331 (in Japanese).

Ware, J. A., Johnson, P. C., Smith, M. and Salzman, W. (1986a). Effect of common agonists on cytoplasmic ionized calcium concentration in platelets. *Journal of Clinical Investigation* **77**, 878–886.

Ware, J. A., Johnson, P. C., Smith, M. and Salzman, W. (1986b). Inhibition of human platelet aggregation and cytoplasmic calcium response by calcium antagonists: studies with aequorin and quin 2. *Circulation Research* **59**, 39–42.

Waters, D., Lesperance, J., Francetich, M., Theroux, P., Reitman, M., Hudon, G., Lemarbre, L., Kamm, B., Joyal, M., Gosselin, G., Dyrda, I. and Havel, R. (1989). A controlled clinical trial to assess the effect of a calcium antagonist upon the progression of coronary atherosclerosis. *Circulation* **80** (suppl. II), II–266.

Weiss, S. J., Young, J., LoBuglio, A. F., Slivka, A. and Nimeh, N. F. (1981). Role of hydrogen peroxide in neutrophil-mediated destruction of cultured endothelial cells. *Journal of Clinical Investigation* **68**, 714–721.

Willis, A. L., Nagel, B., Churchill, V., Whyte, M. A., Smith, D. L., Mahmud, I. and Puppione, D. L. (1985). Antiatherosclerotic effects of nicardipine and nifedipine in cholesterol-fed rabbits. *Arteriosclerosis* **5**, 250–255.

Yanagisawa, M., Kurihara, H., Kimura, S., Tomobe, Y., Kobayashi, M., Mitsui, Y., Yazaki, Y., Goto, K. and Masaki, T. (1988). A novel potent vasoconstrictor peptide produced by vascular endothelial cells. *Nature* **332**, 411–415.

Discussion

Nordin: Dihydrotachysterol you give to the rats may or may not be an essential part of your hypothesis. But dihydrotachysterol in these doses produces hypercalcaemia, and of course in hypercalcaemia you get calcification of soft tissues because of oversaturation of the plasma with calcium phosphate. So you really can't draw any conclusions about the transfer of calcium from bone to blood vessels in normal aging from a model that involves severe hypercalcaemia. Then the second point arising from that is that there may be a link between osteoporosis and atherosclerosis, but you have to exclude all sorts of other possible confounding variables. The most important confounding variable in this situation is the plasma oestrogen level. The osteoporotic people tend to have a lower plasma oestrogen level than normal people, normal women at the same age and, of course, the plasma lipids are also related to the oestrogens. At the menopause, the LDL goes up and the HDL goes down. So, the most likely common factor between atheroma and osteoporosis—if the two are linked, and I am not sure that they are—but the most likely common factor if they are linked is the low oestrogen level and abnormal lipids.

Orimo: I certainly think that a lack of oestrogen is very important, and perhaps the oestrogen protects the shift of calcium from bone to the aorta. Concerning your first question, this is certainly not a model of aging. But what I wish to point out is that I would like to prove a shift of calcium from the bone to the soft tissues. We labelled bones with ^{45}Ca and looked at whether the calcium shift occurs with stress, that's the main point of my experiment. I don't think it is a similar model in humans but just an experimental model to look at this possibility.

Robert: In defence of the theory of Dr Orimo I'd like to say just one word. I do not believe that arteriosclerosis and atheromatous plaques are the same disease and the same process. That's the only point on which I disagree with you. We produced years ago a very good model for arteriosclerosis, you just have to immunize rabbits with elastine peptides, no lipids given, and you have massive calcium deposits. Calcitonin can prevent this event in accordance with part of your hypothesis. Now I don't believe that calcium is really the devil here. I think calcium is not a passive but an active bystander. We could show a few years ago that arterial cells express a specific receptor which is activated by elastine peptides which are all the time produced by degradation of arterial elastic tissue and they can be titrated in the serum. And this receptor is linked to calcium channels and increases steadily calcium influx to the aorta. So I think with this little additive I agree that really calcium influx is important in arteriosclerosis, but I am not convinced at all that it plays an important role in atheromatous plaque formation.

Prediction and Prevention of Osteoporosis

B. E. C. Nordin*† and A. G. Need*

*Division of Clinical Chemistry, Institute of Medical and Veterinary Science, Adelaide, Australia and †Department of Pathology, University of Adelaide, Australia

PREFACE

The term "osteoporosis" denotes a condition in which an insufficiency of bony tissue predisposes to fracture. To be more specific, it is a condition in which there is "too little bone in the bone" (Albright and Reifenstein 1948) signifying a low whole bone density. To be even more specific, osteoporosis may be defined as a whole bone density more than 2 standard deviations below the normal mean at the same site in young adults of the same sex (Nordin 1987). It may result from inadequate consolidation of bone during growth, or accelerated loss of bone during aging—or a combination of the two. In this paper, we shall consider the relative importance of peak bone density and bone loss in the genesis of postmenopausal and age-related fractures.

METHODOLOGY

The method of forearm densitometry used in this paper has been fully described elsewhere (Nordin and Polley 1987). Our procedure for vertebral densitometry by quantitative computerized tomography (QCT) (Cann and Genant 1980) has been described by Nordin et al. (1988). Dual photon absorptiometry (DPA) was performed in the Lunar DP4 scanning

Challenges in Aging
ISBN 0-12-090163-3

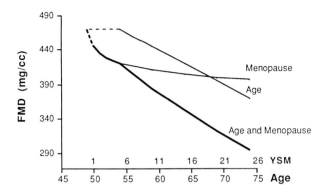

Fig. 1. Diagrammatic representation of the menopausal component in bone loss from the forearm (top line), the age-related component (middle line) and the actual observed value (bottom line).

densitometer using the mean value of L2 to L4 for vertebral density and the value in Ward's triangle for hip density.

Statistical calculations were performed in Minitab Version 7.1.

OBSERVATIONS

Peak Bone Density

It is well recognized that bone density rises during growth to reach a peak value early in the third decade and then remains more or less stationary until the menopause in women and the age of about 55 in men. This was shown by Garn (1970) in the metacarpal but appears to be true of the skeleton as a whole regardless of where the measurement is made. The peak bone density tends to be higher in men than women at most but not at all measurement sites. The pattern of loss is different in the two sexes because the menopause in women accounts for a loss of about 15% of bony tissue in a period of 5–10 years (Seeman et al. 1988, Nordin et al. 1990a). There is also an age-related component in bone loss (common to both sexes) which starts at about age 55, is more or less linear and proceeds at a rate of about 1% of initial value per annum (Fig. 1). Men are less liable to osteoporotic fractures than women for three reasons: firstly because they tend to have a higher peak bone density, secondly because they do not experience the menopause-dependent bone loss, and thirdly—and perhaps most importantly—because they die younger.

Peak bone density is an enormously important concept because it is the

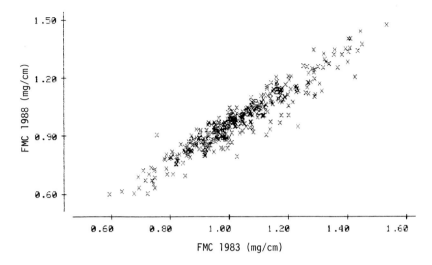

Fig. 2. Forearm mineral content at the beginning and end of a 5-year period in 340 untreated normal postmenopausal women.

main determinant of fracture risk. Although there are interindividual differences in both menopause- and age-related rates of bone loss, the average rate (1–2% per annum) is small compared with the wide range of peak bone densities (at least 20% either side of the mean). As a result, subjects with high peak bone densities tend to remain in the top of the range and those with low peak bone densities to remain low and to be most at risk for fracture for the rest of their lives. This is illustrated in Fig. 2 which shows the forearm mineral densities (FMD) in 340 normal postmenopausal women at the beginning and end of a 5-year period of observation. The high correlation between the first and second values testifies to the relatively small differences that occur in ranking with the passage of time. Despite the tendency for the rate of loss to be related to the initial value (particularly in the first years after the menopause when the pattern of bone loss is exponential in type) the osteoporotic bone density range is reached much more rapidly in those who start with low values than those who start with high values (Fig. 3).

Osteoporosis and Fracture Risk

Age-related fractures can be classified into three groups: non-hip peripheral fractures, vertebral fractures, and hip fractures. Peripheral fractures may occur at any age but are much more common after the menopause than before it (see below). Patients present with vertebral compression ("spinal

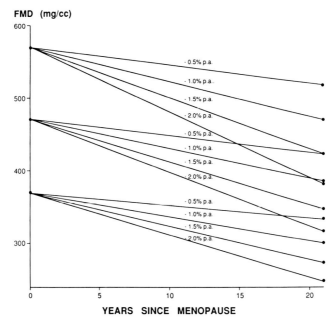

Fig. 3. Diagram to illustrate the effect of different rates of bone loss on bone density after the menopause in women starting at the top, middle and bottom of the normal range.

osteoporosis") at a mean age of 65 years regardless of their age at menopause; the epidemiology of this fracture is not well documented. The hip fracture rates rise logarithmically with age and patients generally present in the eighth decade.

The most common postmenopausal peripheral fracture is at the distal forearm. The incidence of this fracture rises steeply from about age 50 to plateau at about 800 per 100 000 per annum from the age of 60 onwards (Fig. 4). The epidemiology of other non-hip peripheral fractures is very similar to that of the wrist but the absolute rates are greater by a factor of about three because wrist fractures constitute only about 30% of all non-hip peripheral fractures (Nordin *et al.* 1987). Hip fracture epidemiology is quite different in as much as the rate rises much later and continues upwards to the end of life (Fig. 5). They also seem to be increasing from year to year.

These figures are generally derived from hospital statistics, but it is possible to obtain similar information from fracture histories. By questioning a cohort of some 500 normal postmenopausal women about their fractures and the age at which they occurred, we have constructed the non-hip

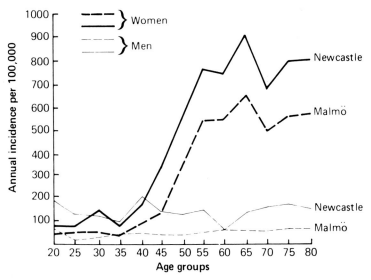

Fig. 4. The annual incidence per 100 000 of wrist fractures as a function of age in men and women in Newcastle and Malmö (from Miller and Grimley Evans 1985).

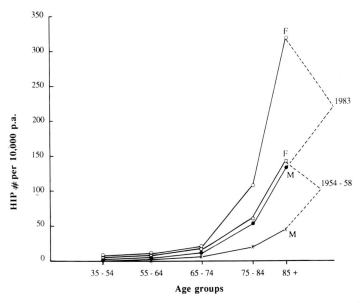

Fig. 5. The annual incidence per 10 000 of hip fractures as a function of age in men and women in the Oxford region in 1950 and 1980 (calculated from Boyce and Vessey, 1985).

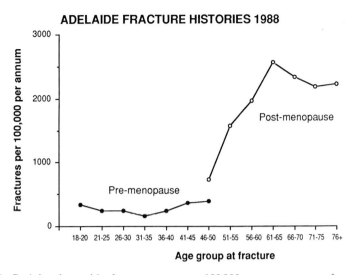

Fig. 6. Peripheral non-hip fracture rates per 100 000 per annum as a function of age at fracture in pre- and postmenopausal women.

peripheral fracture epidemiology shown in Fig. 6. It will be seen that the fracture rates are low and unrelated to age before the menopause, rise immediately after the menopause and plateau at about 2500 per 100 000 per annum from the age of 60 onwards. This pattern is so similar to that in Fig. 4 that the wrist fracture pattern must represent the pattern of non-hip peripheral fractures in general. It is a pattern which reflects the menopausal component of bone loss—rapid at first and then slowing down (Fig. 1) (and is probably mainly trabecular in nature). Hip fracture epidemiology, on the other hand, more closely reflects the age-related pattern of cortical bone loss: continuing loss of cortical bone causes a continuing rise in fracture rate.

The well-known association between wrist and vertebral fractures has led Riggs and Melton (1983) to suggest that these fractures should be grouped together as Type I osteoporosis and hip fractures should be classified as Type II. Unfortunately these categories are not mutually exclusive—many wrist and spine fracture subjects go on to develop hip fractures—and it may be more profitable to think of them as representing different stages in the evolution of trabecular and cortical bone loss.

The relationship between bone density and fracture can be established by measuring bone density in fracture cases and controls either retrospectively or prospectively; the results obtained by the two methods are very similar (Wasnich et al. 1985, Cleghorn et al. 1989a). However, there are at least three measurement sites in current use (vertebrae, femoral neck and forearm)

Table 1
Mean age and forearm mineral densities (SE) in fracture and non-fracture subjects of the same mean age

	n	Age (years)	Density (mg ml^{-1})
Peripheral fracture only	120	66.3 (0.44)	326 (6.6)
Controls	314	66.2 (0.28)	360 (3.7)
P		NS	<0.001
Vertebral fracture (no hip)	117	67.4 (0.36)	278 (5.4)
Controls	107	66.8 (0.42)	314 (7.3)
P		NS	<0.001
Hip fracture (no spine)	65	69.8 (0.97)	288 (9.6)
Controls	150	70.1 (0.34)	340 (5.5)
P		NS	<0.001

NS, not significant.

and there is a tendency for forearm densitometry (which is the simplest and cheapest) to be discounted in favour of densitometry in the spine and femoral neck. Before considering this controversy, we will show the results obtained with forearm densitometry in fracture cases and controls.

Mean forearm mineral density (FMD) in women who have suffered peripheral non-hip, vertebral or hip fractures are shown in Table 1 and compared with non-fracture subjects of the same mean age. In all three types of fracture, the mean FMD is significantly lower than in non-fracture subjects of the same age. The same is true of vertebral mineral density (VMD) measured by QCT, as shown in Table 2, but the magnitudes of the differences are not the same. We therefore decided to compare different densitometric techniques at different sites in the three fracture types by expressing all data in standard deviation units (SDU or Z scores) from the young normal mean. This is done in Table 3. The striking feature of the table is the similarity of the results with different techniques at different sites. Thus the mean values in non-hip peripheral fracture cases range from −1.8 to −2.9 SDU, being lowest in the forearm. In crush fracture cases they range from −3.0 to −3.6 SDU, and in hip fracture cases from −3.2 to −3.6 SDU. There is little to choose between the four different procedures and nothing to suggest that forearm densitometry is inferior to the other techniques in estimating the degree of osteoporosis in fracture cases. Nor do they suggest that measurement of bone density at the fracture site has any particular merit, at least on a group basis and in postmenopausal women.

Table 2
Mean age and vertebral densities (SE) in fracture and non-fracture subjects of the
same mean age

	n	Age (years)	Density (mg ml^{-1})
Peripheral fracture only	89	61.9 (0.81)	103 (3.3)
Controls	129	59.9 (0.68)	113 (2.9)
P		NS	<0.05
Vertebral fracture (no hip)	111	64.4 (0.58)	74 (3.0)
Controls	120	63.8 (0.54)	104 (2.8)
P		NS	<0.001
Hip fracture (no vertebral)	41	68.0 (1.2)	75 (4.0)
Controls	75	67.1 (0.57)	100 (3.5)
P		NS	<0.001

Table 3
Mean Z scores by fracture type and site of measurement

Fracture	Spine		Femur DPA (mg cm^{-2})	Distal radius SPA (mg cm^{-3})
	QCT (mg cm^{-3})	DPA (mg cm^{-2})		
Peripheral (non-hip) only	−2.3 (89)	−1.8 (42)	−2.4 (20)	−2.9 (120)
Spinal (non-hip)	−3.6 (125)	−3.2 (49)	−3.0 (39)	−3.8 (117)
Femoral Neck (non-spine)	−3.4 (41)	−3.2 (47)*	−3.7 (47)	−3.6 (65)

*Calculated from Mazess et al. (1988).

Prevention and Treatment of Osteoporosis

Identifying the Population at Risk

A practical programme for the prevention of osteoporosis must be based on a clear understanding of what one is trying to prevent. Since osteoporosis may be defined as a bone density below the young normal range (Nordin 1987), total prevention of osteoporosis would involve maintaining all women within the normal range to the end of their lives. This is an ideal which is unlikely to be attained in the foreseeable future. A more realistic approach would be to establish what might be achieved in fracture prevention terms if bone density could be held above the −3 or −4 SDU level. This can be

Table 4

Percentage distribution of fracture cases ranked by bone density SDUs from young normal mean

	Forearm mineral density		
	Peripheral fracture (120)	Vertebral fracture (117)	Hip fracture (65)
>Mean	2.5	0	1.5
<Mean to −1	4.2	1.7	3.1
<−1 to −2	22.5	7.7	10.8
<−2 to −3	24.2	8.6	16.9
<−3 to −4	23.3	35.9	29.2
<−4	23.3	46.2	38.5

	Vertebral mineral density		
	(89)	(111)	(41)
>Mean	3.4	0.90	0
<Mean to −1	12.4	3.6	2.4
<−1 to −2	25.8	9.0	12.2
<−2 to −3	28.1	18.9	7.3
<−3 to −4	22.5	36.0	48.8
<−4	7.9	31.5	29.3

estimated from the distribution of bone densities in SDU terms in fracture cases, as shown in Table 4. From this, it emerges that 47% of peripheral fractures, 84% of vertebral fractures and 68% of hip fractures occur in women with forearm values below −3 SDU. Thirty per cent of peripheral fractures, 68% of vertebral fractures and 78% of hip fractures occur in women with vertebral densities below −3 SDU.

Thus the great majority of spinal and femoral neck fractures occur in women with bone densities more than 3 standard deviations below the young normal mean, whether measured in the spine or forearm. The implication is that most of these fractures could (in theory at least) be prevented if bone densities in the female population could be held above (or raised above) this critical level. To prevent a comparable proportion of other peripheral fractures (e.g. at the wrist) would require bone density to be held at or raised above the −2 SDU level.

Because bone is lost more easily than it can be regained, the most realistic way to reduce fracture rates in the future is by preventing bone loss. It may in the future be possible to increase peak bone density by stimulating bone consolidation during growth, but the factors determining this variable are not yet well defined and the time is not ripe for large-scale intervention in childhood. The immediate task must be to prevent the development of osteoporosis by intervention in middle life.

A Practical Programme

Bone density at any particular age after middle life is a function of peak bone density and rate of bone loss since the decline began—which in women means since the menopause. It has already been made clear that of these two factors, peak bone density is by far the more important. Identifying so-called "fast bone losers" (Christiansen et al. 1987) has little merit if these individuals have such a high bone density that they will never be at risk of fracture in their natural lifetime. The first objective, therefore, must be to identify at middle life the individuals in the lower part of the bone density range (say below the 25th centile) who are at highest risk for osteoporotic fractures in later life, even if they lose bone slowly. It is increasingly evident that such women can be identified by forearm densitometry. Even if there were some advantage in measuring vertebral density for the prevention of vertebral fracture and hip density for the prevention of hip fracture (which is highly debatable), the cost-benefit advantage of forearm densitometry (with a capital investment of about $30 000) compared with vertebral and femoral neck densitometry (with a capital outlay over $100 000) makes it the method of choice for screening purposes at least. There is also a purely practical aspect to the matter which points in the same direction. Although vertebral and femoral neck densitometry is becoming increasingly available in major centres, it is difficult to imagine that it will be available in the foreseeble future in small townships far from major centres where many people live in countries like the United States, Canada and Australia—not to mention Third World countries. Nor is it likely that any but the most motivated women would travel considerable distances to undergo a test which may reduce their risk of hip fracture in 25 years' time. An effective screening programme should be available to whole populations and not simply to those with access to major centres.

For these very practical reasons, the programme will need to be based on peripheral bone densitometry which has been shown to be a powerful predictor of vertebral, hip and other fractures (Wasnich et al. 1985, Hui et al. 1989, Cleghorn et al. 1989b, Cummings et al. 1989). The programme we propose would involve screening by forearm densitometry all women at or about the time of the menopause and their classification into three groups. Those above the 75th centile could be reassured that they were very unlikely ever to suffer osteoporotic fractures; those between the 25th and 75th centiles would be asked to return in 2–3 years' time for a further measurement; and those below the 25th centile would be advised about preventive treatment and would have their bone density remeasured at regular intervals to ensure that it had stabilized.

Preventive Regimes

There would be little merit in identifying potential osteoporotics at an early stage if there was not convincing evidence that loss of bone can be delayed or prevented, just as there would be little merit in screening for blood cholesterol and blood pressure if it were not well established that high values can be brought under control. (In this connection it should be noted that the predictive value of bone densitometry in terms of future fracture is stronger than the predictive value of a blood cholesterol or blood pressure measurement in predicting future heart attack or stroke.)

The evidence that oestrogen treatment in adequate dosage prevents bone loss and reduces fracture risk is so strong that it does not need recapitulation here. However, long-term hormone therapy, though extremely valuable not only in prevention of bone loss and alleviation of symptoms but possibly also in the prevention of ischaemic heart disease, is not without risk and side effects and is certainly not at the present time willingly accepted by more than a minority of women. It is therefore important to recognize the mounting evidence that bone loss can be prevented or at least delayed by other therapies, notably calcium supplementation (see below) and possibly also calcitonin (Overgaard et al. 1989) and diphosphonates (Storm et al. 1987).

It is not possible within the scope of this paper to review the effect of calcium supplementation on bone loss in postmenopausal women, which we have reviewed at length elsewhere (Nordin and Heaney 1990). However, the four most recent reports all show a significant, positive effect of calcium in prevention of postmenopausal bone loss (Sinaki et al. 1989, Elders et al. 1989, Dawson-Hughes et al. 1989, Smith et al. 1989). The latest of these (Smith et al. 1989) is a controlled trial in which calcium supplementation was significantly better than placebo at all 12 measurement sites in 44 treated postmenopausal women compared with 38 controls. In our own clinical practice, we regularly prescribe calcium supplements (usually 1 g of effervescent calcium taken at night) to otherwise normal women who have either a low bone density or evidence of rapid bone loss. We prescribe hormone treatment (oestrogen in younger women and progestogen in older women) to those with significant menopausal complaints and/or those with a high fasting obligatory calcium loss. In those with proven calcium malabsorption we use a combination of calcitriol 0.25 μg daily with calcium, even if they do not have crush fractures. The results of this policy are illustrated in Fig. 7a—based on 869 treatment periods in "normal" women, i.e. women without crush fractures. Although this is in no sense a controlled trial but simply an illustration of what happens in clinical practice, the data show that calcium, although probably not as effective as oestrogen in preventing bone loss, is certainly very much more effective than no treatment at all. The mean rate of loss in the untreated subjects is 1.8% per annum and in the calcium-treated 0.93% per annum. At these rates of loss, if linear, a woman reaching midlife with a bone density at the 25th centile would take 13 years to cross the -3 SDU threshold if untreated and 26 years if calcium-treated.

Nor is calcium supplementation the only simple remedy available. We have reported elsewhere (Nordin and Morris 1989) that the high obligatory calcium loss in postmenopausal women is extremely sodium dependent, and that the urinary hydroxyproline is closely related to urinary calcium and therefore to urinary sodium. The importance of this is that urinary hydroxyproline (representing bone resorption) can be reduced by simple salt restriction (Cleghorn et al. 1989b) and increased by salt loading (McParland et al. 1989). It is likely that the same effect can be achieved by administration of a thiazide diuretic which is known to be associated with significantly increased bone mass (Wasnich et al. 1983). There have also been two recent studies showing reduced hip fracture rates in subjects on thiazide diuretics (Holbrook et al. 1988, LaCroix et al. 1990). We also understand that at least two centres have shown, and will be publishing in the near future, evidence that thiazide diuretics delay the rate of bone loss in postmenopausal women.

These proven effects of calcium supplementation and/or urinary calcium reduction can be logically explained. The rise in obligatory calcium loss which occurs at the menopause seems to be tubular in origin, or at least to contain a tubular component (Nordin et al. 1990b) which could reflect the loss of a positive action of oestrogens on tubular reabsorption of calcium, possibly mediated through oestrogen receptors in the kidneys (Hagenfelt and Eriksson 1988). If this is correct, calcium supplementation compensates for increased urinary calcium losses; sodium restriction and thiazide administration actually reduce obligatory calcium loss; and oestrogens (and certain progestogens) also lower excretion of calcium by increasing tubular reabsorption—although they may have a direct action on bone as well.

Treatment of Established Osteoporosis

The treatment of established osteoporosis follows similar lines to prevention but with the one great difference that many of these patients are already below the -3 SDU threshold when they present. Antiresorptive therapy with calcium and/or hormones and/or calcitriol, following the same

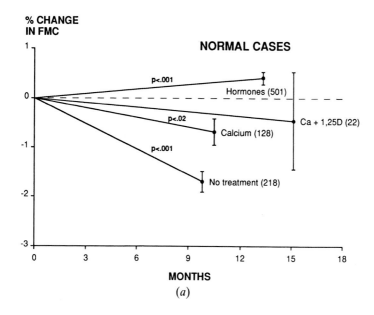

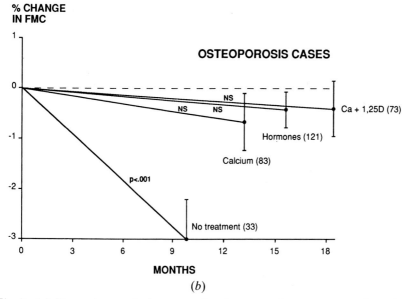

Fig. 7. (a) Mean changes in forearm mineral content (as percentage of starting value) in 869 treatment periods on four different treatments in postmenopausal women without crush fractures. (b) Mean changes in forearm mineral content (as percentage of starting value) in 310 treatment periods on four different treatments in postmenopausal women with crush fractures.

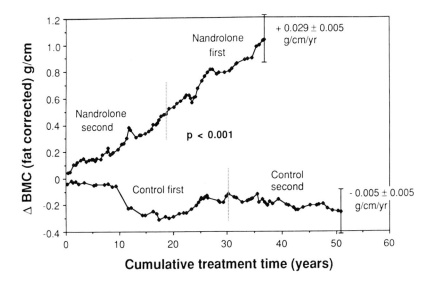

Fig. 8. Cumulative change in fat-corrected forearm mineral content in 50 postmeno-pausal osteoporotic women treated with nandrolone decanoate 50 mg every 2–4 weeks compared with the changes in the same patients before and after nandrolone therapy (Need *et al.* 1989).

indications as were described above, should prevent further bone loss but will not restore lost bone, as illustrated in Fig. 7b. This diagram shows the accelerated bone loss in untreated osteoporotic patients with crush fractures (3.7% per annum) and the greatly reduced rate in those treated with calcium (0.73% per annum). The fact that the combination of calcium and calcitriol (given to malabsorbers of calcium) appears to be more effective than calcium alone given to normal absorbers of calcium may simply mean that we have set our absorption criterion too low. We should perhaps have set this criterion slightly higher than we have done and treated more cases with calcitriol.

Many of these cases are already below the -3 SDU threshold, and one would like to restore their lost bone and so to reduce their fracture risk. At present we know of only one way of doing this and that is with nandrolone decanoate (Need *et al.* 1989) in a dose of 50 mg every 4 weeks. This produces a gain of bone in the forearm at a rate of about 3% per annum after fat correction (Fig. 8). We limit each course of nandrolone to about 6 months to minimize the risk of side effects (mainly huskiness of the voice) but if antiresorptive therapy is given between courses and nandrolone decanoate is given for 6 months a year, it may be possible to produce clinically significant gains of bone over a period of years.

CONCLUSION

The majority of vertebral and hip fractures in postmenopausal women occur in subjects with forearm densities more than 3 standard deviations below the young normal mean, wherever it is measured. There is a strong presumption that these subjects are predominantly recruited from those members of the population whose peak bone density was already low at middle life. It should be a relatively simple matter to screen women at about age 50 to identify those at risk for future fracture and to prevent them ever falling below the critical −3 SDU threshold. In the majority of osteoporotic fractures the result should be seen in declining fracture rates 15–20 years after such a programme was instituted.

REFERENCES

Albright, F. and Reifenstein, E. C. (eds) (1948). "The parathyroid glands and metabolic bone disease". Williams & Wilkins, Baltimore.

Boyce, W. J. and Vessey, M. P. (1985). Rising incidence of fracture of the proximal femur. *Lancet* **i**, 150–151.

Cann, C. E. and Genant, H. F. (1980). Precise measurement of vertebral mineral content using computed tomography. *Journal of Computer Assisted Tomography* **4**, 493–500.

Christiansen, C., Riis, B. J. and Rodbro, P. (1987). Prediction of rapid bone loss in postmenopausal women. *Lancet* **i**, 1105–1107.

Cleghorn, D. B., Nordin, B. E. C. and Need, A. G. (1989a). The relation between peripheral fracture and forearm mineral density in 358 normal postmenopausal women: a 5-year prospective study (Abstract). *Journal of Bone and Mineral Research* **4**(suppl. 1), S327.

Cleghorn, D. B., Need, A. G. and Nordin, B. E. C. (1989b). The effect of salt restriction on urine calcium and hydroxyproline in postmenopausal women (Abstract). *Journal of Bone and Mineral Research* **4**(suppl. 1), S393.

Cummings, S. R., Black, D., Arnaud, C. *et al.* (1989). Appendicular densitometry predicts hip fractures: a prospective study (Abstract). *Journal of Bone and Mineral Research* **4**(suppl. 1), S327.

Dawson-Hughes, B., Dallal, G., Tannenbaum, S., Sahyoun, N. and Krall, E. (1989). Effect of two calcium supplements on postmenopausal bone loss from the spine (Abstract). *Journal of Bone and Mineral Research* **4**(suppl. 1), S390.

Elders, P. J. M., Netelenbos, J. C., Lips, P. and vanGinkel, F. C. (1989). Calcium supplementation reduces perimenopausal bone loss (Abstract) *Journal of Bone and Mineral Research* **4**(suppl. 1), S399.

Garn, S. M. (ed.) (1970). "Nutritional prospective". Thomas Springfield, Illinois.

Hagenfeldt, Y. and Eriksson, H. A. (1988). The estrogen receptor in the rat kidney ontogeny, properties and effect of gonadectomy on its concentration. *Journal of Steroid Biochemistry* **31**, 49–56.

Holbrook, T. L., Barrett-Connor, E. and Wingard, D. L. (1988). Dietary calcium and risk of hip fracture: 14-year prospective population study. *Lancet* **ii**, 1046–1049.

Hui, S. L., Slemenda, C. W. and Johnston, C. C. (1989). Baseline measurement of bone mass predicts fracture in white women. *Annals of Internal Medicine* **111**, 355–361.

LaCroix, A. Z., Wienphal, J., White, L. R. *et al.* (1990). Thiazide diuretic agents and the incidence of hip fracture. *New England Journal of Medicine* **322**, 286–290.

Mazess, R. B., Barden, H., Ettinger, M. and Schultz, E. (1988). Bone density of the radius, spine and proximal femur in osteoporosis. *Journal of Bone and Mineral Research* **3**, 13–18.

McParland, B.E., Goulding, A. and Campbell, A. J. (1989). Dietary salt affects indices of bone resorption and formation in elderly women. *British Medical Journal* **299**, 834–835.

Miller, S. W. M. and Grimley Evans, J. (1985). Fractures of the distal forearm in Newcastle: an epidemiological survey. *Age and Aging* **14**, 155–158.

Need, A. G., Horowitz, M., Walker, C. J., Chatterton, B. E., Chapman, I. C., and Nordin, B. E. C. (1989). Cross-over study of fat-corrected forearm mineral content during nandrolone decanoate therapy for osteoporosis. *Bone* **10**, 3–6.

Nordin, B. E. C. (1987). The definition and diagnosis of osteoporosis. *Calcified Tissue International* **40**, 57–58.

Nordin, B. E. C. and Heaney, R. P. (1990). Calcium supplementation of the diet. *British Medical Journal* **300**, 1056–1060.

Nordin, B. E. C. and Morris, H. A. (1989). The calcium deficiency model for osteoporosis. *Nutrition Reviews* **47**, 65–72.

Nordin, B. E. C. and Polley, K. J. (1987). Metabolic consequences of the menopause. *Calcified Tissue International* **4**, S1–S60.

Nordin, B. E. C., Chatterton, B. E., Walker, C. J. and Wishart, J. (1987). The relation of forearm mineral density to peripheral fractures in postmenopausal women. *Medical Journal of Australia* **146**, 300–304.

Nordin, B. E. C., Wishart, J. M., Horowitz, M., Need, A. G., Bridges, A. and Bellon, M. (1988). The relation between forearm and vertebral mineral density and fractures in postmenopausal women. *Bone and Mineral* **297**, 1314–1315.

Nordin, B. E. C., Need, A. G., Chatterton, B. E., Horowitz, M. and Morris, H. A. (1990a) The relative contributions of age and years since menopause to postmenopausal bone loss. *Journal of Clinical Endocrinology and Metabolism* **70**, 83–88.

Nordin, B. E. C., Need, A. G., Morris, H. A. and Horowitz, M. (1990b). The metabolic basis of osteoporosis. In "Osteoporosis: physiological basis, assessment and treatment" (H. F. DeLuca and R. Mazess, eds) pp. 23–36. Elsevier, New York.

Overgaard, K., Riis, B. J., Christiansen, C., Podenphant, J. and Johansen, J. S. (1989). Nasal calcitonin for treatment of established osteoporosis. *Clinical Endocrinology* **30**, 435–442.

Riggs, B. L. and Melton, J. (1983). Evidence for two distinct syndromes of involutional osteoporosis. *American Journal of Medicine* **75**, 899–901.

Seeman, E., Cooper, M., Hopper, J., Parkinson, E., McKay, J. and Jerums, G. (1988). The effect of early menopause on bone mass in normal women and patients with osteoporosis. *American Journal of Medicine* **85**, 213–216.

Sinaki, M., Wahner, H. W., Offord, K. P. and Hodgson, S. F. (1989). Efficacy of nonloading exercise in prevention of vertebral bone loss in postmenopausal women: a controlled trial. *Mayo Clinics Proceedings* **64**, 762–769.

Smith, E. L., Gilligan, C., Smith, P. E. and Sempos, C. T. (1989). Calcium supplementation and bone loss in middle-aged women. *American Journal of Clinical Nutrition* **50**, 833–842.

Storm, T., Thamsborg, G., Sorensen, O. H. and Lund, B. (1987). The effects of etidronate therapy in postmenopausal women: preliminary results. *In* "Osteoporosis 1987" (C. Christiansen, J. S. Johansen and B. J. Riis, eds) pp. 1172–1176, Osteopress APS, Denmark.

Wasnich, R. D., Benfante, R. J., Yano, K., Heilbrun, L. and Vogel, J. M. (1983). Thiazide effect on the mineral content of bone. *New England Journal of Medicine* **309**, 344–347.

Wasnich, R. D., Ross, P. D., Heilbrun, L. K. and Vogel, J. M. (1985). Prediction of postmenopausal fracture risk with use of bone mineral measurements. *American Journal of Obstetrics and Gynecology* **153**, 745–751.

The Compression of Morbidity: Progress and Potential

James F. Fries

Department of Medicine, Division of Immunology and Rheumatology, Stanford University School of Medicine, Stanford, USA

INTRODUCTION

The future health of our increasingly senior populations depends upon future trends in two critical dates, the onset of time of first major disease, infirmity, or disability, and the time of death. Most lifetime morbidity is concentrated between these dates. Policy initiatives need to be directed at compressing the average period between these dates; the goal of compression of morbidity.

Consider these three possible scenarios with regard to future trends in infirmity (morbidity) and mortality (Fig. 1).

1. *Infirmity begins at the same average age* (for example 55 years) *but life expectancy increases by 5 years* (for example 75 to 80). Under this scenario the increased longevity has added only infirm years to life; the so-called "failure of success".

2. *The average age of infirmity and life expectancy both increase by the same amount*, disability from 55 to 60 years, and mortality from 75 to 80. Under this scenario there are the same number of infirm years per person in the future.

3. *The average age at infirmity increases by more than life expectancy*, for example by 10 years from 55 to 65 while life expectancy increases by only 2 years, from 75 to 77 years. With this scenario, termed the "compression of morbidity" (Fries, 1980, 1988, 1990), the average

Challenges in Aging
ISBN 0-12-090163-3

Scenarios for Future
Morbidity and Longevity

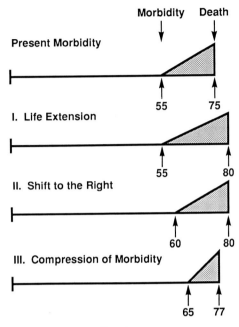

Fig. 1.

period of disability is compressed between an increasing age at disability and a relatively constant age at death. There are fewer numbers of infirm years under this scenario.

Under which scenario is the United States presenting operating? The preponderance of evidence presently suggests, for the most part, the second scenario. Further, data suggest that the first (and worst) scenario was an appropriate model for the first three-quarters of this century, as acute diseases were replaced by chronic ones. What could be? In important areas, the data demonstrate that compression of morbidity is occurring today, and data indicate that the phenomenon of the third scenario can be made to increase in the future by appropriate policy initiatives. For rational policy decisions, it is crucial to understand the complex interrelationships between infirmity and mortality. What is happening to each? What could happen?

Note that the point of first morbidity is a matter of definition, and will vary from study to study. In our work, we have often used the date at which disability index scores become non-zero. In studies of specific diseases, disease points may be appropriate, for example the first symptom of osteoarthritis, of atherosclerosis, or of emphysema. Others may select a particular disability threshold or the first time that a respondent reports poor health. The compression of morbidity model is a broad and flexible one. It is important to recognize that the concept is not restricted to terminal events but is directed at the quality of life in senior years, and that it is the relative dynamic relationship between markers of infirmity and death that determine active life expectancy and total morbidity.

What could cause the average age of first chronic infirmity to arise? First, reduction in risk factors for chronic illness, so that chronic disease occurs later in life or not at all. Second, decrease in cumulative occupational trauma resulting from the shift to employment in the service industries. Third, attention to prevention of the risk factors (such as lack of fitness) which accelerate the senescent (loss of organ reserve) manifestations of human aging.

Why might our past trends of regular increases in longevity change? As life expectancy has increased, the factors of senescence, which genetically determine the optimal life span, begin to exert more control over future advances. It becomes ever more difficult to improve life expectancy. This paper will review some of the lines of evidence which bear upon present and future trends in the two most important markers of national health, the average age at first infirmity and the average age at death.

INFIRMITY

Data on trends in infirmity at specific ages are inadequate. I know of no worker in the field who believes that presently available data allow conclusions to be made with certainty. Indeed, that is one of the lessons to be emphasized: we must have better data if we are to make wise decisions in the future. Nevertheless, data are getting better and there are already a number of lines of evidence which document improvement in health at a given age.

Atherosclerosis, the most common chronic disease in the United States, began to decline over 15 years ago (Stern 1979). The decline, in age-adjusted terms, is now over 40%. Myocardial infarction, the largest component of atherosclerotic mortality, has declined similarly (5). The age-adjusted mortality rates have fallen far more rapidly than the crude rates, indicating a movement of atherosclerotic mortality into later ages. The average age at first heart attacks has been shown in a number of studies to have increased, most probably by about 10 years, over a period when life expectancy increased by less than 2 years (National Center for Health Statistics 1967, Friedman 1979, Gillum et al. 1983, Pell and Fayerweather 1985, Fries 1990).

Lung cancer mortality rates have now begun to decline in American men, reflecting national changes in smoking habits, after a lag (Horm and Kessler 1986). With incidence and mortality separated only by a year in this disease and with survival rates after diagnosis holding constant over the period, it can confidently be stated that these tumours are not only fewer, they are occurring later in life. Indeed, the risk factor models for the major solid cancers *require* that decreased exposure to carcinogens delays or prevents the onset of malignant change.

Atherosclerosis and lung cancer in men combine to make up 51% of total mortality in the United States (National Center for Health Statistics 1989), hence effects in just these two disease categories have larger consequences. While data are less available, similar arguments of the effects of risk factor reduction should apply to chronic obstructive pulmonary disease, diabetes, colorectal cancer, skin cancer, cirrhosis of the liver, and other conditions. It is theoretically possible, by preventive efforts, to cause such conditions to occur later in life. Neither data nor theory currently permit such an optimistic view for certain other conditions, notably Alzheimer's disease (Schneider and Brody 1983).

The scientist's ultimate source of hard data comes from prospective, large, long-term, randomized controlled clinical trials. Such trials of primary prevention of heart disease, whether taken singly or in aggregate, unequivocally document that effects of the study intervention upon morbidity (such as non-fatal heart attacks and strokes, angina pectoris, congestive heart failure, and intermittent claudication) are far greater than effects of the same interventions upon mortality. Effects on morbidity are typically on the order of 20–25%, effects on mortality so far have not been measurable, and are at best, modest (Table 1) (Frick *et al.* 1978, Lipid Research Clinics 1984, Multiple Risk Factor Intervention Trial Research Group 1986, The Steering Committee of Physicians' Health Study Research Group 1988).

Recent work from our group in assessing development of osteoarthritis and musculoskeletal disability is likewise encouraging (Lane *et al.* 1986, 1987). Active individuals with few risk factors for disability (such as obesity or sedentary life style) maintain their physical function far longer, and with a negligible decline for age, when compared to less active individuals. Of interest, those engaged in strenuous or hazardous jobs are of substantially greater risk for premature musculoskeletal morbidity than those in other occupations. Our work clearly identifies risk factors for osteoarthritis and musculoskeletal disability.

Importantly for policy decisions, the presence of risk factors for disease strongly predicts future medical service and hospitalization use (Millman and Robertson Inc. 1987). Our own studies confirm these effects in a retiree population of 1558 individuals. Direct and indirect medical costs are strongly and adversely affected by bad health habits such as cigarette smoking ($842

Table 1
Major randomized trials of primary prevention

	Number of men	Duration (years)	Deaths			Coronary deaths			Morbid events			Morbid/ mortality
			Int.	Cont.	Diff.(%)	Int.	Cont.	Diff.(%)	Int.	Cont.	Diff.(%)	
MRFIT[1]	12866	7	265	260	−5(−2)	115	124	9 (7)	1366	1628	262 (16.1)***	262/−5
LRC[2]	3806	7	68	71	3(4)	44	32	12(27)	906	1112	206(18.5)***	206/3
Physicians[3]	22071	5	110	115	5(4)	5	18	13(72)**	173	239	66(28)**	66/5
Helsinki[4]	4081	5	45	42	−3(−7)	14	19	5(26)	45	71	26(37)*	26/−3

*$P < 0.05$, ** $P < 0.01$, *** $P < 0.001$.

[1] Morbid events angina pectoris, intermittent claudication, congestive heart failure, peripheral vascular disease, stroke, accelerated hypertension, left ventricular hypertrophy, impaired renal function, total non-fatal coronary events.

[2] Morbid events definite or suspect non-fatal coronary, positive exercise test, angina, coronary bypass surgery, congestive heart failure, intraoperative myocardial infarction, resuscitated coronary collapse, TIA, brain infarct, intermittent claudication.

[3] Morbid events non-fatal coronary, non-fatal stroke.

[4] Morbid events non-fatal coronary.

271

Table 2
Health habits and medical costs: 1-year predictions in 1558 Bank of America retirees.
Preliminary multiple regression results

	Hospital days $150	Doctor visits $65	Sick days $54	Estimated cost
Cigarette smoking One pack a day versus none	0.63	0.36	6.4	$842
Alcohol > 2 drinks a day versus ≤ 2	0.37	0.31	1.6	$384
Seat belt use 50% use versus 100% use	0.035	0.005	2.6	$166
Exercise 100-min a week increase	0.05	0.08	4.0	$259

per year), alcohol excess ($384), seat belt use ($166), and lack of exercise ($259) (Table 2).

Morbidity trends over the years have most frequently been estimated in the United States by noting the percentage of respondents reporting fair or poor health, and there has been little change in this percentage until the 1980s when health improvement, most marked in the over-65 population, began to be demonstrated. Unfortunately, with improving health standards the frame of reference changes for what constitutes fair or poor health, rendering these estimates unpersuasive. To avoid this bias and to control for genetic and socio-economic factors, we recently asked some 739 individuals ranging from 55 to 80 years of age to compare their present health status with that of their parent of the same sex at a time when that parent was the same age, and to explain any differences. Respondents estimated their health as a full grade higher than that of their parent at the same age and attributed most of the improvement to life style differences, including exercise, diet, and others. Specific improvements noted ranged from increased physical stamina to differences in dental status (Table 3). Over a generation, these data suggest very marked improvement in health status at any given age.

MORTALITY

Randomized controlled trials of preventive interventions, such as blood pressure control, smoking cessation, and cholesterol reduction have failed,

Table 3
Inter-generational health, 739 subjects

I. Subject's health versus parent (same sex) health at same age (mean 60 years)

Much better	Somewhat better	Same	Somewhat worse	Much worse	(Parent died)
34%	24%	15%	3%	1%	(23%)

II. Child's health (same sex) versus subject's health (same sex) health at same age (mean 38 years)

Much better	Somewhat better	Same	Somewhat worse	Much worse	(Child died) (no child)
7%	14%	39%	14%	2%	(1%) (24%)

when applied to our contemporary society, to demonstrate the life expectancy increases which would have been predicted from the Framingham data of 30 years ago (Frick *et al.* 1978, Lipid Research Clinic 1984, Multiple Risk Factor Intervention Trial Research Group 1986, The Steering Committee of Physicians' Health Study Research Group 1988). Overall, effects on total mortality, in every such study, have been negligible (Table 1). The obvious explanation is that with the greatly increased longevity of the present, further gains in longevity have become more difficult to achieve. We now can change only the cause of death but not the occurrence of death. The biological limits of the genetically determined life span begin to limit benefits in terms of additional longevity, while leaving feasible future gains in terms of morbidity. The ultimate average life expectancy limits are currently best estimated at about 85 years. Our recent estimates by linear regression equations of past longevity trends, using current data and a variety of assumptions (Table 4), are consistent with earlier estimates. Similar estimates using Japanese data yield closely similar results (Fries 1990).

If the forces of senescence actually are beginning to limit gains in life expectancy, we would expect to see this phenomenon occur first in women, who live an average of 7 years longer from birth in the United States and 4 years longer from age 65 than do men. Data from the 1980s clearly demonstrate this phenomenon. Life expectancy for females after age 65 rose rapidly in the 1970s, increasing by 1–3 months each year. Over the past decade, this trend has changed dramatically (Fig. 2). The present

Table 4
Linear regression estimates or maximum average life expectancy

	Males		Females		All	
	Data through 1976	Data through 1986	Data through 1976	Data through 1986	Data through 1976	Data through 1986
From 1900 Mean age	79.2	79.8	83.0	84.2	81.1	82.0
From 1950 Mean age	81.1	83.0	91.7	90.6	86.4	86.8
Last 10 years Mean age	84.4	83.8	92.4	85.9	88.4	84.9
Last 20 years Mean age	83.5	84.3	94.6	89.1	89.1	86.7

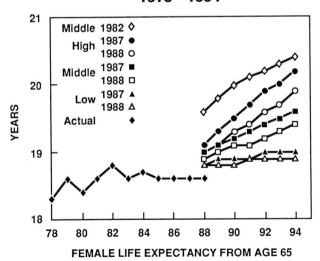

**SOCIAL SECURITY PROJECTIONS
AND ACTUAL VALUES
1978 – 1994**

Sources: Statistical Bulletin, Metropolitan Life Vol. 68 pp. 18-23, 1988.
Statistical Bulletin, Metropolitan Life Vol. 69 pp. 26-32, 1989.
Social Security Area Population Projections, 1987; Actuarial Study No. 99,
   SSA Pub. No. 11-115 46, Actuarial Study No. 102, 1988, Pub. 11-11549,
   Actuarial Study No. 87. SSA Pub. No. 11-11534, 1982.

Fig. 2.

value of 18.6 years for female life expectancy after age 65 was first achieved in 1979 and has been constant over the past 9 years (Metropolitan Life 1987, USDHHS 1988, National Center for Health Statistics 1989).

WHAT COULD BE?

One way to estimate future health would be to ask the consequences of extending the results of the large randomized controlled trials of primary prevention (Table 1) to the entire population. This approach to estimation predicts a large reduction in the morbidity from chronic illness and a very small increase in overall longevity. A policy of prevention thus would be cost effective in both human and economic terms.

A second way of visualizing the future is to ask what the consequences would be if the entire population achieved the health status currently enjoyed by the most favoured members of society. Very strong links between socio-economic status (categorized by education level or by income) with health status have been repeatedly reported. Recent work by our group and others has examined these differences by year of age, using data from the National Health and Nutrition Survey, the Health Interview Survey and other data sets, employing endpoints such as dependency, level of disability, or presence of arthritis diagnosed by a physician. Persons in the highest socio-economic strata have slower increases in disability at every year of age through age 70, after which time they begin to develop ever-accelerating rates of disability and the curves representing the different socio-economic classes rapidly converge. These observations, summarized graphically in Fig. 3, clearly document rectangularization of the morbidity curve (compression of morbidity) in certain favoured subpopulations and suggest that a major future challenge will be to extend these benefits to less advantaged groups.

A third major test of the potential for morbidity compression is documentation of the ability to improve health in the senior years by effecting changes in health risk behaviours. Health promotion programmes directed at seniors were neglected until recently, upon the general belief that changes in health habits late in life were difficult to achieve and, in any event, would be "too little and too late". However, since the magnitude of health expenditures in the senior population is so much greater than at younger ages and the proximity of the intervention and the events to be prevented are so much closer, we and others began to argue that health preservation programmes might be even more effective in seniors than in younger individuals. A recent major study by our group illustrates and documents this contention. Approximately 6000 Bank of America retirees (Leigh *et al.* 1990) were randomized into three groups, one to receive a

Chronic Arthritis, Age,
and Highest Grade Level

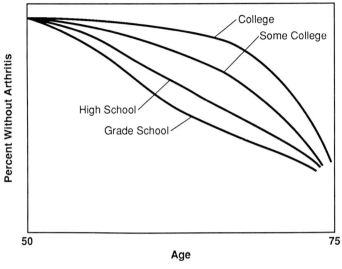

Fig. 3.

low-cost but well-designed health promotion programme, the second to receive survey questionnaires only, and the third to be followed unobtrusively only by measurement of medical claims data. Health habit changes of approximately 10–20% over 1 year were achieved in the experimental group relative to controls (Table 5). Self-reported health status improved by a similar amount. Estimated medical costs and claims data showed cost reductions of over 20% in the experimental group compared with either or both control groups. The dollar savings achieved of $300 per subject per year were 6 or more times greater than the cost of the programme. This particular senior health promotion programme is currently received by several hundred thousand individuals in the United States.

SUMMARY

At present, adding years to life expectancy has conveyed additional years of disability for some and additional years of healthy life for others. Now, it is becoming increasingly difficult to add additional years of life to present levels, whether these years are to be good years or bad years. The effects of preventive programmes in improving health status, decreasing medical

Table 5
The Bank of America retiree study: changes over 12 months (%)

	Experimental Group	Questionnaire Only Group	Claims Data Only
Exercise	−2	−12	
Cigarettes	−21	−9	
Fat intake	−23	−11	
Computed health risk	−4	+1	
Self-reported health	0	+10	
Sick days	−4	+8	
Doctor visits	−7	−3	
Hospital days	−27	+18	
Computed costs	−22	+12	
Computed costs ($)	−132	+18	
Claims costs ($)	−74	+340	+180

utilization requirements, and decreasing health care costs are substantial and are increasingly well documented. It is perhaps utopian, but certainly practically possible, to direct social policies toward "demand reduction"; toward reducing the need for medical services rather than relying upon payment caps or rationing of services in an attempt to control costs.

The predominant health burden of the United States has shifted from acute diseases to chronic ones, and is now in transition from these same chronic diseases to problems of senescence. The national health burden is now overwhelmingly concentrated in the senior years, and in problems of chronic disease and senescent frailty. It is important to treat and to palliate chronic diseases, and to continue and accelerate research into how best to accomplish this. But even more importantly, we must develop policies directed at prevention, at health preservation. Success in achieving an increasingly healthy senior population requires that the age at first permanent disability be raised as rapidly, or more rapidly, than life expectancy. This can only be achieved by interventions which *precede* the development of disability and thus *must* involve preventive efforts. Preventive programmes and services, whether to preserve health or to prevent disease, have not been systematically implemented and this neglect has been a costly one in both human and economic terms.

ACKNOWLEDGEMENT

This paper was supported in part by a grant from the National Institutes of Health (AM21395) to ARAMIS (American, Rheumatism, and Aging Medical Information System).

REFERENCES

Frick, M. H., Elo, O., Haapa, K., Heinonen, O. P. *et al.* (1978). Helsinki heart study: primary-prevention trial with gemfibrozil in middle-aged men with dyslipidemia. *New England Journal of Medicine* **316**, 1237–1245.

Friedman, G. D. (1979). Decline in hospitalization for coronary heart disease and stroke: The Kaiser-Permanente experience in Northern California, 1971–1977. *In* R. J. Havlik and M. Feinleib (eds), "Proceedings of the conference on the decline in coronary heart disease mortality", pp. 116–118. Pub. No. 79–1610, National Institutes of Health.

Fries, J. F. (1980). Aging, natural death, and the compression of morbidity. *New England Journal of Medicine* **303**, 130–136.

Fries, J. F. (1988). Aging, illness, and health policy: Implications of the compression of morbidity. *Perspectives in Biology and Medicine* **31** (3), 407–423.

Fries, J. F. (1990). The compression of morbidity: Near or far? *Milbank Memorial Fund Quarterly* Spring **67** (2), 208–232.

Gillum, R. F., Folson, A., Leupker, R. V. *et al.* (1983). Sudden death and acute myocardial infarction in a metropolitan area, 1970–1980: the Minnesota heart survey. *New England Journal of Medicine* **309**, 1353–1358.

Goldman, L. and Cook, E. F. (1984). The decline in ischemic heart disease mortality rates: An analysis of the comparative effects of medical interventions and changes in lifestyle. *Annals of Internal Medicine* **101**, 825–836.

Horm, J. W. and Kessler, L. G. (1986). Falling rates of lung cancer in men in the United States. *Lancet* **2**, 425–426.

Lane, N. E., Bloch, D. A., Jones, H. H. *et al.* (1986). Long-distance running, bone density, and osteoarthritis. *Journal of the American Medical Association* **255**, 1147–1151.

Lane, N. E., Bloch, D. A., Wood, P. D. *et al.* (1987). Aging, long-distance running, and the development of musculoskeletal disability: a controlled study. *American Journal of Medicine* **82**, 772–780.

Leigh, J. P., Richardson, N., Beck, R., Kerr, C., Harrington, H., Parcell, C. and Fries, J. (1990). Randomized controlled study of a senior health promotion program: the Bank of America Study. (Submitted).

Lipid Research Clinic (1984). Coronary primary prevention trial results. Reduction of incidence of coronary heart disease. *Journal of the American Medical Association* **251**, 351–364.

Metropolitan Life (1987). *Statistical Bulletin* **68**, 10–17.

Milliman and Robertson, Inc. (1987). Health risks and behavior. the impact on medical costs 1987, Control Data Corporation.

Multiple Risk Factor Intervention Trial Research Group (1986). Coronary heart disease death, non-fatal acute myocardial infarction and other clinical outcomes in the multiple risk factor intervention trial. *American Journal of Cardiology* **58**, 1–13.

National Center for Health Statistics (1968, 1968, 1974, 1978). Inpatient utilization of short-stay hospitals by diagnosis: United States. Social Security Administration Series 13, Pub. Nos. 6, 12, 26, 46, Washington, DC.

National Center for Health Statistics (1989). Monthly Vital Statistics Report, vol. 37 (12), 1–15.

Pell, S. and Fayerweather, W. E. (1985). Trends in the incidence of myocardial infarction and in associated mortality and morbidity in a large employed population, 1957–1983. *New England Journal of Medicine* **312**, 1005–1011.

Schneider, E. L. and Brody, J. A. (1983). Aging, natural death, and the compression of morbidity: another view. *New England Journal of Medicine* **309**, 854–856.

Stern, M. P. (1979). The recent decline in ischemic heart disease mortality. *Annals of Internal Medicine* **91**, 630–640.

The Steering Committee of Physicians' Health Study Research Group (1988). Preliminary report: Findings from the aspirin component of the ongoing physicians' health study. *New England Journal of Medicine* **381**, 262–264.

US Department of Health and Human Services (1988). Health United States, 1987. Social Security Administration, DHHS Pub. No. (PHS)88–1232. Washington, DC.

Discussion

Stähelin: If cancer and atherosclerosis are prevented more people might reach a higher age with the risk of AD. Will this increase morbidity?

Fries: I was trying to emphasize the change in life expectancy from age 65 onwards. In fact there is a true plateau and, if it continues as a plateau, then the overall incidence of Alzheimer's disease in women would be the biggest problem, even if there are no other changes and no successful treatments to the extent that increases average age of the over 65. There will be some shifts, but it won't be as bad on the individual probability basis, i.e. looking at yourself *vis-à-vis* your parents. You will individually have a similar risk of Alzheimer's disease and luckily that's still a reasonably low risk. It's a fact that we can't change the incidence age of AD and that plateau of above 65 stops and begins rising again, that in fact you are going to see some of the more sombre conclusions about AD.

Yesavage: Just one more question. On that side you had the reduced cost of health care after the intervention. Was that intervention cost effective in terms of the type of intervention that was involved? What kind of interventions were used?

Fries: The intervention there was a simple low cost intervention of about $30 a year in terms of cost. The savings were depending on how one calculated them, between $150 and $300. So it was highly cost effective. We don't think that you could use an expensive intervention and a cheap cost-effectiveness in all likelihood at the present time.

Summary

H. B. Stähelin

There is no doubt that geriatric medicine and gerontology is a truly interdisciplinary endeavour; it involves prevention, early detection and treatment, it involves on a more aggregate level health policy implications which have to be shifted from medically orientated models to disability or functionally orientated models, but it involves also knowledge of pathophysiological and molecular biological functions, of epidemiology, and the consequence in social life. I think these lessons teach us that there will be a lot of stimulating work for us ahead.

I will not go further but I would like to invite Prof. Danon from Israel to give the general conclusions and his impression of our symposium. As you probably noticed, he is also one of the Sandoz Prize Winners of the Sandoz Prize 1989 and we are very grateful that he took over the task to summarize and draw some general conclusions on this very heavily loaded programme of the last 2 days.

General Conclusions

D. Danon

The Weizmann Institute of Science, Center for the Biology of Aging, Rehovot, Israel

The organizers of the Sandoz Lectures have followed the example of the national and international congresses of gerontology in preparing a multi-disciplinary programme. The advantage of such a programme is in the opportunity of the participants to be exposed and to take part in the discussion of the fields of gerontology that are not usually at the highest priority of their interest. Having no parallel sessions avoids the separation of the various disciplines. It may diminish the level of specialization of every separate lecture, but it does enhance the level of interaction, especially when the number of participants is limited.

Under these conditions the lecturers should keep in mind that a considerable part of the audience is not familiar with their technical terms and initials. We are all familiar with some of the initials like DNA, RNA, SDAT or AIDS. However, when you hear in a lecture which is not in your field "ESR", a clinician may have the tendency to hear the familiar "erythrocyte sedimentation rate" rather than "electron spin resonance". It would also be nice to explicitly mark the units used in the ordinate and the abcissa of graphs. When there are 16 lectures of various disciplines to which everybody is exposed the lecturers should take these considerations seriously.

From the very first lecture by J. E. Birren and the discussion that followed, it was obvious that while a "wide range of behaviours slow with age" these are primarily related to other physiological and psychological factors rather than age alone. Not less important are some pathological events that may precipitate this slowness. The discussion by T. F. Williams pointed out that in some professions, this decline in speed of reaction may not appear until very late in life, if at all. The observation that physical

283

fitness and exercise may serve to maintain optimal levels of performance may inspire the first conclusions:

1. The slowness in behaviour with age is not inevitable.
2. When it occurs, it is related to other physiological factors.

Therefore, this slowness may be delayed or avoided if one or more of these factors do not occur. The fact that in some professionals (pilots, musicians) at least some of the functions are not slowed, indicates that the slowness is not an obligatory part of symptoms of aging. Disease can result in disproportionate slowness and physical fitness can delay slowness. This is indicative of the complexity of the phenomenon, and also that slowness is one of the symptoms of aging that may eventually be preventable. Such a goal can be achieved by a collaborative effort by psychologists, physiologists and biologists.

One of the problems in gerontological research is the insufficient consideration of one discipline by the other. It is a shame to see how often the psychiatrist and psychologist conduct their research without looking carefully into the physiological status of the person studied, like the efficiency of his or her heart, lungs, and blood parameters. It is as regrettable as the immunologist or haematologist who overlook the status of the memory and learning capacity or psychiatric status of their subjects. Obviously different tools and different methods are used in the various studies. One solution is collaboration. Collaboration is a good way of improving the learning from such different branches of research.

Many years ago, when the late Mayer Weisgal was the president of the Weizmann Institute of Science he asked me, "What do you want to discover with such a complex and expensive laboratory?" I answered, "I want to know how do we become old?" He then said to me, "David, don't be a fool. Time alone is enough to make you old." Is it enough? During the discussion in these lectures, there was a proposition to introduce the notion of time into the process of aging. Of course, every biochemical or biophysical process is time dependent.

It is still difficult to clarify what part of the various symptoms of aging is due to what we like to call "normal aging" and what part of the symptoms is due to a previous bacterial or viral disease, or a trauma. We still have a long way to go before we will understand the changes that take place as we advance in age without disease. As B. E. C. Nordin suggested, referring to osteoporosis, "A symptom of aging that becomes preventable is not aging anymore, it is a disease."

Several symptoms of aging are delayed or completely preventable in hypophysectomized experimental animals, as reviewed and discussed by A. Everitt. Most of these symptoms can be delayed or prevented, although to a lesser degree, by the less drastic procedure of dietary restriction. However, there is still a lot to be clarified in this process of prevention. In this sense, H. Orimo opens the hope for prevention and even reversibility of atherogenesis and sclerosis. Is this also a preventable disease? A curable disease? Additionally, M. H. Liang draws our attention to the fact that early diagnosis increases the probability of prevention.

Several speakers in the various sessions mentioned the almost unavoidable consideration of the role of the central nervous system, in this or that symptom of aging. The first lectures related to behaviour and learning are obviously related to brain function. But, referring to a symptom of aging as "brain related" does not explain the mechanism of its occurrence. There was a time when diseases of behaviour were considered diseases of the soul, of the spirit. Let us remember that molecules talk to molecules. Molecules react with molecules. Finally, the more we understand the normal function of neurons and synapses, the better we will understand their dysfunction and what causes it.

In the lectures of G. S. Roth and J. A. Joseph as well as that of C. Bertoni-Freddari we have seen a demonstration of different approaches to the elucidation of the cause of a diminished function at a molecular or subcellular level. Some insight was revealed into the possible natural mechanisms of compensation for these diminished functions.

Again and again, we encounter the notion of "normal and pathological aging". We obviously follow a symptom. Is mild pathology a normal aging? Should we classify an exaggerated symptom of aging as pathological aging? V. V. Frolkis spoke of two systems of information transmission: those regulated by genes and those regulated by the neurohumoral system and their mutual dependence. Again, he uses the term "aging syndromes" and "age-related pathology". Are we dealing with syndromes that have a pathogenic agent that we hope to discover? Is age-related pathology related to advanced age because so many years must pass before the symptom may be expressed, or because so many diseases may interfere with our health during the years until the symptoms are expressed? These questions remain unanswered.

We will be able to answer these questions and gradually reduce the number and severity of the various symptoms of aging if we continue to study the "aging" at the organism level, at the cellular level and at the molecular level. Let some of us concentrate our efforts in the understanding of the process of "normal aging"; others will try to understand the diseases of advanced age; others, still, will try to find their interrelationship. Let us try to understand the impact of genetics on aging at the molecular level, while respecting research into symptoms that occur in advanced age that are not necessarily related to an identifiable gene. The collaboration and exchange of information between these various methods and talents may improve our probability of decreasing and easing the symptoms of aging.